D1001618

Nursing
Staff
Development

Strategies for Success

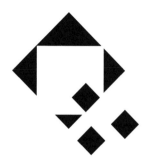

Second Edition

Nursing
Staff
Development

Strategies for Success

Roberta Straessle Abruzzese, RN, EdD, FAAN
Consultant in Continuing Education and Staff Development
The Abruzzese Group
Garden City, New York

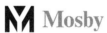 Mosby

St. Louis Baltimore Boston Carlsbad Chicago Naples New York Philadelphia Portland
London Madrid Mexico City Singapore Sydney Tokyo Toronto Wiesbaden

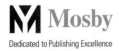 Mosby

Dedicated to Publishing Excellence

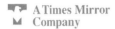 A Times Mirror
Company

Vice President and Publisher: Nancy L. Coon
Executive Editor: N. Darlene Como
Senior Developmental Editor: Laurie Sparks
Project Manager: Linda McKinley
Production Editor: Aimee E. Loewe
Designer Coordinator: Elizabeth Fett
Manufacturing Supervisor: Tony McAllister
Layout Artist: Steve Cavanaugh

Second Edition

Copyright ©1996 by Mosby–Year Book, Inc.

Previous edition copyrighted 1992 by Mosby–Year Book, Inc.

Printed in the United States of America

Composition by Mosby Electronic Production, Philadelphia
Printing/binding by R.R. Donnelley & Sons Company

Mosby–Year Book, Inc.
11830 Westline Industrial Drive
St. Louis, Missouri 63146

Library of Congress Cataloging in Publication Data

Nursing staff development : strategies for success / [edited by]
    Roberta Straessle Abruzzese.—2nd ed.
        p. cm.
    Includes bibliographical references and index.
    ISBN 0-8151-0053-1
    1. Nursing—In-service training. 2. Nursing—Study and teaching
(Continuing education)   I. Abruzzese, Roberta Straessle.
[DNLM: 1. Education, Nursing, Continuing—organization &
administration.   2. Nursing Staff—education.   3. Staff
Development—methods.   WY 18.5 N974 1996]
RT76.N87   1996
610.73′ 071′ 55--dc20
DNLM/DLC
for Library of Congress   95-49884
                                                                    CIP

96 97 98 99 00 / 9 8 7 6 5 4 3 2 1

Contributors

Robert S. Abruzzese, RN, EdD, FAAN

Consultant in Continuing Education and
    Staff Development
The Abruzzese Group
Garden City, New York

Adrianne E. Avillion, MS, RN, CRRN, CNA

Director, Training and Development
    Center
University Rehabilitation Network
University of Maryland Medical Center
Baltimore, Maryland

Jane Kreplick Brody, RN, PhD

Assistant Professor in Nursing
Nassau Community College
Garden City, New York

Betty Cody, MSN, RN C, CNA

Chairperson, Nursing Staff Development
University of Texas, MD Anderson Cancer
    Center
Houston, Texas

Janet Meyer-Desnoyer, BS Ed, BSN, MSN

Manager, Professional Development
BJC Health Systems
St. Louis, Missouri

Patricia Frost-Hartzer, RN, MS, PNP

Nurse Educator
Lucile Salter Packard Children's Hospital
    at Stanford
Palo Alto, California

Alice Gianella, RN, MA

Director, Nursing Education
Memorial Sloan Kettering Cancer Center
New York City, New York

**Carol Green-Hernandez, PhD, FNS, RN,
    CS, ANP/FNP-C**

Associate Professor and Director, Nurse
    Practitioner Program
University of Vermont, School of Nursing
Burlington, Vermont

Gary Herrmann, MS

Learning Resource Center Coordinator
BJC Health System
St. Louis, Missouri

Kim S. Hitchings, RN C, MSN

Manager, Professional Development
Lehigh Valley Hospital
Bethlehem, Pennsylvania

Jacqueline M. Katz, MS, RN

Vice President, Development
  Division of Continuing Education and
  Training
Mosby
St. Louis, Missouri

Donna S. Leroux, MEd, MSN, RN

Instructor in Maternal Child Health
Mesa Community College
Mesa, Arizona

Carol A. Mottola, RN, PhD

Assistant Professor
Nassau Community College
Garden City, New York

Barbara K. Penn, PhD, RN, C

Colonel, U.S. Army Nurse Corps (Retired)
Consultant in Education
Fairfax, Virginia

Terry O'Grady, RN, MS

Director, Community and Physician
  Relations
Lucile Salter Packard Children's Hospital
  at Stanford
Palo Alto, California

Beth Quinn-O'Neil, RN, MEd, CNA

Director, Hospital Education
Holy Name Hospital
Teaneck, New Jersey

Lori Rodriguez, RN, MA, MSN

Director, Organization and Leadership
  Development
Sequoia Hospital
Redwood City, California

**Donna Richards Sheridan, RN, MS, MBA,
  PhD**

Chief Nurse Executive
Saint Francis Memorial Hospital
San Francisco, California

**Patricia S. Yoder Wise, RNC, EdD, CNAA,
  FAAN**

Professor and Dean
Texas Tech University Health Sciences
  Center
Lubbock, Texas
Editor
*The Journal of Continuing Education in
  Nursing*

To the memory of my husband,
Thomas Joseph Abruzzese,
who taught me how to play.

Foreword

You will enjoy reading this book.

It is written in clear, down-to-earth English—not stuffy, turgid academese. But more than that, it is written by people who are enthusiastic about their subject, who care about the people they are writing for, and who take joy in sharing their discoveries and experiences with others. They are all professional nurses who love nursing and know what it's like to be a nurse with responsibility for staff development. You will recognize yourself on many pages.

Above all, you will get a lot of help from this book.

It is full of bright ideas and practical suggestions. But it is not preachy. It is not a how-to-do-it book, but a how-we-do-it and how-others-do-it and how-it-could-be-done book. It respects your right to choose how you want to do it, but helps you to choose wisely by providing you with a range of alternatives. More than that, it provides a sound foundation of philosophical and theoretical concepts and principles for making your choices. When you finish, you will feel confident that you know what you are doing and why—that you are a real "pro" in staff development.

For more than 50 years I have perceived the nursing profession as being the leader of all the professions in promoting the continuing professional (and personal) development of its members. This book certifies that this is still the case.

MALCOM S. KNOWLES
Professor Emeritus of Adult Education
North Carolina State University

Preface

Nurses involved in staff development face enormous challenges in the 1990s because of changes in health care delivery, increased use of technology, risk of communicable diseases, and acuity of illness among an aging population. These factors and others increase the need for ongoing education to ensure that the knowledge and skills of practicing nurses are current. The responsibilities of staff development departments include such crucial and diverse activities as orientation, competency assessment, cross-training, new product and technology training, specialty practice preparation, management and leadership development, research program development, and continuing education for nurses in the community. The trends toward downsizing, subacute care, home care, managed care, and HMOs have dramatically increased the importance of staff development departments that measure success by cost-effectiveness and continuous quality improvement. Never was it more important for staff development educators to demonstrate competence in achieving educational outcomes based on the organization's goals and quality patient care outcomes.

This book was written to help staff development educators excel in the crucial aspects of their teaching/learning activities. This second edition expands and updates the concepts and strategies presented in the first edition, provides new concepts and strategies, and enhances their use. This book is a practical guide for nurses who are new to staff development and a resource for experienced nurse educators. Nurses in graduate programs who are preparing for a career in staff development will find the book useful because its historical basis, in-depth and broad coverage of all topics, and extensive references provide crucial directions in the rapidly changing health care system. Staff development educators preparing for certification will find extensive review for all areas of the certification exam.

This is the first book to integrate the literature from nursing education, business and industry, and adult and continuing education into practical and innovative strategies for staff development. Updated references from the four major journals pertinent to staff development are integrated throughout this edition; thus educators do not need to do literature searches in *The Journal of Continuing Education in Nursing, Journal of Nursing Staff Development, Training and Development,* or *Training: The Human Side of Business* from January 1992 through June 1995 on any chapter. These updated concepts and strategies, as well as many from the most recent book publications pertaining to adult continuing education, make this edition a must for every staff development educator. In addition, this is the first book for nursing staff development that thoroughly uses the adult education strategies of Malcolm Knowles as its basis.

As with the first edition, this second edition is divided into four sections—foundations, management, process, and professional issues. The first section, "Foundations of Nursing Staff Development," presents an expanded and updated history of staff development including the 1994 standards for nursing professional development: continuing education and staff development. Since the focus and changes expected to affect staff development educators in the latter half of the 1990s have changed drastically, the predictions of leaders such as Margaretta Styles are discussed along with futurists such as John Naisbitt. Cultural diversity and human caring in this age of uncertainty are considered in relation to their effect on staff development.

The Chapters 3 and 4 on the conceptual foundations for adult learning and the role of philosophy and goals for structuring learning experiences are updated and enhanced by Chapter 5, a completely new chapter on learning styles. This new chapter clarifies many erroneous ideas about the ramifications of learning styles.

The second section, "Managing Nursing Staff Development," describes many management strategies and their practical application to the activities of staff development educators and departments. Chapter 6 details the advantages and disadvantages of various organizational structures for staff development departments; additional emphasis is placed on hospital-wide and matrix organizations in restructuring. Chapter 7 presents an overview of the development of staff development educators and evaluation strategies to ensure continuing competency. Chapter 8 describes the way to present cost-effective budgeting for educational activities and reflects all the budgeting ideas presented in the four major staff development journals and other pertinent sources. Chapter 9 contains many innovative ideas for increasing participation in staff development learning activities even in this time of changing personnel ratios. Chapter 10 updates efficient ways to use the computer as educational and management tools.

The third section, "The Process of Nursing Staff Development," describes activities surrounding the teaching/learning process from the assessment of learner needs to the evaluation of outcomes. Determining the needs of different types of learners is updated in Chapter 11. These needs are translated to curriculum planning in Chapter 12, and in-depth explanations and updated examples of this often-neglected aspect of learning facilitation are also provided. Chapter 13 integrates effective strategies for maximum learning into time-saving patterns. Important new evaluation strategies are added to Chapter 14, including the Cervero Model and Kirkpatrick's four levels of evaluation. Chapter 15 presents the challenges of planning and implementing orientation programs more creatively now that new hiring policies, cross-training of different types of personnel, time constraints, and exact documentation of competence are so important.

The fourth section, "Professional Issues in Nursing Staff Development," explores ethical and legal issues, continuous quality improvement, and research. For the first time, ethical, legal, and continuous quality improvement ideas have been synthesized into models for staff development departments. Chapter 16, which focuses on ethical and legal topics, has been rewritten by a new author and has expanded each section. Chapter 17 includes the latest recommendations from Joint Commission on Accreditation of Healthcare Organizations (JCAHO) about quality improvement in staff development. Chapter 18 presents an overview of the research process with new examples focused on staff development; suggestions for current topics that need to be investigated by staff development educators are also included.

The appendix contains an expanded and updated list of educational resources for staff development educators, which includes journals, books, organizations, and national continuing education opportunities. These references provide many ideas for new teaching strategies and networking among educators.

Many people have influenced the content of this book. I would like to acknowledge the contributions of some people who have been important in the development of my staff development ideas. Edna Danielson, "Danny," who was my advisor for my master's degree in in-service education at Teachers College, Columbia University, had a profound effect on my life. Danny believed in me before I believed in myself, and she encouraged me to read literature on training and development in business and industry if I wished to be on the cutting edge in staff development.

I also owe a debt of thanks to Cynthia Vaughn Gordan, who obtained her master's in in-service education with me and has remained a best friend over the years. Cynthia and her husband, Gilbert, have provided a refuge for me in San Francisco for much needed rest and relaxation. There are no adequate words to thank Leanore Romm, who was my partner in staff development activities from the early 70s until her retirement.

A special thank you to the following staff development educators who were with me during the years that I was Director of Staff Development at St. Luke's Hospital in New York City: Gerri Allerman, Ellen Wilgus Bell, Nancy Clayton, Suzanne Concato, Joanne Elliott, Judith Evans, Jean Pieri Flynn, Ruth Kippax Clark, Hilda Koehler, Leena Rinaldi, Kathy Ryaby, Daisy Scott, Elizabeth Hofstetter, and Edna Zebelman. Those years remain some of my most productive as we brainstormed educational strategies for the 850-bed hospital.

Many thanks to the staff development educators on Long Island who attended Adelphi University's continuing education programs for staff development, served on the advisory committee, and belonged to the Inter-County Society of Nursing Inservice Educators (ISNIE). Over the years they heard many of the ideas in this book, provided critiques, and shared their insights. They kept me reality based, welcomed me to their staff development departments, and contributed greatly to my success as Director of Continuing Education at Adelphi University.

A special debt of gratitude goes to Jay and Jackie Katz of Mosby educational services for their invitation to Lee Romm and me to coordinate the annual Staff Development Conference. It has been a joy and a great satisfaction to interact with some of the best and brightest staff development educators on the continent. Many of them are authors of chapters in this book, and many others have critiqued the content for the book.

Lastly, there are some people who were vital to this book and without whom the book would not have been written. A special thanks to Antoinette Wrighton Mason, who typed every word of the first edition; to my editors Darlene Como, Laurie Sparks, and Aimee Loewe; and to my statistician, research consultant, and dear friend Carol Mottola. Lastly, I owe a debt of gratitude to my assistant, Nicole Harris Butler, who made this book possible with her diligence and persistence.

ROBERTA STRAESSLE ABRUZZESE

Contents

II Managing Nursing Staff Development

III   The Process of Nursing Staff Development

IV Professional Issues in Nursing Staff Development

Foundations of Nursing Staff Development

I

ROBERTA S. ABRUZZESE ◆ PATRICIA S. YODER WISE

◆ ■ ◆ ■ ◆ ■ ◆ ■ ◆ ■

Staff Development: Our Heritage, Our Visions

Staff development comprises a field of practice in nursing that helps shape the future of the profession and of nursing services. Staff development is a key to quality nursing care and has been a concern of nursing leaders since the beginning of organized nursing.

The current roles of staff development educators are strongly influenced by the nursing heritage and prior efforts to facilitate the competence of nurses in practice. This chapter provides a brief overview of the heritage and visions that have shaped current staff development efforts.

THE HERITAGE OF STAFF DEVELOPMENT IN NURSING

Staff development began with Florence Nightingale's efforts during the Crimean War when she worked with "nurses" to improve the care they were providing. Part of her responsibility as a supervisor or director of nursing care was to ensure that the nurses met her standards of care. She also encouraged them to continue to learn, saying "Let us never consider ourselves finished nurses...we must be learning all our lives."[21]

Despite Nightingale's efforts, no staff development programs existed in the early hospitals in the United States. Every hospital sought to establish its own training school for nurses, and hospitals were staffed by students. Graduate nurses primarily functioned in private duty situations or, to use modern terminology, as independent service providers.[5] The few graduate nurses hired by hospitals had no need for orientation classes because they had been students in those hospitals and were well versed in the procedures and policies. As late as 1932, 73% of hospitals did not have general staff nurses; only 15% of hospitals had four or more general staff nurses.[13]

Although the educational emphasis during the early 1900s was placed on improving the schools of nursing rather than on maintaining and improving the competencies of graduate nurses, early leaders recognized the need for graduate nurses to learn continuously. To facilitate continued learning, public health nurses often carried two or three reference books with them as they made their home visits.[13]

In 1912, Edna L. Foley, superintendent of the Visiting Nurses' Association of Chicago, urged nursing leaders to realize that the expansion of knowledge necessitated a program of both continuing education and in-service education.[8] In 1928, Blanche Pfefferkorn,[22] executive secretary for the National League for Nursing Education (now called the *National League for Nursing*), traced the history of staff development. Pfefferkorn stated that in its broadest meaning, in-service programs for nurses were as old as organized nursing. In fact, many early hospital training programs were more similar to on-the-job training than to Nightingale's schools of nursing.

After 1929, articles in nursing journals about in-service education became more numerous. Nursing organizations also turned their attention to the training of unlicensed personnel, such as aides and orderlies, who assisted nurses in patient care. Although the main concern of nursing organizations was to establish schools to prepare individuals to become licensed practical/vocational nurses, their recommendations included one stipulating that "ward helpers and orderlies should be prepared on the job for the specific tasks they are to perform within the institution employing them."[9]

As nurses moved from independent practice during recessions and the Great Depression of the 1930s to hospital employee status, they were often provided with "postgraduate" courses. Sometimes these courses were provided for a small fee, but often they were offered in exchange for nursing services. The best of these courses resembled current staff development courses that prepare nurses for practice in specialty care units.[7] Sometimes these courses were made available to nurses who were not employed by the hospital offering the course.

During the Great Depression an estimated 8000 to 10,000 nurses were unemployed.[13] Many nurses offered to work for hospitals in exchange for room, board, and laundry, but most hospitals were already staffed by either students or attendants. "Of the hospitals with schools, 73% did not have a single graduate nurse on floor duty..."[13] Some administrators, however, permitted graduate nurses to work as staff nurses in specialty areas, thereby providing postgraduate training.

By 1937 the number of graduate nurses working in hospitals had risen from 4000 in 1929 to 28,000.[13] At this time the 8-hour workday was instituted for all workers, and the 1937 *Curriculum Guide for Schools of Nursing*[13] declared that the primary function of nursing schools was to educate students and not to provide service for hospitals. These events had a profound effect on the need for in-service education within hospitals.

In-Service Needs Increase

During the 1940s, orientation programs for new employees, nurse refresher course graduates, and aides were common for nursing service departments.[18] In

July 1941, Congress passed the Labor-Federal Security Appropriation Act, which provided $1.8 million for nursing education. This included monies for nurse refresher courses. These courses were an important means of ensuring the availability of inactive nurses for patient care during a time when one out of four nurses volunteered for military service.[13] These inactive nurses needed in-service education because many of them had not been in clinical nursing practice since their graduation from nursing school.

Two types of aides were oriented to hospital practice during the war years. The American Red Cross initiated an extensive program to train volunteer aides to assist nurses during the war shortages. By 1944, paid auxiliary workers performed 42% of the nursing care in hospitals without nursing schools and 17% of the care in hospitals with nursing schools.[13]

The shortage of nurses continued after the war because increases in technology and expanding opportunities for nursing practice created a greater need for nurses. In 1950 the W.K. Kellogg Foundation in Chicago funded programs "designed to upgrade nursing practice and keep nurses informed of new developments in the field of nursing."[17] Among other aims the program intended to "enlarge curriculum offerings of in-service education to nurses employed in hospitals through institutes, workshops, work conferences, seminar discussion and through direct contact with individual nurses in their respective hospital situations."[17]

In-service education began to be separated from other head nurse and supervisory responsibilities. By 1953 one hospital administrator said that "with the establishment of a Division of Inservice Education within the Nursing Service Department...[we have] given this important part of nursing education the recognition and status it deserves."[18]

In March 1953 the Joint Commission for the Improvement of Care of the Patient noted that in-service education should be established for all levels of nursing personnel—professional nurses, practical/vocational nurses, and auxiliary workers. This committee later became the Department of Hospital Nursing of the National League for Nursing (NLN). Mary Annice Miller was appointed as a consultant. Her primary responsibility was to develop materials and methods for in-service programs within hospitals. In 1965 her manual of in-service education was published.[17] This department of the NLN, in cooperation with the American Hospital Association (AHA) and the Public Health Service, developed the Nursing Service Aide In-Service Training Project. They estimated that in 18 months, they had influenced the training of 72,000 nursing aides through train-the-trainer programs. Two NLN staff members trained 199 teacher-trainers, who trained 2576 instructors, who trained 72,000 aides on the job.[16]

In the 1950s and 1960s the increase in baccalaureate and associate degree programs, which provided less exposure to clinical practice than traditional diploma programs, made it imperative for hospitals to offer in-service education to guarantee a safe transition from student to registered nurse performance. Another innovation that fostered the growth of in-service teaching was the proliferation of intensive care units in the 1960s. With the publication in 1965 of

Meltzer, Pinneo, and Kitchell's findings in intensive coronary care,[15] the number of courses preparing nurses to function as coronary care nursing specialists rapidly increased.

Resources for In-Service

By the mid-1960s large hospitals had well-developed in-service education programs. This is evidenced by the publication of Miller's *Inservice Education for Hospital Nursing Personnel*[16] in 1965 and Sommer's *Inservice Education Manual for Nursing Service*[27] in 1966. A survey by *RN* magazine in 1970 showed that 93% of responding hospitals had nursing in-service programs.[11] However, the 1970 report from the National Commission for the Study of Nursing and Nursing Education[20] states that "Of the more than 7,000 hospitals in the United States...no more than 300 have a professional training specialist to direct their in-service program. All too frequently, responsibility has devolved upon nursing service...." In other words, too many hospitals still considered in-service education to be an additional responsibility of head nurses and supervisors.

The study recommended that "Health care facilities, including hospitals, nursing homes, and other institutions, either individually or collectively through joint councils, provide professional facilities, and organizational support for the presentation of in-service nursing education as well as that for other occupations."[20] The study expected that regional medical programs, which were designed to ensure continuing education for physicians and others through their educational activities, would help some nurses increase their abilities to provide in-service education.

Between 1964 and 1972 significant study on in-service education was conducted by the Hospital Continuing Education Project of the Hospital Research and Educational Trust. The purpose of the project was to expand staff development opportunities for health care personnel by emphasizing the concept of hospital-wide education and training. *Training and Continuing Education: A Handbook for Health Care Institutions*[10] was published in 1970 and served as a practical guide for hospital education. This book became one of the early reference texts for in-service education departments.

In 1970 the Board of Trustees of the AHA approved the formation of a new personal membership organization, the American Society for Health Manpower Education and Training (ASHET). Many nurses interested in in-service education joined this group and took advantage of the newsletters and other opportunities to gain information about hospital education and employee training.

Another opportunity to learn arose when the Hospital Research and Educational Trust of AHA obtained another 5-year grant from the W.K. Kellogg Foundation for the years 1972 through 1977. This project enabled the AHA to clarify the roles of employee education and training. A total of 11 regional conferences reached approximately 1000 people with various models for organizing hospitalwide education.[18]

Esther Lucille Brown, in her famous study entitled *Nursing Reconsidered: A Study of Change*,[6] said that the development of formal in-service education departments was needed because of the increase in nursing assistants and practical and graduate nurses, which was one of the most widespread developments since World War II. She also noted the need for in-service classes to teach nurses the way to engage in therapeutic conversations with patients. Furthermore, she acknowledged the effect that in-service education can have on the recruitment of qualified nurses, saying that "Various hospitals in an attempt to attract educationally qualified nurses attempted to solve these problems by expanding the inservice program to include continuing education."[6]

Organizations and Journals for Staff Development

Continuing education programs in colleges and universities provided still more opportunities for in-service educators to learn about teaching. In 1969 the First National Conference on Continuing Education for Nurses was sponsored by the Medical College of Virginia's Health Sciences Division of Virginia Commonwealth University.[26] Of the 82 participants, 46 represented colleges, 19 came from regional medical programs, and 7 were from hospitals. This 5-day conference was the beginning of annual fall meetings for educators interested in continuing education.

One of the discussion topics at the second conference, which was held in 1970 and sponsored by Syracuse University, was the development of a national organization for nurses interested in providing continuing education.[14] In 1973 the Council on Continuing Education of the American Nurses Association (ANA) was organized and held its first meeting at the Fifth National Conference on Continuing Education for Nurses sponsored by the Ohio State University School of Nursing.[25] Because the term *continuing education* was meant to include all education that takes place beyond basic nursing school, in-service educators and college continuing educators were encouraged to join the new council. In the first year, 305 nurses became members. The fall conferences continued to be sponsored by university continuing education programs and participants were primarily college continuing educators. As more hospitals developed departments of staff development (formerly called "in-service departments"), they also sent participants to the conferences. The fall conferences of The Council on Continuing Education provided major networking opportunities for nurses interested in the education of adult providers of health care.

Even the annual business meetings of The Council on Continuing Education were held at the fall conferences rather than at the ANA biennial conventions because more educators attended the fall conferences. Many forms of collaboration and sponsorships of the fall conferences have been used since 1975. These have varied from complete sponsorship by the ANA to combined sponsorship by colleges and service agencies. In the 1980s almost as many hospital staff development educators attended these conferences as college continuing educators. The Council's name was changed to the Council on Continuing Education and

Staff Development in 1988 to recognize the involvement of hospital staff development educations.

Many changes were taking place within the ANA regarding the 15 councils and their relevance to the structure of the ANA as a federation of state nurses' associations with renewed emphasis on clinical practice. The Council on Continuing Education and Staff Development was at risk of being eliminated, as were most other councils. Although it did not happen, there was much discussion about the council reverting to an independent organization of continuing educators. In 1994 the ANA decided to reorganize the council into a continuum of educators from basic nursing programs through doctoral and continuing education programs. The new council was named *Council on Professional Nursing Education and Development (CPNED)*. The fall conferences have continued with the collaboration of colleges, hospitals, and other service agencies.

The staff development educators, on the other hand, chose to form an organization of their own and established a steering committee in 1989. This committee led to the National Nursing Staff Development Organization (NNSDO), which fosters the art and science of nursing staff development and provides a forum to discuss matters of interest to the group. They offered an annual national conference for their members in conjunction with other regional and national conferences of interest to staff development educators. In July 1994 the first independent conference by NNSDO was held in Chicago. Similar national programs are planned for the future.

In addition to the three organizations mentioned, more written resources such as pamphlets, standards, journals, and books have become available since 1970. Charles B. Slack, Inc. began publishing the *Journal of Continuing Education in Nursing (JCEN)* in 1970, a landmark year for staff development educators. *JCEN* and the published proceedings of each fall conference through 1976 provided valuable references for staff development educators through the turbulent 1970s. Of special interest to staff development educators were the discussions and articles about trends in accreditation of continuing education and staff development programs, mandatory continuing education for renewal of license to practice nursing, and certification to document continued competence in a specialty area of practice.

Accreditation of Staff Development Programs

The movement toward accreditation of staff development programs arose from the realization by the ANA that it must control the education and practice of its own members. The usual ways to do this entail approval of preparatory programs, control of licensure, standard setting, and assurance of continuing competence of its members. The desire of regulatory bodies to ensure that the public has competent practitioners was a high priority in the early 1970s. There were many national discussions and debates about the need for professionals to retake their licensure test periodically or to demonstrate that they have continued to learn and remain safe practitioners. To demonstrate continued competence, many professional organizations and the general public proposed a system of mandatory education for nursing practitioners to renew their license to practice.

A system of mandatory education required standards to judge educational programs. The ANA knew that these standards should be set by a professional organization. In 1975 the ANA established an accreditation system for judging the quality of noncredit courses and programs that could be used to document continued competence. Staff development educators served on all accreditation committees with people from colleges, state nursing associations, specialty nursing organizations, federal agencies, clinical practice groups, and consumers.

Many staff development education departments in large hospitals quickly applied for approval of their continuing education programs. One of the first questions that arose was related to distinguishing in-service education classes (that is, orientation and new product information specific to one setting) from continuing education classes (that is, nursing practice information useful in any setting). These and many other questions have been asked since the accreditation program began. The answers to these questions have evolved from the standards set for staff development and continuing education by the Council on Continuing Education (box). The accreditation process and the certification programs were integrated into a subsidiary of the ANA called the *American Nurses Credentialing Center (ANCC)* in 1991.

ANA PUBLICATIONS INFLUENCING STAFF DEVELOPMENT STANDARDS

1974
   Continuing Education Guidelines for State Nurses' Associations
1974
   Standards for Continuing Education in Nursing
1975
   Accreditation of Continuing Education in Nursing
1976
   Guidelines for Staff Development
1975
   Guidelines for State Voluntary and Mandatory Systems
1978
   Revision of Guidelines for Staff Development
1983
   Peer Review in Nursing Practice
   Self Directed Continuing Education
1984
   Revision of Standards for Continuing Education in Nursing
   CE in Nursing: a Consumer's Guide
1990
   Revision of Standards for Nursing Staff Development
1994
   Standards for Nursing Professional Development: Continuing Education and
      Staff Development

HALLMARK DOCUMENTS AFFECTING THE HISTORY OF STAFF DEVELOPMENT

1966

American Nurses Association: *Statement of functions and qualifications for inservice educators,* developed by the Nursing Service Administrators Section, Kansas City, Mo, The Association.

1970

American Nurses Association: Landmark statement on inservice education, *Journal of Continuing Education in Nursing,* 1(1):23-25.

1972

American Nurses Association's Council on Continuing Education: Landmark statement on continuing education, *Journal of Continuing Education in Nursing,* 3(6):21-23.

1973

American Nurses Association Council on Continuing Education: Landmark statement on the continuing education unit, *Journal of Continuing Education in Nursing,* 4(1):28-31.

1975

American Nurses Association: *Standards for continuing education in nursing,* Kansas City, Mo, The Association.
National League for Nursing: *Position statement on NLN's role in continuing education,* New York, The League.

1976

American Nurses Association: *Guidelines for staff development,* Kansas City, Mo, The Association.
American Nurses Association: *Reference resources for research and continuing education in nursing,* Kansas City, Mo, The Association.

1978

American Nurses Association: *Accreditation of continuing education in nursing: the site visit process,* Kansas City, Mo, The Association.
American Nurses Association: *Self-directed continuing education in nursing,* Kansas City, Mo, The Association.

1979

American Nurses Association: *Continuing education in nursing: an overview,* Kansas City, Mo, The Association.

STANDARDS FOR STAFF DEVELOPMENT

In 1965 a landmark document published by the NLN contributed to standard setting for in-service education. Miller[17] stated that the emphasis on improving the performance of employees was a recognition of human resources as a valuable asset in institutions. In addition, she stated that in-service education should focus on four aspects of employees' needs: introduction to the job, training in both the manual and behavioral skills, leadership and management abilities, and continuing investigation of nursing. She saw these needs as program areas of orientation, skill training, leadership and management development, and continuing education.

Drusilla Poole[24] helped make some of these programs available in the military. She created a milestone standard by encouraging nursing service administrators to assign the function of in-service education to an assistant administrator instead of continuing to make in-service education one more responsibility for managers.

The National Advisory Commission on Health Manpower[19] cited the need to examine relicensure practices and perhaps require some measure of continued competency. *The Report on Licensure and Related Health Personnel Credentialing*[31] and *An Abstract for Action*[20] reiterated the need for some assurance of continued competency for health care personnel. Both reports called for opportunities for health care personnel to maintain their competency through continuing education and staff development. The Western Interstate Commission for Higher Education[32] expressed concern about the probability that many nurses would not pursue planned programs to remain competent. The ANA's Council on Continuing Education also focused attention on the need for high standards in continuing education of health care personnel to provide quality patient care. From its inception in 1970, the *Journal of Continuing Education in Nursing* has also provided valuable resources for high-quality staff development, thereby enhancing the quality of education in these departments. These events influenced an increase in the number of in-service education departments and enhanced the expertise of the educators.

From the late 1960s to the late 1970s many hallmark statements and publications by the ANA[1,2] contributed to raising standards of staff development (boxes on pp. 9 and 10). Two editors of *The Process of Staff Development* by Tobin et al[28,29] also helped raise the standards.

The movement in the 1970s that had the greatest impact on the standards of staff development was the drive to require continuing education for reregistration of licensure. Between 1971 and 1979, states either proposed or passed legislation requiring mandatory continuing education. Some states rescinded their mandatory continuing education regulations in the 1980s; others never enacted them. There is continuing debate as to the value of mandatory continuing education, but the growing number of states requiring mandatory continuing education for all professional licenses reflects the trend of consumers demanding competence. It is difficult to keep up with the status of mandatory continuing education in each state. One source of information is the *Journal of Continuing*

**AREAS OF PRACTICE CITED IN THE ANA'S STANDARDS FOR STAFF
DEVELOPMENT, 1990 REVISED[4]**

1. Organization and administration	7. Records and reports
2. Human resources	8. Evaluation
3. Learner	9. Consultation
4. Program planning	10. Climate
5. Education design	11. Systematic inquiry
6. Material resources and facilities	

Education in Nursing, which publishes a yearly summary of state requirements in its January issues.

The trend toward mandatory continuing education and the system of accreditation or approval of continuing education programs have had a major impact on the quality of staff development departments. The standards and guidelines created the expectation of peer review and led to the 1990 revisions of the ANA's *Standards for Nursing Staff Development.* The box above lists the 11 areas of practice for staff development cited in the 1990 standards. These 11 areas provide the norms for excellence in staff development. They were developed from the landmark statements and the earlier publications of the ANA and were influenced by the expectations of related groups, such as the Joint Commission on Accreditation of Healthcare Organizations (JCAHO) and state approval bodies. Even in the early 1970s, Standard V of the Joint Commission standards stated that, "There shall be continuing training programs and educational opportunities for the development of nursing personnel."[12] The standards for nursing staff development coincided with the establishment of standards by other groups committed to the educational and training development of employees, such as the ASHET and the American Society for Training and Development (ASTD).

In 1994 the standards for staff development and the standards for continuing education were integrated into one publication—*Standards for Nursing Professional Development: Continuing Education and Staff Development.*[3] This publication's emphasis is on nursing professional development and on the following six standards: administration, human resources, material resources and facilities, educational design, records and reports, and professional practice.

STRUCTURE OF STAFF DEVELOPMENT DEPARTMENTS

The structure of staff development departments has also evolved and varies widely among health care organizations. In rural areas, small community hospitals may not have a formal staff development program; the provision of education remains a part of the job responsibilities of nurse managers. Another common structure is for one person, usually a nurse, to provide staff development for all departments of small hospitals.

Many small community hospitals, however, have found innovative ways to provide staff development through regional consortium arrangements. A consortium of urban and rural hospitals can provide programmatic support for one-person staff development departments. Through the consortium, staff development educators can share resources and provide many more classes on a wider variety of topics than they could if they were working alone. In addition, teleconference technology allows numerous sites to access a course that might otherwise be unavailable or would allow relatively few staff members to attend.[23]

In contrast, staff development departments in large, university-based health science centers may be directed by a doctorally prepared nurse. The responsibilities of these departments often include continuous quality improvement, coordination of nursing students, and research activities, in addition to orientation, in-service classes, continuing education, and short courses to prepare nurses for practice in specialty areas. Usually the director of staff development has a title commensurate with other top managers of nursing specialty areas and is a valued member of the nurse executive team. In some instances these large staff development departments are structured as small business units within the larger health care organization and are expected to generate revenue. Many of these large departments provide hospital-wide education to enhance their importance and better serve their hospitals' needs as a whole. Most staff development departments fall somewhere between these two extreme types of structures.

The current structure of staff development is influenced by the ingenuity of staff development educators and reflects the diverse ways to provide staff development for an organization's personnel. Further examples of such structures are described in the *Journal of Nursing Staff Development*, which began publication in 1985.

The importance of staff development departments can never be overestimated. Cooper and Hornback said, "The cessation of learning is as real a threat to professional life as the cessation of pulse is to life itself. One of the ways by which the practicing nurse may continue learning is through educational opportunities...provided by the employing agency or institution."[7] Ulschak[30] considers staff development departments extremely important because they must provide the foundation for creative adjustment to change in the twenty-first century.

SUMMARY

The heritage of staff development includes many leaders from Nightingale to dynamic contemporary leaders. Standards for what staff development should be and visions for what staff development can be have transcended the evolution of standards and structure. Regardless of the structure, which responds to or shapes the changes in nursing staff development, nurses with a responsibility for this function have accepted the charge to focus nursing's visions and make the nursing care of tomorrow reflect the standards, research, technology, and human caring of today.

REFERENCES

1. American Nurses Association: *Guidelines for staff development*, Kansas City, Mo, 1978, The Association.
2. American Nurses Association: *Standards for continuing education in nursing*, Kansas City, Mo, 1984, The Association.
3. American Nurses Association: *Standards for nursing professional development: continuing education and staff development*, Kansas City, Mo, 1994, The Association.
4. American Nurses Association: *Standards for nursing staff development*, Kansas City, Mo, 1990, The Association.
5. Ashley JA: *Hospitals, paternalism, and role of the nurse*, New York, 1976, Teachers College, Columbia University.
6. Brown EL: *Nursing reconsidered: a study of change*, Philadelphia, 1970, JB Lippincott.
7. Cooper SK, Hornback MS: *Continuing nursing education*, New York, 1973, McGraw-Hill.
8. Dolan JA: *Nursing in society: a historical perspective*, Philadelphia, 1978, WB Saunders.
9. Flanagan L, editor: *One strong voice: the story of the American Nurses Association*, Kansas City, Mo, 1976, American Nurses Association.
10. Hospital Research and Educational Trust: *Training and continuing education: a handbook for health care institutions*, Chicago, 1970, Hospital Research and Educational Trust.
11. Inservice education: how it really is, *RN* 34(2):36, 1971.
12. Joint Commission on Accreditation of Hospitals: *Nursing services: accreditation manual for hospitals*, Chicago, 1971, Hospital Accreditation Program.
13. Kalish PA, Kalisch BJ: *The advance of American nursing*, Boston, 1986, Little, Brown.
14. McHenry RW: *Ends and means: the national conference on continuing education in nursing, 1971, Syracuse University*, Syracuse, NY, 1970, Publications in Continuing Education.
15. Meltzer L, Pinneo R, Kitchell R: *Intensive coronary care: a manual for nurses*, Philadelphia, 1965, Charles Press.
16. Miller MA: *Inservice education for hospital nursing personnel*, New York, 1965, National League for Nursing.
17. Miller MA: Trends of in-service education. In Cowan MC, editor: *The yearbook of modern nursing: 1956*, New York, 1956, GP Putnam's Sons.
18. Munk RJ, Lovett M: *Hospitalwide education and training*, Chicago, 1977, Hospital Research and Educational Trust.
19. National Advisory Commission on Health Manpower: *Report*, Washington, DC, 1967, US Government Printing Office.
20. National Commission for the Study of Nursing and Nursing Education: *An abstract for action*, New York, 1970, McGraw-Hill.
21. Nightingale F: *Notes on nursing: what it is, and what it is not*, Philadelphia, 1946, Lippincott (originally published in 1859).
22. Pfefferkorn B: Improvement of the nurse in service: an historical review, *Am J Nurs* 28(6):700, 1928.
23. Phillips CY, Hagenbuch EG, Baldwin PJ: A collaborative effort in using telecommunications to enhance learning, *J Cont Educ Nurs* 23(3):134, 1992.
24. Poole DR: In-service education reaches a milestone, *Am J Nurs* 53:1456, 1953.
25. *Proceedings Book of the Fifth National Conference on Continuing Education for Nurses*, Ohio State University School of Nursing, Columbus, Ohio, Sept 24-27, 1973.
26. *Proceedings Book of the First National Conference on Continuing Education for Nurses*, Medical College of Virginia Health Sciences Division of Virginia Commonwealth University, Williamsburg, Va, Nov 10-14, 1969.
27. Sommer D: *Inservice education manual for nursing service*, St Louis, 1966, Catholic Hospital Association.
28. Tobin HM et al: *The process of staff development: components for change*, St Louis, 1974, Mosby.
29. Tobin HM, Wise PSY, Hull PK: *The process of staff development: components for change*, St Louis, 1979, Mosby.

30. Ulschak FL: *Creating the future of health care education*, Chicago, 1988, American Hospital Publishing.
31. US Department of Health, Education and Welfare: *Report on licensure and related health personnel credentialing*, Washington, DC, 1971, US Government Printing Office.
32. Western Interstate Commission for Higher Education: *Continuing education in nursing*, Boulder, Colo, 1969, The Commission.

DONNA RICHARDS SHERIDAN ◆ ROBERTA S. ABRUZZESE
TERRY O'GRADY ◆ CAROL GREEN-HERNANDEZ

Nursing Staff Development in the 1990s

Nursing staff development naturally follows the patterns set by health care. Although forecasting is inherently risky, health care trends in the last half of the 1990s are not difficult to identify. Since the early 1980s, finding nursing management and nursing education literature that does not address the cost constraints of the health care environment is rare. The fiscal issues of the 1980s have intensified in the 1990s as all attention focuses on health care reform. Health care organizations are required to cut costs and further increase efficiencies. Some organizations merge with their competition for financial stability, whereas others are forced to cut back on services to manage fiscal constraints.[4]

To add stress to an already financially burdened health care system, society is faced with many health care and societal challenges, all of which affect the future of nursing and staff development. First, the much debated and much delayed health care reform is creating strange combinations and permutations in the delivery of health care. Second, the reorganization of health care delivery is creating problems in staffing ratios and quality improvement efforts. Third, there are multiple problems in caring for patients with communicable diseases. There is a worsening of the acquired immunodeficiency syndrome (AIDS) crisis that has been building throughout the 1980s and 1990s. Added to that are the problems related to a reemergence of tuberculosis, hepatitis, and strange new entities such as fulminating fasciitis. Fourth, exploding technology in terms of diagnostic equipment, treatment modalities, and computer advances make change and flexibility a necessity. Fifth, cultural diversity in the workforce and in patients necessitates a new sensitivity and respect for diversity. Last, there is a surge of humanistic caring and respect for individuals. In response to these and other challenges, the health care industry will see major changes in the last years of the twentieth century.

As health care's contribution to the gross national product (already more than 15%) continues to increase, rationing of health care is not a concept of the future but a consideration (and in some states an actuality) of the present. The contemporary focus in health care must be placed on access to health care, efficient quality, and cost containment to manage increased demands. Both high-quality processes and high-quality outcomes are demanded and must be provided in a cost-conscious manner. Accomplishing "more with less" is a challenge to all health care providers, nurse clinicians, administrators, and educators.

In the 1990s more than ever, nursing staff development departments must become increasingly effective to justify their existence. Staff development educators must creatively balance increased needs with limited resources. The agenda for the latter half of the 1990s includes the alignment of educational goals with hospital goals and the quantification of costs versus benefits.[19]

With consumer education currently expanding to include not only nursing staff but also other department personnel, managers, and administrators, flexibility will be a crucial skill for future successful staff development educators. Functions of staff development must be directed at the organization's learning needs, unit learning needs, and support of organizational goals.[18,19]

Gundlach[16] contends that it will be organizational needs that determine the nature and setting of staff development activities. These challenges will set the stage for nursing staff development in the final years of the twentieth century.

TRENDS AFFECTING STAFF DEVELOPMENT

Choosing the trends evident today and projecting that these trends will affect the lives of staff development educators through the year 2000 is a daunting task. Among the futurists or those brave enough to voice projections for the future, there is a considerable overlap of ideas. For example, Margaretta Styles[31] emphasized in a 1992 lecture to staff development educators that she saw two roles for the future—to build bridges and to freshen the vital growing group of care givers through knowledge, skills, motivation, and perceptions. In other words, she saw staff development educators as the people who would build bridges to all types of caregivers.

As Peggy Chinn[11] looked at the future, she saw four trends: explosion of technology, drastic diseases, scarcity of resources, and dramatic increase in complexity in all arenas of life. In the books *Megatrends 2000*[23] and *Megatrends for Women*,[2] John Naisbitt and Aburdene made many projections for trends that will affect lives in the United States. The projections that may influence health care in particular relate to providers of goods and services tailoring their products to the needs of individual consumers, cost-control and prevention dominating health care reform, and numbers of on-line information systems increasing exponentially.

Virgina Trotter Betts,[5] the president of the American Nurses Association (ANA) in 1995, said one of the purposes of the ANA is to forecast trends in health care that will have a large impact on nurses. She predicted that the work of nurses will probably change as much as the health delivery systems, that more nursing care will be in the community, and that nursing care will focus on primary health care and prevention.

Curtin,[12] in her discussions on future trends, emphasized that caregivers should not defend and try to hold onto functions and roles that are obsolete. They should "give time and attention to the emotional and relationship aspects of role changes." She believes the future is about developing "strong, competent, first-line nurse managers." Argyris, Kanter, Peters, Senge, and other perspicacious thinkers in business and industry concur and predict that the future is about building learning organizations. Argyris[3] says "awareness that high-performance work systems, with an emphasis on learning, hold the key to future competitive success and represents a tremendous opportunity for the training profession—but only if the profession reinvents itself." They stress that educators must constantly help others to "continually challenge prevailing thinking."[3] Wheatley[3] suggests that "learning will be ubiquitous, unavoidable, constantly challenging, and frequently chaotic."

Effects of Health Care Reform on Staff Development

While Congress wrangled over legislation for health care reform, the industry transformed itself. Cost cutting, intensive competition, and the growing role of large, profit- seeking corporations have forever changed care delivery systems in the United States. The following are some of the results[14]:

- Privately insured people have joined managed care plans.
- For-profit health management organizations (HMOs) have preempted non-profit HMOs as the major force in health care.
- At least 75% of all physicians have signed agreements with managed care groups.
- Nothing has been done to ease the plight of the uninsured, which now includes more than 39 million people.
- Most post–acute care is shifting to long-term and home care.
- Quality care and ethical dilemmas are major concerns.
- Prevention of hospitalization is a major goal that can be effected only by consumer education.
- HMOs want medical care that centers around a family physician and is oriented toward prevention.

The effects of health care reform on staff development educators has varied. In an effort to cut costs, entire education departments have been transformed to unit based operations in which the educator is quickly consumed with providing patient care. At a time when patients need to take charge of their own health care, they are receiving less education than ever. Staff nurses are finding it almost impossible to document patient outcomes regarding whether patients are ready to return home. Conferences that used to provide for patient education are no longer available. Patient education teaching aides are being neither developed nor purchased. Some education departments have expanded responsibilities for all personnel training, so these departments do not have time for anything other than mandatory classes and cross training.[8]

Effects of RN Substitution on Staff Development

One effect of hospital restructuring is the need to be more cost effective in delivering care. As hospitals close beds and units, reorganize into patient-focused units, and lose revenue, provision of more cost effective care is vital. Because nursing makes up the largest part of personnel costs, it is logical to examine savings in that department. As in every crisis, less expensive patient caregivers are one answer to cost reduction. The days of the all RN staff and primary care as envisioned in the 1980s are gone. That has been replaced by cross-training nursing personnel so that they can provide safe care in more than one unit. This has added more orientation hours to teach specific competencies for additional aspects of patient needs.

The use of more sophisticated equipment has led to hiring and training technicians who have a narrow range of technical activity. Sometimes these activities border on the professional practices of nursing. At other times, unlicensed assistive personnel are taught in short classes to take over many tasks that were formerly carried out by RNs or LPNs. These assistive personnel are ill prepared to manage patients with complex nursing problems, but educators are being asked to prepare more of these workers. Some educators are questioning the ethical issues of preparing nurse replacement workers who they know are unsafe.

In many organizations the down-substitution of nurses has resulted in more layoffs and greater responsibilities for the remaining RN staff. Educators have difficulty providing management classes that would ameliorate some of these problems. Managers say that the down-substitution of nurses is not unsafe because few patients stay in hospitals longer than 24 hours and the number of people in ambulatory units and home care are increasing. Nurses need to stop thinking in terms of bedside care and realize that most nursing care of the future will not take place in hospitals. Nurses should think in terms of being *beside* their patients, wherever these patients are, and not think so much about being at the *bedside*.[7] For staff development educators, this means an expanded opportunity to provide education for home care agencies. Some educators have established a business that practices independently to provide educational services for home care, long-term care, and other agencies providing home health services.

Effects of Communicable Diseases on Staff Development

Once again, communicable diseases are a major problem for nursing care. The human immunodeficiency virus/acquired immune deficiency syndrome (HIV/AIDS) epidemic is in its second decade. Prevention of the spread of this disease depends on community education and on educating patient care personnel who are often anxious about their own safety and the safety of their families.

Staff development educators can present many classes on universal precautions and monitoring of compliance. They also can be involved with other educators in the community to offer educational programs for nurses who would have no other opportunity to learn about new aspects of this disease.[21] These efforts at community education should be extended to businesses that need to develop educational programs and policies for this epidemic. Staff development educators could have a consulting business that provides this service.[25]

Hepatitis is another infectious disease that requires much education. As with HIV the teaching responsibilities relate to safe practices for all caregivers and extended patient education related to rest, nutrition, and hygiene practices. The staff development education role is to assist managers with teaching material for staff and patient education. A vigilant quality improvement program is an important adjunct in prevention.

Tuberculosis is another communicable disease that provides problems for caregivers and requires patient education and caregiver prevention programs. It is another topic to be added to orientation and yearly mandatory updates. The common occurrence of drug-resistant strains of tuberculosis and the use of special masks provides another teaching topic and monitoring for compliance. Prevention and patient education programs need to be offered continuously.

Effects of Increased Technology on Staff Development

Naisbitt and Aburdene, in *Megatrends 2000*,[23] identified a shift toward an information society in which both high technology and high touch necessarily coexist. Increased technology increases requisite knowledge and skills to be learned. Learning is absolutely central to the information age. As the twenty-first century approaches, an estimated 75% of the U.S. workforce will require retraining to retain current jobs.[3] New knowledge will lead to new applications of that knowledge; therefore the need for health care professionals to learn will also continue. An estimated 10% of a professional's knowledge in a high-technology–related field such as health care becomes obsolete each year.[13] The United States' information society is becoming computer literate. Computers are used for record keeping, word processing, message sending, and data retrieval. Most important to nurses is the computer's ability to monitor and document patient information. The use of computers in education will be increasingly common in the current decade. Research reveals that computer-assisted interactive instruction (CAII) promotes a significant increase in both learning performance and satisfaction. This learning occurs in less time than with traditional instruction.[15] However, computers have yet to reach their full potential. Future uses of the computer include problem solving and the monitoring and guiding of both professional conduct and the delivery of more components of patient care. The possibilities of information exchange on the Internet and other similar connections is limitless.

The proactive nursing staff educator should be computer literate and become a "user-friendly" resource to both management and staff. A common staff development function should be computer training, especially during orientation.

Changes in health care, such as early patient discharge, mean that many patients who need a high level of technology are being cared for in the home. The home care nurse will be able to access information via a small, portable computer.

Effects of Cultural Diversity on Staff Development

The idea that America would become the "melting pot" of the world was an unrealistic concept that failed to acknowledge the deep psychological need for people of similar backgrounds to be together. Today there is an acute awareness that effective nursing care requires an understanding of various cultures and "their values, beliefs, behaviors, perspectives, language, culture, and ways of thinking."[26] The major cultures in the 1990s in the United States are Hispanic Americans, African Americans, Asian Americans, and Native Americans. Valuing and managing cultural diversity requires cultural transformation within health care organizations. This cultural transformation requires commitment by top management and ongoing strategies to heighten the awareness of cultural diversity. The aim of cultural diversity is to treat all consumers by the platinum rather than the golden rule. The golden rule says treat others as you would want to be treated; the platinum rule says treat others as they would wish to be treated.

Ongoing classes and experiential learning are the two strategies most frequently used to change people's perceptions of other cultures. A commitment is needed from staff development educators to include aspects of cultural diversity in all learning activities. Some of the classes specifically related to cultural diversity focus on interview techniques, nutrition preferences, religious beliefs, ideas about health and illness, and death. In this way, nurse clinicians can gain an understanding and respect for cultural beliefs and plan nursing care to meet their patients' needs. These understandings are especially needed in planning patient education before discharge.

This emphasis on cultural diversity is not only for interacting with patients; it is also important for learning to treat all employees equally. An outgrowth of affirmative action seeks to value diversity and should lead to managing diversity so that work teams are more productive. Diversity is a long-term project that belongs in every organization's strategic plan.[9,32]

Effects of Caring on Staff Development

As the essence of nursing, caring is receiving much attention during this era of high technology. People are caring in the traditional sense of touch, sensitivity to pain, and empathy for others, as well as in the contemporary sense of caring about the environment, the planet, social activism, and political awareness.[10]

Perhaps Carol Green-Hernandez[17] best expresses caring in nursing in her theoretical framework that describes caring. Building on Mayeroff's work,[22] Green-Hernandez[17] says that natural caring is a human process in which one person assists another in growth and actualization. This experience also supports selfacutalization in the caregiver. Giving care to patients is made possible and more effective if the caregiver is also a care receiver. Because caring cannot always be reciprocated by a patient, care needs to be reciprocated by colleagues. A nurse's ability to give care is enhanced if that nurse has experienced caring in personal life. If nurses learn how to give care and have confidence in their technical and professional competence, Green-Hernandez[17] says that they can be effective caregivers. That is, learning + competence + confidence = caring. Further, Green-Hernandez believes there are seven concepts that guide caring in today's world of high technology—being there, supporting, empathizing, communicating, helping, giving time, and reciprocating. By being there for the consumer, nurses can provide comfort and security. This may be expressed verbally or nonverbally but should be expressed, predictable, and nonjudgmental. In this way, nurses can transmit support through nurturing. Empathy comes from life experience and is a necessary skill for caregivers to communicate effectively. Helping others while providing physical care is enhanced by nurses' perceptions that time is available to do holistic care. To practice nursing in a caring manner necessitates reciprocity of caring; this prevents burnout of the caregiver.[16,17]

Whatever theory of caring is personally subscribed to, educators need to weave the concepts of caring into all learning experiences. If staff development educators truly care, caring will become a part of the educational endeavors.

INCREASING IMPORTANCE OF CREDENTIALS AND CREDENTIALING

With the growing demand for quality care, consumers have great interest in the credentials of their caregivers. Government agencies, including state boards of nursing, are requiring certain certificates, courses, and credentials for some advanced nurse practitioner roles. Appropriate roles demand appropriate credentials. Academic credentials commensurate with college teachers are normally expected of staff development educators if they are to be respected in their roles as educators.

Appropriate Credentials and Roles for Staff Development

A graduate degree in nursing is currently necessary for educators in nursing staff development. Roberta Abruzzese[1] contends that advanced degrees are necessary for the ability to manage systems, solve problems, and motivate others in the turbulent environment in which health care leaders and educators must function. In the service setting, clinical nurse specialists are prepared at the master's degree level. Similar preparation must be expected of the nursing staff development educator if equal peer status is to be maintained. Staff development educators must be prepared to assess needs, develop appropriate curricula within budgeted realities, implement innovative learning methodologies, and evaluate outcomes regarding quality and cost effectiveness. Skills required for staff development educators, such as proposal and grant writing, require basic critical thinking, organized writing, and budgeting skills.

Some graduate nursing programs offer a tract in staff development within the education specialty. If the program does not offer such an emphasis, the choice is usually between a clinical specialty or nursing administration. Although either avenue can offer appropriate preparation for educators, nursing administration is more beneficial to staff development educators who are interested in managing hospital unit programs and hospital projects. If a clinical specialty or nurse practitioner tract is chosen, a few administrative courses should be incorporated for educators who want to be effective in today's health care organizations. Clinical specialty courses also enhance nurse educators who are in the administrative tract.

Nursing staff development departments must build support within the administration. An excellent way to accomplish this is by understanding the management perspective and setting mutual goals. A background in administration is also helpful when structuring a management development program, which is strongly needed by all hospitals at this time.

To promote the mission of the organization, current nurse educators need to understand and teach (or facilitate the teaching of) systems, change theory, interpersonal relationships, organizational behavior, and health care economics and politics. In *Megatrends 2000*, Naisbitt and Aburdene[23] emphasize the importance of "people" skills rather than "task" skills. These authors predict that the most exciting breakthroughs of the twenty-first century will shift from technology to an expanding concept of what it means to be human.

It is also essential for health care organizations to provide management development, especially to first-level and middle-level managers. The question is, who should provide this management development? Executive managers are generally not educators, and the concept of mentors (as found in the business world) is not prevalent in the health care industry. It is too time and energy consuming for these managers to focus on basic management development. Therefore classes on management development are best taught with an educator-manager team to incorporate theory and practical examples. Several other approaches for management development include self-study or group-study programs based on management theory as applied to nursing practice. The National League for Nursing (NLN) offers this approach through its management development series.[27,28] This series is a competency-based approach that covers economics, accounting, finance, people, policies, politics, quality improvement, risk management, and law for administrators and vice-presidents of nursing. Using good resources, team teaching and group discussions provide simple but effective basic management development programs. Nursing staff development educators who are well versed in administrative theory have an organizational advantage. Such educators can facilitate not only management development but also strategic retreats, meetings, projects, and proposals. A management understanding broadens both the scope and worth of educators' services to the organization. In addition to the administrative focus in the role of nursing staff development educators, clinical experience is essential. Even staff development educators who focus on administration should have a background of strong clinical experience and recognized competence. Most staff development educators are responsible for multiple and diverse areas of clinical practice, but it is difficult to be a clinical expert in all areas. Therefore contemporary nursing staff development educators must function as coordinators of education and integrate both staff nurses with clinical expertise and clinical nurse specialists into program planning and teaching. Spalt and Moellering[30] support the system in which the staff development educator plays a facilitative role by providing high-quality education in this era of rapidly advancing technology. In this system a staff nurse is selected, developed, and supported in the assessment, planning, implementation, and evaluation of education for each unit within the hospital. Alternatively, a nurse educator may be counted as a staff member 20% of the time. This provides the opportunity for the nurse educator to maintain competencies and credibility, readily assess the learning needs of staff nurses, and function as a role model by demonstrating excellent clinical skills.

In many systems, each nurse educator is responsible for several specific hospital units and stays in touch with the real needs of staff nurses and these units. Co-chairing a staff development unit-based task force with a staff nurse helps ensure that staff development classes and projects are based on need. In addition to providing necessary education, this facilitation results in effective networking among nursing staff, management, and educators. This facilitation also provides an opportunity to develop the staff nurse who acts as co-chairperson.

Certification for Nursing Staff Development Educators

According to Piemonte,[24] "The certification process enables a profession to design and articulate for its members the new knowledge required for practice." The certification for nursing staff development educators validates the knowledge and expertise required in a specific clinical or functional area of nursing.[6]

Certification is not a new concept to nursing. Many nursing organizations have certified clinical nurses for years. Piemonte[24] reports that the advent of "advanced clinical specialties influenced steady movement toward certification of individuals prepared to practice beyond a minimum level of competence." Certification recognizes advanced practice, enhances prestige, and provides opportunities to upgrade performance.[20]

The interest in certification for nursing staff development is recent. This interest emerged when the ANA offered certification for nursing administration. Certification provides a mechanism to ensure that educators have the knowledge, skills, and credentials necessary for nursing staff development. Education is a specialty practice area. As Harris asked, "How can we value continuing education, orientation, and inservice education without recognizing that certain expertise must be present among those who are planning, implementing and evaluating such programs?"[20] Certification promotes recognition for staff development educators. This recognition exists among professional peers and other professional groups that equate certification with credibility and status. In addition, certification encourages interprofessional consultation and mutual problem solving.[20]

The first certification examination for staff development and continuing education was offered in the fall of 1992. This examination tests foundations of nursing practice, educational process, management of offerings and programs, and roles of manager, consultant, and researcher.*

Accreditation of Nursing Staff Development Programs

Accreditation is another credentialing issue affecting staff development departments in the 1990s. As the resurgence of interest in mandatory continuing education for renewal of RN licensure sweeps the United States again, there is renewed interest in accreditation of nursing staff development programs. The American Nurses Credentialing Center (ANCC) provides several options for staff development departments to become accredited or approved. First, the department may choose to submit a detailed report to be evaluated by site visitors and if judged worthy to be accredited for 6 years. Second, the department may choose to apply to an accredited state nurses' association for a 2-year program approval. Third, the department may choose to submit only certain courses for approval by the state nurses' association or a specialty nurses' association. Whether the department seeks accreditation, program approval, or course approval, the purpose is to document high standards and to award contact hours for continuing education. Ordinarily, classes that provide in-service education specific to only one organization are not eligible for contact hour approval.

This system of credentialing by the ANCC is often complicated by additional regulations determined by some states that have mandatory continuing education through their state boards of nursing. Some states with mandatory continuing education recognize and accept the high standards of ANCC, whereas other states maintain their own system of credentialing. Conscientious staff development directors must decide which rules apply in a given state and which credentials have the greatest return for the investment of time and money.

When mandatory continuing education is instituted within a state, the nursing staff development department is often expected to provide more continuing education courses. These courses may compete with in-service classes for both time and resources of the staff development department. Whenever an inservice class is at least an hour long, an attempt should be made to elevate it to the level of continuing education if, in fact, it is continuing education.

CAREER DEVELOPMENT

The career development role of the staff development educator is an ongoing, helpful resource. It can provide career advancement counseling, resources for educational advancement, study techniques, publications, and grant writing.

---

*Applications for the blueprint of the examination can be obtained by writing the American Nurses Credentialing Center, 600 Maryland Avenue SW, #100W, Washington, DC 20024-2571 or by calling 1-800-284-2378.

Career Advancement Counseling Service

The counseling role of the nursing staff development educator is varied and needs to be innovative and individualized for each situation. For example, a nurse facing an ethical dilemma in the intensive care nursery may be directed to the ethics committee or helped to form an ethics committee. A nurse who has written an excellent care plan on a unique patient problem may need help organizing and presenting a conference or class about the case. A nurse who has shown interest in patient-controlled analgesia may be willing to help in the product evaluation of related equipment being purchased for the hospital. An obstetric nurse who is an exceptional speaker may be enticed to speak to a community group about the specialty. Assisting with the funding and development of research proposals would be wonderful support for several nurses interested in a more formal approach to a nursing care problem. Nursing staff development educators need to play a major role in identifying these individual growth opportunities for more advanced staff nurses.

Resources for Educational Advancement

As the trend toward higher education for nurses continues, one counseling goal for staff development educators is to encourage nurses to pursue academic advancement. This is especially important for nurses holding diplomas and associate degrees because new legislation threatens to change the value of their status. Returning to school for a master's or doctorate degree is also an area that needs staff development support.

Staff development departments can assist and encourage further academic pursuits in several ways. The first step is to offer information about returning to school, thus increasing awareness and interest. Inviting colleges and universities to participate in a "school fair" that provides pamphlets, posters, and representatives to answer questions is a good start. Flyers and one-to-one efforts to increase class attendance are also essential, as is a central location and time for class. A "library" of school catalogs with sample applications may be helpful if it is done before enrollment dates and provides enrollment information. This information could be located in the education department or on a poster that rotates from unit to unit. Some academic programs may be offered "on-site"; that is, a university holds the classes at an agency. Enrollment may be from one hospital only or open to nurses of neighboring hospitals; this helps achieve a minimum number of learners and extends goodwill. On-site programs work best for baccalaureate of science in nursing (BSN) programs. The on-site design allows classes to be scheduled at times when the staff is most available.

After nurses have begun to pursue degrees, the staff development department may further help these nurses by organizing a student support group. For example, once a month, nurses could have brown-bag lunches and listen to a speaker who would briefly discuss topics such as "managing the stress of job, school, and life" and then have a few minutes for sharing coping perspectives. Another support is to recognize each nurse in an in-house newsletter or to send a personal letter of recognition from the director of nursing.

The agency could assist its students by finding placements within that agency for a residency or school project; this benefits both the student and the organization. Using staff development networks to find the right "fit" for this is worth the time and energy required.

Educational advancement may also take the form of continuing education. Encouraging nurses to attend professional programs in their areas of expertise supports their professional development.

In addition, the staff development department can encourage and assist nurses to run for political office or for an office in a professional association, to make a presentation, or to respond to calls for abstracts. This may be done by sharing information. Individuals may need to be identified and encouraged or mentored one-to-one as they move from a position on a local association committee to regional or national offices. Again, recognition of these accomplishments in an in-house newsletter or local newspaper, an awards ceremony, or a letter from the director of nursing will encourage others to pursue professional activities.

Techniques for Studying and Test Taking

When assisting staff nurses as they "move ahead," whether through academic preparation or certification, the staff development department can assist them in relearning studying and test-taking skills.

Some nurses may not have attended formal education courses for many years and need help with study techniques. Reminders of how to read faster, how to take notes effectively, and how to reinforce learning can make the difference between success and failure.

A brief program or self-study module covering the basics of outlining and the use of study groups, stress reducers, memory aids, and other available resources may benefit some nurses. Other helpful resources for nurses who are studying include information on review courses and access to computer lines for literature searches.

Test taking often provokes anxiety in nurses who have not taken tests recently. Providing mock tests that illustrate a variety of multiple choice and essay questions prepares nurses for success in academic courses or on certification examinations. The nursing staff development department should have sample questions, outlines, and recommended references for all certification examinations. The introductory pages of some National Council Licensure Examination (NCLEX) review books contain many helpful hints for successfully answering multiple choice questions. These hints are as helpful for tests in a baccalaureate program or certification examination as they are for NCLEX examinations.

Providing Assistance with Manuscripts

Many nurses have a potential manuscript for publication within them; some have several. The increasing number of journals on health care topics creates an opportunity for many new writers to become published. Setting up a publishing support group and helping nurses get started is of benefit to the nurses' development. A "kickoff" event, such as a speaker on the topic of writing, is helpful to begin a writing support group. Each group session should offer an opportunity to review progress on individual manuscripts after a brief presentation given by a staff development educator about some aspect of publishing. Examples of discussion topics include the following: ideas for publication, finding a journal, writing a query letter, conducting computer searches, and using peer reviews. *How to Write and Publish Articles in Nursing*[29] offers many tools for step-by-step writing and publishing, including numerous "tips of the trade" from leading nurse authors who were surveyed as part of the book's development.

Developing Grants for Nursing Service

Another increasing trend is the pursuit of grant monies. Facilitating the development of grant proposals is increasingly becoming a responsibility of the nursing staff development department. Whether setting up a distinguished lecture series, a nursing research center, or a reentry nursing education program, the nursing staff development department routinely finds funding outside the organization. Staff development educators are ideal facilitators for the development of grant proposals. A relationship should be established between the hospital development office and community relations department (if these departments exist) to work together to seek funding.

SUMMARY

For nursing staff development departments to survive in the turbulent health care arena of the 1990s, educational processes must be consistent with the needs and expectations of the organization and the employees. Desired outcomes must be defined and clearly measurable.[33]

The nursing staff development department of the future must be aware of the organization's direction. This department must also be a major and supportive force in achieving high-quality patient care in a cost-effective way while maintaining a satisfied, competent, productive nursing staff. Nurse educators must be integrated into the organization that supports and develops nurse managers, staff nurses, and all levels of personnel in the differentiated practice of nursing. Nurse educators must have educational, clinical, and business skills. They should use these skills to help create the health care organization of the future through the development of innovative projects and programs that are visible, valued, and necessary for organizational excellence.

REFERENCES

1. Abruzzese R: Counterpoint: against certification of staff development educators, *J Nurs Staff Dev* 2(1):9, 1986.
2. Aburdene P, Naisbitt J: *Megatrends for women*, New York, 1992, Villard Books.
3. Argyris C et al: The future of workplace learning and performance, *Train Dev* 48(5A):s36, 1994.

4. Bergman RR: Reengineering health care; *Hosp Health Networks* 68(3):28, 1994.
5. Betts VT: Defining our future, dividing our resources, *Am Nurse*, Mar 1995, p 3.
6. Brunt B: Continuing education and megatrends, *J Nurs Staff Dev* 4(4):174, 1988.
7. Byers B: AONE exec talks about restructuring issues, *Am Nurse*, Mar 1995, p 21.
8. Camin LR: Health care reform: initial implications for continuing education in nursing, *J Contin Educ Nurs* 26(2):53, 1995.
9. Carnevale AP, Stone SC: Diversity beyond the Golden Rule, *Train Dev* 48(10):22, 1994.
10. Chinn PL: Anthology on caring, New York, 1991, National League for Nursing.
11. Chinn PL: Looking into the crystal ball: positioning ourselves for the year 2000, *Nursing Outlook* 36(6):251, 1991.
12. Curtin LL: Designing new roles: nursing in the '90s and beyond, *Nurs Manage* 21(2):7, 1990.
13. Dahmer B: When technologies connect, *Train Dev* 47(1):52, 1993.
14. Eckholm E: While Congress remains silent, health care transforms itself, *New York Times*, Dec 18, 1994.
15. Gonce-Winder C, Kidd RO, Lenz ER: Optimizing computer-based system use in health professions' education programs, *Comput Nurs* 11(4):199, 1993.
16. Green-Hernandez C: A phenomenological investigation of caring as a lived experience in nurses. In Chinn PL, editor: *Anthology on caring*, New York, 1991, National League for Nursing.
17. Green-Hernandez C: Professional nurse caring: a conceptual model for nursing. In Neil RM, Watts R, editors: *Caring and nursing: explorations in feminist perspectives*, New York, 1991, National League for Nursing.
18. Gundlach AM: Adapting to change: reconsidering staff development organization, design, and purpose, *JCEN* 25(3):120, 1994.
19. Hard R: Inside track: hospitals link education with hard numbers, *Hospitals* 64:46, 1990.
20. Harris H: Point: for certification of nursing staff development educators, *J Nurs Staff Dev* 2(1):5, 1986.
21. Lachat MF, Cowen ER: Developing a community-wide HIV/AIDS nurse education series: a strategy for success, *J Contin Educ Nurs*, 24(6):255, 1993.
22. Mayeroff M: *On caring*, New York, 1971, Harper & Row.
23. Naisbitt J, Aburdene P: *Megatrends 2000*, New York, 1990, William Morrow.
24. Piemonte R: Point-counterpoint: certification of staff development educators—the credentialling process, *J Nurs Staff Dev* 2(1):2, 1986.
25. Pincus LB, Trivedi SM: A time for action: responding to AIDS, *Train Dev* 48(1):45, 1994.
26. Price JL, Cordell B: Cultural diversity and patient teaching, *J Contin Educ Nurs* 25(4):163, 1994.
27. Sheridan DR: *NLN nursing management skills: a modular self-assessment series. Module no. 1: Economics, accounting, and finance*, New York, 1989, National League for Nursing.
28. Sheridan DR: *NLN nursing management skills: a modular self-assessment series. Module no. 3: Quality assurance, law, and risk management*, New York, 1991, National League for Nursing.
29. Sheridan DR, Dowdney R: *How to write and publish articles in nursing*, New York, 1986, Springer Publishing.
30. Spalt S, Moellering J: The education connection: a staff development concept, *J Nurs Staff Dev* 5(3):116, 1989.
31. Styles MM: Macrotrends in nursing practice: what's in the pipeline, *JCEN* 24(1):7, 1993.
32. Thomas VC: The downside of diversity, *Train Dev* 48(1)60, 1994.
33. Weeks L, Spor K: Hospital nursing education: dispelling the doomsday prophesies, *J Nurs Adm* 17(3):34, 1987.

◆ ■ ◆ ■ ◆ ■ ◆ ■ ◆ ■

Conceptual Foundations of Nursing Staff Development

3

The primary task of nursing staff development educators is to help the nursing staff translate the knowledge, principles, skills, and theories learned in nursing school into practice. Sometimes this requires assistance with immediate problem solving such as learning a new procedure; other times this requires assistance with planning and implementing long-range career goals. Nursing staff development educators work with nurses of different educational backgrounds and varied interests. In addition, their clinical practice levels may range from advanced beginner to expert clinician.

Currently, the health care environment requires staff development educators to demonstrate their worth to the entire organization rather than exclusively to the department of nursing. Clients of the staff department are not only members of the nursing department but also staff from other departments. The prevailing emphasis on interdisciplinary, patient-centered health care mandates that staff development educators fulfill the roles of educational consultant and clinical resource. Educators must be recognized as experts in the educational process. As staff development educators help others translate their knowledge, skills, and attitudes into practical problem solving, they most often use the guidelines for adult learning, as popularized by Malcolm Knowles,[12] and the Dreyfus model of skill acquisition, as popularized by Patricia Benner.[2]

The emphasis on problem solving in clinical practice requires the incorporation of critical thinking skills into all aspects of nursing staff development programming. Learners must be encouraged to question long-held beliefs and explore new ways of interpreting situations, especially situations based on cultural customs.

Humanistic education emphasizes that adult learners are self-determining and capable of identifying their own learning needs. Educators of adults should be "learner centered." That is, these educators should acknowledge the emotions and feelings of adult learners and understand the importance of personal fulfillment[8] while remaining focused and competent on the job. A humanistic viewpoint does not discount the importance of accurately performing certain tasks such as cardiopulmonary resuscitation (CPR) or intravenous management. Rather, humanistic education stresses the partnership of learners and educators. In such a relationship, educators function as resources and support people, whereas learners in the health care profession assume responsibility for learning the skills necessary to provide high-quality patient health care. Humanism can be incorporated into a program by meeting individual needs to be treated as adult learners, to attend classes specifically directed to the appropriate level of practice, and have opportunities to use and improve critical thinking skills. These aspects of humanistic education form the foundation for staff development departments that emphasize individuality, caring, and competence. These aspects also reflect a concern for the psychosocial development of adults and its impact on adult learning.

KNOWLES' CONCEPTS OF ADULT LEARNING

Knowles[13] stated that "At its best, an adult-learning experience should be a process of self-directed inquiry, with the resources of the teacher, fellow students, and materials being available to the learners, but not imposed on them." Knowles' name is linked with andragogic concepts of learning. Andragogy is "the art and science of helping adults learn"; pedagogy is "the art and science of teaching."[12] Knowles believed the primary and immediate mission of every adult educator should be to help adults satisfy their learning needs and achieve their goals. In his opinion, educators are most effective when they act as catalysts for learning. As learners proceed through a process of self-directed inquiry, educators become facilitators and resources.

According to Knowles, andragogy can be explained as a set of learning assumptions and a series of recommendations for planning, implementing, and evaluating learning.[14] The following lists assumptions about learning[14]:

1. Adults have a need to know the reason they should learn something.
2. Adults have a need to be self-directed.
3. Adults have a greater amount and different quality of experience than people who are younger.
4. Adults become ready to learn when they need to know or be able to do something so that they can perform their tasks more effectively and satisfyingly.
5. Adults enter into a learning experience with a task-centered, problem-centered, or life-centered orientation to learning.
6. Adults are motivated to learn by extrinsic and intrinsic motivators.

In andragogy the series of recommendations or implications for educating adults has a different focus than pedagogy. Pedagogic educators focus on transmitting the content; andragogic educators focus on facilitating the learners' acquisition of the content.[14] Knowles' series of recommendations relates to the following[14]:

1. Setting the atmosphere
2. Creating a mutual planning mechanism
3. Diagnosing the participants' learning needs
4. Translating learning needs into objectives
5. Designing and managing a pattern of learning experiences
6. Evaluating the extent to which the objectives have been achieved

Although refined and slightly different from earlier statements by Knowles,[12,13] these concepts have exciting implications for nursing staff development educators. These concepts enhance the educational programs of nursing staff development departments and make educators and learners equal partners in maintaining previously learned competencies and attaining new competencies for high-quality patient health care.

Need to Know

Professional nurses have strong beliefs about what educational offerings are needed to enhance clinical practice. As with other adult learners, nurses may weigh the value of participating in a learning experience before committing their time. Encouragement from a manager about the program is rarely reason enough to attend. Therefore staff development educators should structure learning experiences through simulation or role playing so that reasons to learn and the value of learning are experienced.

Need to Be Self-Directing

Adults are individuals who have accepted the responsiblity for their own lives. Adults are self-directed, making decisions and facing the consequences of those decisions.[13] Although adults can be very self-directed in other facets of their lives, most adults have been conditioned by previous educational experiences to assume that learners should be passive and dependent. Adult learners may approach an educational setting with the attitude that teachers are responsible for the direction and success of learning experiences. Knowles points out that adult educators need to help learners discover that they can and should take responsibility for their own learning, in addition to being accountable for their own professional development.

Several implications for nursing staff development practice may be derived from the need of adults to be self-directed. The learning environment should be conducive to adult learning by establishing an atmosphere of mutuality, respectfulness, collaboration, and informality. The physical environment of the classroom should be arranged comfortably and informally. Acoustics and lighting need to accommodate any adult who may have difficulty hearing or seeing. If traditional classroom seating arrangements are altered, group participation may be enhanced. For example, chairs or desks may be arranged in a circle or around a table with the educator seated with the learners. If this is not possible, the educator can give learners a feeling of partnership by using good communication skills, such as maintaining eye contact, encouraging and respecting student input, and acknowledging that adult learning is self-directed.

These skills correlate with the most important aspect of learning—the psychologic environment. Adults need to feel accepted, respected, and supported. The crucial component of the psychologic environment is that adult learners should feel free to express themselves without fear of punishment, censure, or ridicule.

Differences in Experiences

Adults primarily derive their self-identity from their experiences. They have different types and amounts of experience than children. Regardless of the amount of "formal" education, an adult's experiences should be valued; to devalue a person's experience is to show that person disrespect.[14] When teaching adults, educators must acknowledge the experiences of their learners and provide experiential learning exercises that capture the learner's knowledge and skills. Experiential methods such as case studies, simulation, group discussion, and role playing are effective. For example, many practice settings require mandatory attendance at programs that review emergency situations. Instead of a simple lecture and discussion format, a variety of simulated situations can be used in which learners must respond by performing interventions and using equipment. Such an approach is more practical, involves group participation, and may actually be "fun" for the participants. Attendance may also improve.

Educators should remember that adults have acquired a number of habits and ideas that may tend to be unaccepting of some new concepts or proposals for change. To counteract these negative attitudes toward learning experiences, educators should try brain storming, enacting a worst or best case scenario, and working on "future-gazing" exercises with the participants.

Readiness to Learn

Adults need to be involved in assessing their own educational needs and planning ways to meet those needs. Adults are more committed to activities that they have helped plan and implement. Nursing staff development educators conduct endless needs assessments and inquiries regarding the nursing service department's educational needs. Unless the results of these surveys are shared with the respondents and acted on in an appropriate time, participation in learning experiences will be adversely affected. Nursing service staff will not necessarily remember that a particular class was formed in response to a 6-month-old needs survey.

When adult learners are "sent" to a class by their managers or assigned because the class is mandatory, they may exhibit negative attitudes and show a lack of attention. One way to counteract this is to openly acknowledge the dissonance and involve all learners in some form of self-diagnosis of their learning needs. The use of a competency rating scale or pretest may demonstrate the class' value in terms of necessary knowledge or skills.

Survey results and self-diagnosis of learning needs may also be valuable tools for retention of nurses. Often the needs surveys provide clues about long-range career plans. Staff development educators may use these clues to foster professional development and retention of valuable employees by helping nurses and organizations identify mutuality of goals and ways to meet the goals that will benefit employees and employers.

Orientation to Learning

A development task is one that takes place at a certain period in an individual's life. Task achievement leads to satisfaction and success with later tasks; task failure leads to failure with future goals and endeavors.[13] Each developmental task produces a readiness to learn. A learning situation has its best chance of success if approached developmentally. Adults' readiness to learn and "teachable moments" occur as a result of social roles. Education that is needed to succeed in a specific adult role (for example, as a parent, worker, or spouse) must be presented at the appropriate time. Adult educators and adult learners must learn to recognize and prepare for these teachable moments.

Another factor that stimulates adults' readiness to learn is the immediate applicability of the educational information to life situations. Nurses enter the staff development or continuing education setting seeking solutions to problems they encounter on the job or in career planning. They must be able to see the usefulness and applicability of the educational content to their clinical performance and professional growth. This problem-solving orientation of adult learners means that the staff development specialist must understand every learning experience from the viewpoint of the learners and must take into account the learners' concerns in their professional environments.

Extrinsic and Intrinsic Motivators

Children are often motivated to learn by pressure from their parents and teachers, competition for grades, desire to earn a degree, or other external motivations. Adults also respond to external motivators for learning, such as a pay raise or promotion, a permanent day-shift assignment, or no obligation to work on weekends once they advance to a higher level of competence. However, professional people are more likely to seek learning because of intrinsic motivation such as self-fulfillment, responsibility, achievement, or a desire to better perform their tasks.

Staff development educators can capitalize on both extrinsic and intrinsic motivators when publicizing course offerings. Educators can involve learners in identifying the benefits of a class, setting personal and work objectives, and choosing between two different methods of presenting course content. For example, learners could choose between role playing and a written examination to demonstrate competence in a particular area.

Implications for Staff Development

Knowles' concepts of teaching from the andragogic perspective offers guidance for teachers of adults. Nursing staff development educators are facilitators and resource people. Staff development educators expose learners to new possibilities for self-fulfillment and help learners clarify their educational needs as a means of achieving professional goals. Educators are responsible for providing appropriate physical and psychologic environments for the educational experience. The atmosphere must be one of mutual support. Adult learners should be encouraged to express their views and feelings without fear of condemnation or ridicule.

Learners must realize that they are accountable for their own learning experiences and that they have a responsibility to the educational process and their own professional development. Educators and learners should evaluate learning experiences together after developing mutually acceptable criteria for success.

PSYCHOSOCIAL DEVELOPMENT AND ADULT EDUCATION

Nursing staff development specialists must be able to link the conceptual foundations of adult education to psychosocial development, or to the ways adults grow and develop throughout their lives. A great deal of the work in adult learning is based on psychosocial developmental paradigms.[16,17] However, these paradigms have often been based on traditional theories of psychosocial development that have been derived primarily from studies of men.[5] These traditional theories describe adult development as a universal experience with specific periods or stages through which all adults must pass. Success is measured by accomplishing particular tasks within each stage, and the ultimate goal of life is to achieve autonomy.[9,15]

The majority of nurses with whom nursing staff development specialists interact are women. It has been proposed that women's psychosocial development is different from that of men in the following three key ways: (1) women's development is diverse and discontinuous, (2) relationships are of critical importance to women throughout their lives, and (3) women strive to achieve both identity and intimacy.[5,6] Educators must find ways to design adult education programs with consideration of a variety of psychosocial foundations.

The humanist philosophy of adult education provides a framework for such educational design.[5] Relational learning can be facilitated by stressing collaborative inquiry and a democratic approach to learning.[11] Diverse and discontinuous patterns of development require a staff development specialist to be aware of the possibility for periods of stability and transition that will influence their learners' needs, values, and goals.[5] Identity and intimacy requires collaboration, respect, and awareness of the principles of adult learning and adult psychosocial development. The challenge remains for staff development specialists to grasp the essentials of the impact of psychosocial development and design an educational framework that allows for the development of the beneficial teaching/learning experience for educators and learners.

Belensky et al[1] agree with Caffarella[5] that women have different ways of knowing as a result of their psychological development. Women may lack confidence in their learning activities and require support from their teachers. Treating women learners as intelligent and respecting the knowledge they have gained from their nurturing roles helps women connect present learning to previous experience. Respect for other women's ideas and conclusions provides a "voice" for many women who have previously been silent. Developing a voice helps adult women learners develop a sense of self as a respected learner whose mind is capable of facing many challenges.[1]

BENNER'S CONCEPTS OF PRACTICE LEVELS

The promotion of professional growth and development among nurses is contingent on educational needs being recognized and met throughout their careers. By analyzing observations reported by nurses in actual clinical practice, Patricia Benner[2] was able to identify various levels of clinical nursing practice. She noted that as clinical practice skills develop, nurses change their intellectual orientation, integrate their knowledge, and refocus their decision-making processes based on perceptual awareness rather than on process-oriented foundations.[2] Benner describes five levels of clinical nursing practice—novice, advanced beginner, competent, proficient, and expert.

The recognition of five distinct levels of clinical nursing practice has significant implications for nursing staff development educators. Within realistic time, personnel, and budgetary limitations, educational programs should be planned to meet the needs and promote the professional growth of nurses at all levels of expertise.

Novice and Advanced-Beginner Levels

Benner uses the term *novice* to refer to beginning nursing students who have no background or understanding of clinical situations. She notes, however, that students who have functioned as nurse assistants are not novices in basic skills. In Benner's opinion, "it is unusual for a graduate nurse to be a novice...the newly graduated nurse will perform at the advanced-beginner level."[2]

The common practice of referring to new graduates as novices when they are really performing at advanced-beginner levels has adverse implications for staff development education. The knowledge of new nurses is devalued, and they receive instruction appropriate for first-year nursing students rather than for newly graduated nurses. Because newly graduated nurses feel insecure about their clinical practice skills, they are often happy to hide behind the label of novice thereby having a more sheltered introduction to the work world of nursing.

In contrast to the context-free rules taught to novices, advanced beginners require extensive, guided experiences with patients so that they can readily identify components of recurring patient situations. These recurring components provide cues that enable nurses to make judgments and predictions about patients who are becoming more ill, are improving, or are ready to learn about their health problems.

Nursing staff development educators are responsible for facilitating a successful transfer from acquiring context-free knowledge as students to performing effectively in the new role of professional nurses. Orientation to the practice setting should be based on measurable, reliable, and valid methods, such as performance simulations, role playing, and games that provide opportunities for new nurses to perform technical procedures and begin functioning within the rules and regulations of the practice setting.[7] Educational interventions that concentrate on the enhancement of organizational skills, priority setting, and technical skills are appropriate. Performance simulations, rehearsals, and return demonstrations of technical skills are critical aspects for the development needs of advanced beginners.

The term *novice* is not exclusive to beginning students. Benner points out that nurses entering a clinical setting in which they are not experienced may function at the performance level of novices if the patient health care goals are unfamiliar. For example, a nurse who transfers from a rehabilitation unit to a high-risk neonatal unit will be at the novice level. This is an important concept for staff development because rule-governed orientations may be appropriate for experienced nurses if the experienced nurses are entering a completely unfamiliar area of practice. Staff development educators have a responsibility to assess levels of expertise and initiate appropriate educational opportunities.

The Competent Level

The competent level of practice is usually demonstrated by nurses who have been in the same or a similar clinical practice situation for 2 or 3 years. Competent nurses are consciously aware of managing clinical practice in terms of long-range goals or plans.[2] Competent nurses develop nursing plans based on a conscious, abstract, and analytic assessment of the problem. They also set priorities, meet the most urgent needs, and identify the aspects of patient care that may safely be addressed after critical interventions are performed. They do not have the speed and flexibility of proficient practitioners, but they are able to cope with many facets of clinical nursing.

Staff development learning opportunities for this level of nursing practice should include decision-making games and simulations based on targeted competencies. Patient management problems may be simulated to permit learners to make decisions about patient care management and cope with the consequences of their decisions.[10]

At the end of 3 or 4 years of practice in the same or a similar patient care setting, competent nurses are often restless. This is frequently the time when they return to school for a higher degree or change to a different area of practice. As one nurse described the process, "I've been on the neurosurgical floor for 3 years. There aren't any new procedures; there aren't any new surgeons. They do the same procedures every week and the nursing care has become routine. I can't see myself doing this for the rest of my life. There's nothing new to learn. I'm bored."

Many competent nurses spend their nursing careers changing from one clinical area of practice to another. As soon as they become competent in one area, they move to another to keep themselves stimulated by new challenges. In this way, nurses are denying themselves the opportunity to advance to the proficient and expert levels of practice. As a result, they are less likely to contribute to nursing theory through research and advanced practice patterns and to attain doctoral degrees.

Staff development educators play a major role in helping competent nurses increase their opportunities for self-fulfillment by providing information about advanced education, inviting them to help teach classes or to be preceptors, and helping them write books for publication or become involved in research projects. In these ways, competent nurses are stimulated to learn and share with others their insights about their particular area of practice. This is also the time to encourage nurses to become more interested in the patients and individual coping strategies of each family. No two patients experience the same surgical procedure in the same way. Each patient is unique and requires particular adjustments to the illness. Nurses need to find satisfaction in helping and teaching families. This satisfaction can compensate for the stimulation that was previously found in learning about new procedures and proving competent in emergency situations. These nurses can then progress to the proficient and expert levels of practice.

The Proficient and Expert Levels

The term *perception* is key when describing proficient nurses. Proficient nurses perceive clinical situations as wholes rather than components; they base decisions on experience and recent events. Proficient practitioners understand the clinical situation in relation to long-term goals. From their own experience, they can anticipate the events to expect in a given situation and the way that care should be planned in response to these events.[2] For example, a proficient nurse is able to assess a patient's readiness to learn by observing subtle clues in that patient's behavior. These nurses use rules as a guide but are able to assess situations as a whole before intervening. For instance, a proficient nurse evaluates an elevation of systolic blood pressure in terms of the entire patient picture, not simply by establishing norms of blood pressure ranges. A proficient nurse considers whether the patient is in pain or anxious and then looks for factors that may be contributing to the elevated reading.

Benner believes that proficient nurses benefit from inductive staff development activities that begin with clinical situations requiring identification of ways to cope with the situation and problem solving. Staff development educators may find that case studies and self-learning modules are helpful educational tools that combine theoretical and practical applications. These methods must contain complexities and challenges similar to actual clinical situations to be effective.

Expert nurses have extensive experience and possess an intuitive grasp of clinical situations. They identify critical problem areas without wasting time reviewing multiple alternatives, and they are quick to initiate correct interventions. Expert clinicians have a perceptual acuity that characterizes their clinical judgment and ability. Their management of complex clinical situations is recognized by colleagues and patients as expert. However, attempts to objectively measure the perceptual abilities that characterize these clinicians is difficult. Experts need to document their decision-making steps so that these steps can be available for further study and can help other nurses move from the proficient to expert level of practice.

The implications of these needs for staff development are complex and challenging. These nurses should be assisted to explore career pathways such as clinical teaching and administration. Educational options such as certification and graduate degrees should be facilitated. These nurses should be lecturing at national meetings, publishing their patient care experiences, writing books, and participating as principal investigators in large grants. For some expert nurses, this will never happen unless they receive encouragement and assistance from nursing staff development educators.

One role frequently assigned to expert nurses is that of preceptor. This is advantageous only if they are preceptors for nurses at the competent or proficient levels of practice. Most expert nurses have already forgotten the many steps and cues that led to decision making at the advanced-beginner level of practice, so they often become impatient with nurses at that level. The advanced-beginner nurse also becomes frustrated because the expert seems to make decisions with little objective data, and the expert's decision is based on intuitive data that the expert may not be able to quantify easily.

Implications for Staff Development

Benner's application of skill acquisition steps to levels of nursing practice has important implications for nursing staff development educators. The professional development and job satisfaction of nurses are enhanced by investigating the educational needs of nurses at each practice level and by planning learning experiences that meet those needs. Likewise, the effectiveness of staff development educational endeavors may increase when learning is tailored to different practice levels. The staff development department also benefits by incorporating the talents of nurses at higher levels of practice into learning experiences.

BROOKFIELD'S CONCEPTS OF CRITICAL THINKING

In addition to using guidelines to facilitate adult learning and to structure learning activities differently for various levels of practice, today's staff development educators attempt to infuse critical thinking skills into all learning experiences. This is not easy because of the negative connotations attached to the term *critical*. Critical connotes criticism, which is often thought of as negative, hurtful, harmful, or unfriendly. This word implies some failure on the part of the person being criticized.

Critical thinking, on the other hand, comprises "two interrelated processes: identifying and challenging assumptions, and imagining and exploring alternatives."[3] The importance of engaging in both of these processes is evident in everyday nursing practice. Managers often experience the first process without the second. Intellectually gifted new nurses are often extremely critical of systems and procedures on a patient care unit, but they do not suggest alternatives to improve the situation. Managers interpret the criticism as a personal devaluing and react negatively to this criticism and all other statements from that nurse. New nurses become frustrated because their ideas are not valued. These are major communication problems that staff development educators can improve by incorporating aspects of critical thinking in all learning experiences.

Components

Brookfield envisioned four components of critical thinking: (1) identifying and challenging assumptions, (2) challenging the importance of context, (3) imagining and exploring alternatives, and (4) allowing reflective skepticism.[4] The first component is to examine the values, beliefs, rationale, and appropriateness of ideas that influence actions. Many of the ideas that influence actions are based on ethnic values, cultural customs, influential teachers, or policies and procedures learned in nursing school. Some examples of these ideas on patient health care units are that bathing every patient everyday is important, that physical activities such as measuring vital signs or changing dressings should be completed before intellectual activities such as diabetic teaching or discharge planning are performed, and that providing oral reports of the status of patients at a shift change is adequate.

The second process of critical thinking implies an examination of the circumstances surrounding an action such as the factors related to a patient's complaints or reactions to illness. Interpreting actions without considering the context with which that action occurred is seldom appropriate. "Appropriate" conduct is a function of time and culture.

The third process of critical thinking involves imagining alternatives and then exploring the feasibility of those alternatives. Anyone can think of alternatives to present systems, but finding *feasible* alternatives is a more difficult process. For example, it is easy to propose the latest fad in nursing care delivery as an alternative to the present system, but to structure the new system as a cost-effective alternative is extremely difficult to achieve.

The fourth process of critical thinking permits individuals to question ideas that claim to be the answer for all problems or the ultimate explanation of all behavior. Some examples of ideas that were supposed to be the answer to the problems of all health care organizations include management by objectives, quality circles, and primary care. These ideas are excellent and effective in some situations, but they are not solutions for every organization.

Brookfield's experiences[3] with critical thinking led him to believe that critical thinking is experienced differently by different people and is influenced most by a person's personality and background. Emotions are often a part of the critical thinking process. For example, grief or loss, as in the death of a spouse or in divorce, sometimes prompts a person to examine long-standing assumptions. The aim of incorporating critical thinking into all teaching is to promote critical thinking as a routine way of thinking and not only as a response to life crises. Usually there are both extrinsic and intrinsic motives for engaging in critical thinking. An external factor, such as a new nurse manager, may trigger an intrinsic dissatisfaction that leads to a reevaluation of working relationships or life goals. Brookfield[3] also believed that critical thinking led to critical insights, which are often serendipitous and may result from speculation on a totally different topic from the one related to the insight. For example, the discussion topic may be the way Maslow's hierarchy of needs relates to orientation of nurses to a new patient care unit. The insight may be about a child's problem adjusting to a new school. Critical thinking is most likely to occur and continue when supported by others. That is the reason all staff development educators must be familiar with the processes of critical thinking and the strategies for facilitating critical thinking in adult learners.

Facilitating Critical Thinking

There are many ways to encourage learners to be critical thinkers, that is, to encourage learners to identify and challenge assumptions and to explore alternative ways of thinking and acting. This often occurs during experiential learning strategies such as case studies, role playing, critical incident techniques, brain storming, games, and simulations. Critical thinking is also encouraged by using metaphors and analogies in teaching.

Staff development educators can facilitate the acquisition of critical thinking skills by affirming the self-worth of learners, listening attentively, supporting learners' efforts to think critically, and reflecting what seems to be the learners' perspective. Being a role model for critical thinking by examining alternative ways of interpreting events is helpful to learners. This latter opportunity often arises in patient grand rounds or case conferences in which health care professionals attempt to understand patients with difficult problems. Opportunities to model critical thinking also occur when interacting with nurses who are new to the organization. These interactions create opportunities to inquire about procedures or protocols used in other settings, discuss patient health care policies used in this setting, and explore typical problems encountered when adjusting to a new work setting.

Caffarella[4] notes that learning does not happen in a vacuum. Helping adults think critically and become self-directed is not just a "nice" idea but essential for survival in a constantly changing world. When teaching management skills to nurses who are being promoted to manager roles, staff development educators can role play situations in which employees are encouraged to voice complaints only if they also present alternative solutions and an evaluation of which solution has the best chance of success. This is one way to teach managers to encourage critical thinking on their units. It is also a problem-solving method at the lowest level of decision making. Such solutions often have the greatest success.

Implications for Staff Development

Staff development educators today are encouraged to integrate critical thinking skills into learning experiences so that learners are able to think new thoughts, question underlying assumptions that may no longer be effective, and respect each other and patients as unique individuals. Analyzing the process and components of critical thinking allows staff development educators to devise methods of structuring learning experiences so that learners are encouraged to identify and challenge assumptions and explore alternative ways of thinking and acting.

SUMMARY

The emphasis on providing self-worth, self-direction, and a respectful, supportive learning environment is evident in each of the preceding discussions. In nursing staff development the emphasis on assisting learners to translate knowledge, principles, skills, and theory into clinical practice is stressed through the pragmatic application of ideas.

Knowles' guidelines for adult learning provide a foundation for the development of the physiologic and psychologic environments necessary to promote learning. His educational guidelines depict nurses as self-directed professionals. The importance of linking psychosocial development to the practice of adult education allows for a more collaborative teaching/learning environment. Benner identified five levels of clinical practice. She describes nurses at each level and recommends teaching strategies that acknowledge the importance of nurturing nurses as they mature professionally. Brookfield advocates the fostering of critical thinking so that adults may gain control over their lives through a critical evaluation of their underlying beliefs. He espouses the empowerment of adults as they seek to challenge long-held beliefs and encourages them to consider alternatives to those beliefs. Each author advocates components of humanistic education, which emphasizes concern for the individual.

Staff development educators must analyze their own educational concepts to promote effective professional growth and development for themselves and others. Success in staff development is marked by a humanistic emphasis on individuality, caring, and competence.

REFERENCES
1. Belenky SB et al: *Women's ways of knowing*, New York, 1986, Basic Books.
2. Benner P: *From novice to expert: excellence and power in clinical practice*, Menlo Park, Calif, 1984, Addison-Wesley.
3. Brookfield S: *Developing critical thinkers*, San Francisco, 1987, Jossey-Bass.

4. Caffarella RS: On being a self-directed learner, *Adult Learning* 5(5):7, 1994.
5. Caffarella RS: *Psychosocial development of women: linkages to teaching and leadership in adult education*, Columbus, Ohio, 1992, ERIC Clearinghouse.
6. Caffarella RS, Olsen SK: Psychosocial development of women: a critical review of the literature, *Adult Educ Q* 43:125, 1993.
7. del Bueno D et al: The clinical teacher: a critical link in competence development, *J Nurs Staff Dev* 6(3):135, 1990.
8. Dolphin P, Holtzclaw BJ: *Continuing education in nursing*, Reston, Va, 1983, Reston Publishing.
9. Erikson EH: *The life cycle completed: a review*, New York, 1982, Norton.
10. Evans ML: Simulations: their selection and use in developing nursing competencies, *J Nurs Staff Dev* 5(2):65, 1989.
11. Hayes E: Insights from women's experiences for teaching and learning. In Hayes E, editor: *Effective teaching styles: new direction for continuing education*, San Francisco, 1989, Jossey-Bass.
12. Knowles MS: *The modern practice of adult education: andragogy versus pedagogy*, New York, 1970, Association Press.
13. Knowles MS: *The modern practice of adult education from pedagogy to andragogy*, Chicago, 1980, Follett.
14. Knowles MS: Adult learning. In Craig RL, editor: *Training and development handbook: a guide to human resource development*, ed 3, New York, 1987, McGraw-Hill.
15. Levinson DJ: A conception of adult development, *Am Psych* 41:3, 1986.
16. Merriam SB: *Adult development: implications for adult education*, Columbus, Ohio, 1984, ERIC Clearinghouse.
17. Merriam SB, Caffarella RS: *Lifelines: patterns of work, love, and learning in adulthood*, San Francisco, 1991, Jossey-Bass.

Guiding Principles: Vision, Values, Mission, and Goals of Staff Development

In this fast-paced and competitive world of constant change, organizations must have a framework providing a set of principles and guiding practices, "which bind people together around a common identity and sense of destiny."[19] These principles, as expressed in the organization's vision, values, and mission,[20] become the guide for the structure and activities of the staff development department.

Current health care management texts and periodicals are filled with the importance of articulating and transmitting vision, values, mission, and goals of organizations to all employees. In reviewing use and effectiveness, Trexler[22] says that "statements of philosophy, purpose, and objectives can be viewed as threads that relate individual nursing care units to one another, to the nursing departments as a whole, and to the organization and environment in which that nursing department is located." Kanter[12] describes the self-reflective examination of values by corporate leaders and others as "an important starting point for corporate renaissance." In addition, Kanter[12] states that there is "a growing trend toward self-conscious corporate examination of purpose and philosophy."

Pascarella and Frohman[14] describe the direction and commitment that results in a "purpose-driven organization" when "organizations define where they are going amid what they stand for in order to achieve organizational viability and encourage employee commitment." Senge et al[20] further emphasize the importance of a never-ending process of building shared vision "whereby people in an organization articulate their common stories—around vision, purpose, values, why their work matters, and how it fits in the larger world."

DEFINITIONS

In a discussion of vision, values, mission, and goals, definitions are important to clarify the meaning of these words as they are used in this field:

44

A *philosophy* is a statement of the values and beliefs that direct an organization in its attempt to achieve a purpose. An organization's philosophy explains the reason procedures and tasks are carried out in the way that they are. A philosophy serves as a directive to the way a purpose is achieved.

A *mission statement* is "an articulated, written purpose that reflects the [organization's] value core. It defines an acceptable direction and a target for the [organization's] energies, and provides a guideline that allows educators to go about the business of education."[23]

A *purpose* is the reason for an organization's existence; it is the "why" of the organization.[6] The terms *purpose* and *mission* are often used interchangeably.

Goals "are broadly stated terminal or long-term outcomes of a program/process."[9]

Objectives are "specific, operational terms that signify significant points necessary for eventual goal attainment."[9] Objectives are statements that direct activity toward the achievement of the organization's purpose.

Vision is an "image of our desired future...it shows where we want to go, and what we'll be like when we get there."[20]

Values describe the way that an organization intends to operate daily while pursuing its vision.

PHILOSOPHY/VALUES
Uses of a Philosophy

A philosophy articulates the beliefs and values that direct all the work of the staff development department. Bevis[5] says that a philosophy "answers the question *why* and queries the worth of an experience...science answers *how*, *when*, and *where*." These values become the rationale for selecting one form of action over another. A staff development philosophy can be described as the following:

1. A guide to the mission and values of the organization and the division of nursing
2. A guide to the nursing profession
3. A guide to the establishment of the department's purpose, goals, and objectives
4. Grounds for the conceptual framework
5. The basis for the staff development curriculum

Guide to the Mission and Values of the Institution and Division of Nursing. Because the staff development department operates within the broader context of the organization and the nursing division, the philosophy must reflect the values of the organization and nursing division served. The staff development philosophy should reflect a commitment to fulfill obligations outlined in the organization's operational documents. For example, the philosophy of the Division of Nursing at the University of Texas, MD Anderson Cancer Center states that "We aim to combine the activities of patient care, education, rehabilitation, prevention, and research for the benefit of those currently receiving care and also for future generations" (box below). This value is articulated in the staff development philosophy as the focus of staff development activities toward "the enhancement of nursing care given to individuals with cancer...to promote a high standard of safe, effective nursing practice" (box on p. 47).

Guide to the Profession. Bevis[5] outlines the progressive power that evolves from the development and implementation of a philosophy:

PHILOSOPHY OF NURSING

Our institution is a specialized center whose primary mission focuses on providing comprehensive care to patients with cancer while simultaneously striving to eradicate malignant diseases. We aim to combine the activities of patient care, education, rehabilitation, prevention and research for the benefit of those currently receiving care and also for future generations.

As oncology nurses, we value our commitment to establish and maintain an exceptional relationship of caring for and about individuals wherever we encounter them in the health continuum. Our partnership with patients, their families, and all of our multidisciplinary colleagues seeks to promote optimal health potential for everyone we are privileged to support.

Principle 1
Evolving scientific knowledge and the nursing profession's high standards govern and influence the development, application, and evaluation of our practice. These standards provide a flexible framework for delivering competent and compassionate services for which we are accountable.

Principle 2
We accept patients, their families and our associates without regard to differences in physical or emotional health, age, socioeconomic condition, cultural background, or spiritual belief. This acceptance forms the cornerstone of our partnership with others and affords a foundation for mutual trust.

Principle 3
In our unique roles as patient advocates and managers of care, we strive to reach the best possible outcome from the patient's perspective. We value our collaboration with physicians and other health care team members in the shared goal of achieving continuity of comprehensive patient care.

Principle 4
As nurses concerned with the full spectrum of malignant diseases, we recognize that, while cure is not always possible, care is. Inherent in this case is our promise to nurture the hope that gives our patients strength to contend with the various stages of their illness.

Principle 5
Because we strongly believe that patients and families have a right to participate in the decision-making process, we seek to involve them in formulating their own plan of care. Within each plan, we may encounter differing values that challenge us to implement and support patient and family goals.

Continued.

A unification of some common philosophical elements for all nursing may be a source of power that will help nursing make sense of the world and nursing's place in that world. It will be a foundation for a sense of identity, security, and confidence and ultimately will enable a clear or a better identification of purpose, evolution of a system to achieve that purpose, and creation of new approaches to nursing problems.

If there is to be unity and a common philosophy, it is imperative that the philosophic concepts come from the entire nursing staff, not just managers or educators.

Guide to the Establishment of Purpose, Goals, and Objectives. A sound and well-articulated philosophy provides the foundation for a sense of identity, security, and confidence. Ultimately, the philosophy enables a "clear or better identification of purpose, evolution of objectives to achieve that purpose, and creation of new approaches to nursing problems."[5]

PHILOSOPHY OF NURSING—cont'd

Principle 6

Continual education is important for us, as well as for patients and families as a means of independence. The ongoing teaching process guarantees that we can assist patients in achieving the highest level of control in their health care and also fulfills our responsibility for promoting cancer prevention and earlier diagnosis among the larger community in which we live.

Principle 7

We acknowledge that research supplies the methods for validating and improving our practice, and we take pride in our contribution to the multifaceted scientific investigations that are an integral mission of this institution.

Principle 8

Believing that our staff is our most valuable resource, nursing administration pledges to work for a physically safe environment and to provide support services essential for professional and personal problem solving. A visible and responsive administration facilitates a growth-oriented milieu in which individuals have the freedom to flourish and, in return, expects the nursing staff to influence decisions impacting their practice.

Principle 9

With continual changes in the health care system, we recognize the need for proactive responses and the prudent use of all resources to assure quality in the delivery of care.

Principle 10

Peer support, which we place at a high priority, involves sensitive, active listening and a commitment to respond to the expressed needs of our colleagues. We encourage a balance of personal and professional responsibilities through the investment of time for self to promote healthy, productive caregivers.

Courtesy University of Texas, MD Anderson Cancer Center, Division of Nursing, Houston.

PHILOSOPHY

The Department of Nursing Staff Development is an integral part of the Division of Nursing and embraces the philosophy of the Division. The Department also has the following beliefs:

The focus of the Department of Nursing Staff Development is the development of employees of the Division of Nursing, all professional nurses employed by the Cancer Center, and the nursing community at large for the enhancement of nursing care given to individuals with cancer. Educational activities should be designed and implemented to promote a high standard of safe, effective nursing practice and to increase job enrichment through life-long learning. Emphasis should be on application of knowledge to the actual work environment. The impact of programs should be directed to the learner, the system and the patient and his family.

The educational environment should be non-threatening and should acknowledge the individuality of its learners. It should also encourage application of learning, free exchange of ideas and creativity.

Teaching-learning is a dynamic, collaborative, shared process between teacher and learner. It proceeds best in a relationship characterized by mutual trust and acceptance with varying degrees of independence, dependence, and interdependence. The process should result in a change in the cognitive, psychomotor and affective behavior of the individual.

Mastery learning assists learners in achieving an acceptable level of performance and should be utilized to provide a basis for accountability to the client, to the Institution and to the profession of nursing.

Nursing Service, Nursing Education and Nursing Research must collaborate to effectively solve problems and to facilitate divisional goal attainment.

Courtesy University of Texas, MD Anderson Cancer Center, Division of Nursing, Department of Staff Development, Houston.

Grounds for the Conceptual Framework. The conceptual framework is the structure guiding all decisions that are relevant to the curriculum, including objectives, content, implementation, and evaluation. Bevis[5] states that the "philosophy influences the concepts and theories selected to comprise the conceptual framework." The philosophy "provides the value system for ordering priorities and selecting from among the various data." Bevis warns that a conceptual framework built on philosophy alone results in a framework based solely on the values and beliefs of the faculty. Other concepts, theories, and facts that influence curriculum decisions are important to include.

Basis for the Staff Development Curriculum. As the staff development department designs learning activities to meet specific educational goals, the philosophy directs not only the content but also the types of learning activities and the methods of evaluation. The "emphasis should be on application of knowledge to the actual work environment" (box). This concept becomes an important part of the conceptual framework as the learner and setting are further defined and the focus of staff development is centered on problem solving and knowledge application in the work setting. The philosophic statement takes on practical meaning in the curriculum design when the selection of content is based on relevance to the work setting, the teaching methods that are implemented progress beyond traditional lectures to simulation and clinical practice, and evaluation is measured by the learner's ability to apply the content in the work setting.

Attributes of a Philosophy

If a philosophy is to be vital and meaningful, it must possess certain characteristics. The characteristics of an effective philosophy should be as follows:
- Unique and descriptive of the setting's values
- Simple, clear, and meaningful to the reader
- Applicable and pragmatic
- A basis for structure, direction, and action
- Nonrestrictive
- A shared vision among employees and managers
- Practiced as it is stated

In discussing the importance of values in the strategic planning process, Bean[3] states that "working and agreeing on a set of shared values not only galvanizes the team, but releases the flow of creative, channeled, congruent energy...."

Development of a Philosophy

For a philosophy to be pervasive in the organization and reflected in the actions and words of the departments, those affected by the philosophy must be committed to it. To earn this commitment, individuals must feel a sense of ownership toward the stated values. Individuals must believe that they are involved in the development of the philosophy statement.[7] Peters[15] suggests that those responsible "look inward, work with colleagues and customers—work with everyone—to develop and instill a philosophy and vision that is enabling and empowering."

The first step of philosophy development should be the appointment of a small task force to determine a plan of action. This group should address the following issues:
1. Who are the claimant groups from whom input should be sought?
2. What structure or information should be given to the claimant groups?
3. Who will determine the component characteristics of the philosophy?
4. How will the input be gathered from claimant groups?
5. Who will write the philosophy?
6. What final approval is required for the philosophy statement?
7. How will the philosophy be implemented?

It is critical that those who have a vested interest in the services of the staff development department should be given an opportunity to contribute to the development of the philosophy. The following individuals or groups should be considered for their input when developing a philosophy:
- Education advisory committees

- Staff development department managers
- Staff development department instructors
- Nursing managers
- Nursing executives

In seeking input from claimant groups, the following two approaches can be used. First, groups are allowed a free and unprejudiced discussion of ideas when they are not given predetermined philosophic concepts. This gives claimant groups the important message that all ideas are valued and will be considered, in addition to helping those who are providing input to feel ownership of and commitment to the philosophy. Participants should be given a copy of the organization's and nursing division's current philosophy and/or mission statement before beginning such sessions. This facilitates congruency between staff and organizational values. The second approach to the process gives participants an opportunity to relate their values and ideas to predetermined components of the philosophy. These components should be determined by the staff development management and education advisory committee. These components should include concepts such as the following:

- Relationship of the philosophy to the organization and the nursing department's current philosophy
- The nature of nursing and health care
- The nature of the teaching and learning process
- The nature of the learner
- The learner's responsibility for learning
- The organization's responsibility for learning
- The relationship between staff development continuing education and academic education
- The staff development's relationship to the nursing department and organization
- The focus of education
- The role of the educator

Input from claimant groups can be obtained in a number of ways. Brainstorming sessions allow many individuals to give verbal input and build on one another's ideas. If all participants' ideas are written on flip charts and a value of good or bad is not placed on the statements, participants believe their ideas are valued and being considered for the final draft. Concepts can also be gathered in writing from claimant groups by asking open-ended questions about concepts such as those listed earlier. Then these concepts can be combined into a philosophic statement that reflects the major values and beliefs of the group. This task is best done by a small group that works to perfect the statements expressed by the majority of the group. The final philosophic statement should be accepted by the staff development managers and the nursing administration.

The philosophy is the key to building an organization's guiding principles. Senge et al[20] emphasize that "when values are made a central part of the organization's shared vision effort, and put out in full view, they become like a figurehead on a ship: a guiding symbol of the behavior that will help people move toward the vision."

MISSION AND PURPOSE

Whether the staff development department labels the statement as a "mission" or "purpose" is not important, but the department must clearly explain the reason the statement is necessary. The department's statement of purpose provides a clear direction to achieving departmental goals and objectives, a way to measure progress, and a definition to employees. This mission statement is a "connecting bridge between where you are currently and where you want to be in the next two to three years."[3] The purpose should be an operational statement rather than an idealistic one. The statement should reflect the following:

- Who we are
- What we are
- Why we exist
- Whom we serve

In a description of organizational integrity, Ulschak[23] describes the importance of a clearly articulated purpose, as stated by James Farr:

The essence of an organization is its purpose. Without the organizing force of purpose, there is no organization, there are merely people and things in random arrangement. The integrity of an organization, therefore, lies in the extent to which it operates on-purpose. With full integrity, an organization acts with total commitment, precisely toward its purpose. With decreasing integrity, actions are off-purpose, nonsupportive, or even destructive of progress.

Two examples of mission statements that provide the fundamental reason for the existence of their organizations are from MD Anderson's Staff Development Department and Texas Children's Hospital (boxes).

Ulschak[23] further states that although Farr's reference is to the overall organization, the implications are significant for any department within the organization. "Until there is agreement about purpose, a department has no direction, no tool to measure progress, no real reason to be motivated, and no clear focus for its energy."

VISION

Peters[16] says "In a time of turbulence and uncertainty, we must be able to take instant action on the front line. But to support such action-taking at the front, everyone must have a clear understanding of what the organization is trying to achieve." "Vision is our ideal, our image of what we want to become. Vision connotes emotion, commitment, passion, momentum; it [vision] binds people together around a common identity and sense of destiny."[8] Vision differentiates between long-term success and mediocre performance.

Peters[15] describes the "what" of effective visions as the following:

- Inspiring
- Clear and challenging—and about excellence
- Making sense in the market place…and standing the test of time in a turbulent world
- Stable but constantly challenged—and changed at the margin

STRATEGIC BLUEPRINT: TEXAS CHILDREN'S HOSPITAL

Department
The Center for Nursing Development

Purpose
To support operations by:
- Providing services that facilitate the ongoing development of nursing personnel
- Collaborating with other clinical departments to facilitate the delivery of competency-based patient care

Product
Performance improvement

Core Processes
- Staff development
- Continuing quality improvement support
- Community education support

Vision
Competent and empowered patient care providers who have access to timely, outcome based, user friendly learning resources that stimulate the desire for continuous learning and continuous quality improvement

Customers
- Managers of patient care providers
- Educators of patient care providers
- Patient care providers

Values
- Quality
- Teamwork

Services
Staff development services
- Needs analysis
- Competence assessment and validation
- Inservice education
- Continuing education
- Orientation of newly hired, transferred, and promoted employees
- Consultation regarding performance improvement and staff development
- Coordination and approval of continuing nursing education (CNE) contact hours
- Program/project design, implementation, and evaluation
- Consultation regarding design and development of teaching and learning aids
- Coordination of CPR training program
- Management of multidisciplinary training center (MDTC)

Continued.

STRATEGIC BLUEPRINT: TEXAS CHILDREN'S HOSPITAL—cont'd

Continuous quality improvement (CQI) support services
- Automated data processing and report generation
- Consultation regarding development of data collection tools
- Consultation regarding use of CQI tools and techniques

Community education support services
- Coordination of student nurse affiliations
- Coordination of observation and preceptor experience for visiting nurses
- Coordination of nurse externship program
- Coordination of nursing outreach programs

Courtesy Texas Children's Hospital, Center for Nursing Development, Houston.

STATEMENTS OF PURPOSE: THE UNIVERSITY OF TEXAS MD ANDERSON CANCER CENTER

Mission

As nurse educators specializing in cancer care, we are dedicated to promote excellence in nursing practice by contributing to the development of competent providers and managers of patient care. We achieve this commitment through the education, consultation, and mentoring of:

- Nursing personnel throughout UTMDACC
- Nurses external to the institution
- Professional and vocational nursing students and high school students

Vision

To be the international leader of professional staff development dedicated to excellence in oncology nursing practice

Goals
1. Promote competence in cancer nursing practice by providing individuals with superior education
2. Provide an environment that stimulates inquiry, learning, and conversion of knowledge into action
3. Optimally manage Nursing Staff Development Department's resources (human, physical, and fiscal)
4. Provide a faculty who are international leaders of professional staff development in oncology nursing practice

---

Courtesy University of Texas, MD Anderson Cancer Center, Division of Nursing, Department of Staff Development, Houston.

- Beacons and controls when all else is up for grabs
- Empowering our own people first, customers second
- Preparing for the future, but honoring the past
- Living in details, not broad strokes

Leaders must live, communicate, and inspire the vision if it is to be a shared vision with their staff. A clear vision creates value for employees and customers, in addition to empowering them. James Belasco gives excellent guidelines for the development and use of vision in *Teaching the Elephant to Dance.*[4]

GOALS

The terms *goals, purpose, mission,* and *objectives* cause much confusion because their meanings overlap. For the sake of clarity the term *goal* is defined within this text as a broadly stated or long-term outcome resulting from staff development activities, that is, what the department hopes to achieve. Some people refer to these as "broad" or "general" objectives (as opposed to "specific" objectives) rather than as goals.

Goals are the first product of the planning process and set the direction for department activities. Goals are derived from the philosophy, vision, and purpose of the parent organization and nursing division. These goals are a translation of the mission into broad, proactive statements of intent that direct the following:

- Staff development objectives and strategies for action
- Curriculum building
- Designation and allocation of resources
- Priorities for action
- Organizational structure

For example, the goal to "promote competence in cancer nursing practice," as stated in the box found on the bottom of p. 53, requires a plan for regular inservice programs to introduce new technology. In a research and teaching hospital the introduction of new technology and equipment is constant. Although the timing of these events is rarely scheduled far in advance, a system must be devised to provide a classroom, a schedule of in-service education times convenient to all staff, an instructor, and necessary supplies to teach the use of this equipment. This important priority of the staff development department requires proactive planning to meet this goal.

Building a curriculum for the nursing staff in a health care setting is an important yet often overlooked process. O'Connor[13] states that "curriculum for nursing staff development or continuing education provides organizing themes that prescribe audiences to be served, content to be presented, outcomes to be achieved, and approaches to be used in conducting the education program."

In describing curriculum building in patient education, Redman[18] explains that a curriculum "implies an integrated effort adequately differentiated for learning success with various individuals, toward a societal goal." The staff development goals derived from the philosophy and mission give a clear direction to curriculum building, including a definition of the population to be served and the intended outcomes.

Designation and allocation of resources is guided by the departmental goals and the priority of the goals. When stated, goals should be placed in order of their importance.

As Rakich, Longest, and Darr[17] state, "The organization's [or the staff development department's] structure is effective if it facilitates individual contribution toward attaining the organization's objectives with a minimum of cost." The networking of tasks should be dictated by the department's goals and must determine the department's structural characteristics, including the allocation of authority (that is, who has which responsibilities and the nature of superior and subordinate relationships), the grouping of work activities, and the coordination, communication, information, and control mechanisms. A conflict often exists between long-term proactive goals and immediate needs requiring the manager's attention. "These problem-dictated, resolution-seeking intentions are goals in a practice sense...They stem from the day-to-day pressures that direct [the manager's] actions and choices."[2] The importance of balancing these two different dimensions of the job become a challenge for staff development managers and instructors.

In these "crazy times" described by Tom Peters,[15] staff educators must be open to imaginative, creative approaches to meet the mission, vision, and goals of the organization. Although the structures will change, educators can remain centered by focusing on the guiding principles and goals of the organization.

OBJECTIVES

The objectives for the staff development department are the "operational terms that signify significant points necessary for eventual goal attainment."[9] The objectives direct the selection and determine the priority of activities to achieve the purpose of the department. Drucker[10] states the following:

Objectives are the basis for work and assignments. They determine the structure of the business, the key activities which must be discharged, and above all, the allocation of people to tasks. Objectives are the foundation for designing both the structure of the business and the work of individual units and individual managers.

Objectives are derived not only from the value, vision, mission, and goals of the organization, but from the relevant environment and all conditions related to that environment.

Development of Organization Objectives

A helpful model for objective gathering and the analysis of information to be used for developing staff development department objectives is Stufflebeam's context, input, process, and product (CIPP) program evaluation model.[21] Stufflebeam states that the purpose of context evaluation is to provide a rationale for determining objectives. This rationale is achieved by doing the following:

1. Defining the relevant environment
2. Describing the actual versus the desired environmental conditions
3. Identifying unmet needs and unused opportunities
4. Diagnosing the problems preventing needs from being met and opportunities from being used
5. Describing the system to be evaluated, which is the basis for developing objectives and identifying potential strategies

Stufflebeam[21] further suggests that a series of questions about the rationale's context be addressed as follows:

1. What are the overall goals and purpose of the organization or department?
2. What is the need or discrepancy? Does the goal differ from what is actually happening?
3. Who are the interested parties or claimant groups?
4. Are the goals of the claimant groups congruent to the organization's or department's stated goals?
5. What current community standards are relevant to the goal?
6. What current professional standards are relevant to the goals?
7. What societal, political, economic, and technologic trends are related to this program?
8. What are the current means of meeting the goals?
9. Are the current systems and policies congruent to the goals?

Answering these and other questions will give the information needed to write the staff development department objectives. The context evaluation process is best done by a task force made up of representatives from the staff development department and customers of the department's services. The objectives resulting from the context evaluation will result in the selection of strategies, an organization structure, and resource allocation procedures needed to meet the departmental goals; a means to monitor the system to indicate how well the strategies, structure, and resources are meeting the departmental goals; and an outcome evaluation, indicating how effectively the objectives are being accomplished.

Categorizing Objectives

Categorizing objectives into the following topics can be helpful. First, operation (routine) objectives that are related to the regular operations of the staff development department should be chosen. Second, program objectives should state the specific programs and courses to be held throughout the fiscal year, the number of times these courses will be offered, and the projected number of participants. Third, innovative objectives should be directed toward the development of new programs or activities designed to meet future needs. The American Nurses Association uses the following categories in *Standards for Nursing*

Professional Development: Continuing Education and Staff Development[1]:
- Administration
- Human resources
- Learners
- Material resources and facilities
- Educational design
- Records and reports
- Professional practice

Characteristics of Effective Objectives

Objectives that are merely good intentions are worthless. Drucker[10] states that objectives "must degenerate into work. And work is always specific, always has—or should have—clear, unambiguous, measurable results, a deadline, and a specific assignment of accountability."

An example of an operations objective is shown in Table 4-1. This objective, or standard, is integrated into departmental policies and procedures. The attainment of this objective is measured by a review of documentation completed by assigned persons who are given a defined due date. Program objectives outline the specified educational programs to be implemented, the target population and number of participants to be served, and the number of courses to be held (Table 4-2).

Innovative objectives include objectives related to the design of new programs or use of new technology, for example, the development of an interactive video program on the care of immunosuppressed oncology patients. The inclusion of innovative objectives each year forces the staff development personnel to challenge themselves, experiment, and think in new and creative ways.

STRATEGIC PLANNING TO ENHANCE PHILOSOPHY, GOALS, AND OBJECTIVES

To react quickly to the rapidly changing forces in health care, many organizations, divisions of nursing, and staff development departments have implemented a strategic planning process to regularly review organizational goals, objectives, and strategies. An example of a strategic decision-making process is shown in Figure 4-1. Most approaches to strategic planning follow a process involving the following:
1. View of the future
   a. Development of mission
   b. Development of vision
2. Assessment of the present and past
   a. Internal assessment
      (1) Organization and management
      (2) Current activities

  (3) Current resources
  (4) Historical and current resource requirements
 b. External environmental assessment
3. Strategy formulation by developing goals, objectives, and strategies
4. Prioritization of critical strategies
5. Review and approval
6. Evaluation and control

Strategic planning gives the staff development unit a process to examine the elements of the organization, (that is, the organization's culture, philosophy, goals, and objectives) and develop plans to guide the organization through changes. The steps of this process and the interrelationships of the philosophy,

Table 4-1   Standard 4: educational design*

Standards	Outcome	Responsibility
Structure criterion		
An educational design based on adult learning principles and focusing on application is valued and utilized.	Adult learning principles are utilized in all educational offerings. a. The learner is represented in identifying learning needs. b. Content is relevant to an identified need. c. Learning activities are planned to facilitate mastery of identified needs. d. The learner participates in the evaluation process. e. Learning is applicable in the clinical setting.	Instructor
	The design for each offering includes needs assessment, behavior objectives, content outline, teaching methods, learning experiences, resource utilization plan, and evaluation	Instructor

Courtesy University of Texas, MD Anderson Cancer Center, Division of Nursing, Department of Staff Development, Houston.
*The educational design for each program consists of planned, organized, and evaluated learning activities based on the principles of adult learning and focusing on application learning in the clinical area.

goals, and objectives are vital to any staff development department. The steps are not a sequential process but a series of actions that occur and interact simultaneously.[11]

SUMMARY

The process of developing a philosophy, goals, and objectives for the staff development department is a critical step that provides a foundation for all department activities. This process prepares the staff development professional to act proactively in harmony with the larger system. The philosophy, mission, vision, and goals must be "living" documents, not just words on a sheet of paper

Assessment	Frequency	Validation
Evidence of: 1) Assess/analyze need of target 2) Planning with learner to meet identified need 3) Behavioral objectives and content related to those objectives 4) Relevant knowledge to nursing practice 5) Appropriate teaching methods; adequate resources are included in the lesson plan 6) Evaluation incorporates learner's ability to apply content in the work setting	Every program	Employee conference record orientation (Phase I) master file CNE application file Offering file Peer/supervisor evaluation Unit education program file

Every program	Every program	As above
		Curriculum committee review
		  CNE application file
		  Phase I—orientation
		  CPR file
		Director reviews
		  Peer/supervisor evaluation
		  Unit education program book
		  Central offering file
		  Employee conference record

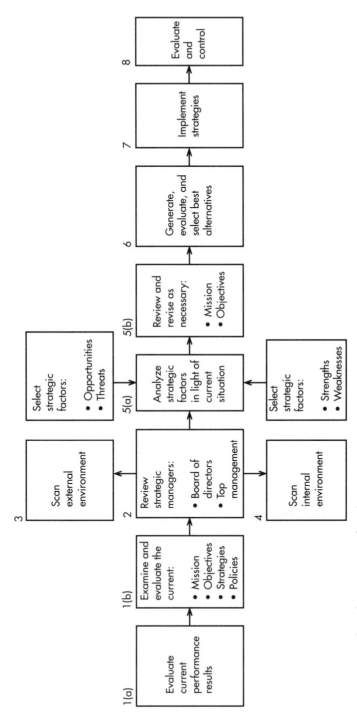

Fig. 4-1   Strategic decision-making process. (From Wheelen T, Hunger JD: *Strategic management and business policy*, ed 2, Reading, MA, 1986, Addison-Wesley.)

NOTE: Steps 1 through 6 are strategy formulation.
Step 7 is strategy implementation.
Step 8 is evaluation and control.

Table 4-2   Program objectives: 1994–1995

Programs	Offerings projected
Entry level programs	
New employee orientations	25
Basic critical care program	2
Basic operating room program	2
Continuing education programs	
Advanced medical surgical nursing	2
Code blue/CPR	6
Critical care	2
Management	
Seminars	2
Focus sessions	6
Head nurse orientation	5
Medication technician	4
Oncology nursing clinical conference	11
Oncology I	4
Oncology II	3
Oncology specialty modules	4
Professional issues forums	4
Preceptor course	3

Courtesy University of Texas, MD Anderson Cancer Center, Division of Nursing, Department of Staff Development, Houston.

that are tucked away in a file. They must be regularly reviewed to accurately reflect the context of the setting and nursing practice. These relevant and usable concepts become the framework for the curriculum and operations of the staff development unit and, more important, the basis for the experimentation and innovation necessary to keep up with a rapidly changing world.

REFERENCES

1. American Nurses Association: *Standards for nursing professional development: continuing education and staff development*, Washington, DC, 1994, American Nurses Publishing.
2. Barnum BS, Mallard CO: *Essentials of nursing management*, Rockville, Md, 1989, Aspen.
3. Bean WC: *Strategic planning that makes things happen*, Amherst, Mass, 1993, Human Resource Development Press.
4. Belasco JA: *Teaching the elephant to dance: empowering change in your organization*, New York, 1990, Crown Publishing.
5. Bevis EO: *Curriculum building in nursing: a process*, New York, 1989, National League for Nursing.
6. Cantor MM: Philosophy, purpose, and objectives: why do we have them? *J Nurs Adm* 3(4):21, 1973.
7. Cody B: Developing a philosophy of nursing, *J Nurs Adm* 20(1):16, 1990.
8. DePree M: *Leadership is an art*, New York, 1989, Doubleday.
9. Dienemann JA: *Nursing administration: strategic perspectives and application*, Norwalk, Conn, 1990, Appleton & Lange.
10. Drucker PF: *Management: tasks, responsibilities, practices*, New York, 1985, Harper & Row.

11. Grolerud E: Strategic planning in health care organizations. In Dienemann JA, editor: *Nursing administration*, Norwalk, Conn, 1989, Appleton & Lange.
12. Kanter RM: *The change masters*, New York, 1983, Simon & Schuster.
13. O'Connor AB: *Nursing staff development and continuing education*, Boston, 1986, Little Brown.
14. Pascarella P, Frohman M: *The purpose–driven organization*, San Francisco, 1989, Jossey–Bass.
15. Peters T: *Thriving on chaos*, New York, 1987, Alfred A Knopf.
16. Peters T: *The Tom Peters Seminar: crazy times call for crazy organizations*, New York, 1994, Vintage Books.
17. Rakich JS, Longest BB, Darr K: *Managing health services organizations*, Philadelphia, 1985, WB Saunders.
18. Redman BK: Curriculum in patient education, *AM J Nurs* 79:1363, 1979.
19. Senge PM: *The fifth discipline: the art and practice of the learning organization*, New York, 1990, Doubleday.
20. Senge PM et al: *The fifth discipline fieldbook: strategies and tools for building a learning organization*, New York, 1994, Doubleday.
21. Stufflebeam DL: *Educational evaluation and decision making*, Itasca, Ill, 1971, Peacock Publishers.
22. Trexler BJ: Nursing department purpose, philosophy, and objectives: their use and effectiveness, *J Nurs Adm* 17(3):8, 1987.
23. Ulschak FL: *Creating the future of health care education*, Chicago, 1988, American Hospital Publishing.

BARBARA K. PENN

Learning Styles in Staff Development*

The notion of learning styles has been popular in education for many years. Research in this area was particularly prevalent in the 1970s and 1980s when many authors advocated using learning styles as prescriptions for changing the teaching-learning environment. One particularly popular suggestion was to match teaching strategies with learning styles to improve learning outcomes. Research did not support this approach, and educators are no longer burdened by the mandate for matching these strategies and styles. Although learning styles were initially attractive, educators have realized that this method did not always take education in the proper direction. Educational literature describes the teaching-learning process as complex with many interacting variables. One variable is the different ways learners prefer to learn. This is certainly an important variable but not a remedy for the teaching-learning environment. As a whole, learning style research is fragmented and the literature is contradictory, thereby making practical application difficult.

Learning style information is useful to staff development educators, however. The concept of learning style demonstrates that each adult learner brings a unique approach to any learning opportunity. Each adult has different strengths and weaknesses. Each views life and interacts with the environment differently. Knowledge of learning styles in staff development heightens awareness of learner diversity and gives educators a reason to offer a variety of teaching-learning strategies. Most educators intuitively know that teaching all learners with the same method is doomed to fail. However, educators may not be fully aware of the way to capitalize on individual differences to enhance the teaching-learning process. If allowed or encouraged to do so, most adult learners use a variety of techniques to master new knowledge and skills. Adults particularly welcome

---

*The views expressed by Dr. Penn are her own and do not reflect the official policy or position of the Department of the Army, Department of Defense, or the U.S. government.

opportunities to use personally selected learning methods according to their own needs or preferences.

Dozens of theories and instruments describe the different ways individuals respond to their environment, interact with others, and approach learning. For example, Myers and Briggs identify 16 personality types based on Jungian psychology.[32] Kolb[24] describes four learning styles according to his experiential learning theory. Witkin[47] separates individuals into two cognitive styles based on field dependence-independence theory. Use of these tools may be helpful in teaching leadership or management seminars, preparing nurses to function as teachers, or increasing awareness of individual differences when appropriate. New staff development educators may find it helpful to study learning styles to expand their repertoires of teaching strategies. However, the routine use of instruments to measure learning styles is probably inappropriate in most staff development settings. Regardless of the specific theories or tools an educator prefers, recognition and encouragement of learner diversity enriches the learning environment and may enhance learning itself.

CONCEPTS OF LEARNING STYLE, COGNITIVE STYLE, AND PERSONALITY TYPE

Three major concepts that describe differences in learning approaches are learning style, cognitive style, and personality type. These terms are inextricably linked in the literature. Personality type is the clearest of the three interrelated concepts. This term refers to the categorization of normal human behaviors and attitudes that make people individuals. The Myers-Briggs Type Indicator (MBTI) is a particularly popular and reputable instrument to measure personality type. The MBTI describes individuals on four independent continua—extraversion-introversion (attitude), sensing-intuition (perception), thinking-feeling (judgment), and judgment-perception (orientation to the world). An individual is placed into 1 of 16 personality type categories. Each category has distinctive characteristics, strengths, and weaknesses. The MBTI may be used in a variety of instructional, counseling, and management applications.[32]

The terms *learning style* and *cognitive style* are often used interchangeably. Numerous authors acknowledge that these concepts are *not* equivalent, but few clearly differentiate between them.[2] Although disagreement exists, learning style is generally thought to be the broader term and thought to encompass cognitive style. This chapter will also treat these terms in this way.

Learning style can be broadly defined as "the characteristic way in which a learner operates within the learning situation"[3] and "the means by which an individual prefers to learn."[9] Learning style is considered malleable and amenable to conscious and purposeful change by individual learners. This makes learning style an aspect of applicability to educators.

In contrast, Witkin[47] defines *cognitive style* as "the characteristic, self-consistent modes of functioning which individuals show in their perceptual and intellectual activities." Cognitive style, which is possibly an aspect of personality structure, refers to many basic aspects of perception and cognition including problem solving, decision making, and remembering. Cognitive style characterizes an individual's relatively fixed patterns for viewing the world and, like personality type, is less vulnerable to environmental influences.[8] Although numerous instruments measure aspects of cognitive style, Witkin's field dependence-independence theory measured by the embedded figures test (EFT) dominates the literature.[2] The EFT, a nonverbal test, reflects the extent to which individuals can differentiate patterns from their backgrounds, thereby indicating perceptual and psychologic functioning.[47] Learning style, as opposed to cognitive style, will be discussed further in this chapter because it specifically focuses on learning environments, which makes it more practical to educators.[2]

Learning Style

Aspects of learning style can be traced to 1892 in research literature.[23] Learning style underlies the popular notion in education that much instruction can and should be individualized according to students' strengths or styles.[9,12] The box shows varied uses of learning style information suggested by different authors. The study of learning style was particularly intense in the 1970s and 1980s but seems to be less frequently reported now. This is unfortunate because the cessation of study left conceptual confusion, incomplete investigation, and unclear application.[8] Despite the enormous popularity of the subject, learning style does not have a generally accepted definition, a unified perspective, a common paradigm or theoretical framework, or clear characteristics.[2] This confusion is compounded by the lack of clear differentiation between cognitive style and learning style in the research literature. Many components of learning style have been identified, including cognitive style, cognitive processing, cognitive personality style, student response style, learning preference, instructional preference, and information processing.[7,8,36] These diverse ways of viewing learning style have resulted in so many theories and tools that a single theory or instrument does not completely dominate this body of literature.[2] Dozens of models for mea-

---

VARIOUS USES FOR LEARNING STYLE INFORMATION

- Acknowledge student diversity
- Identify appropriate teaching strategies
- Perform preentry assessment
- Predict academic or clinical achievement
- Improve teaching in specific subjects or programs
- Heighten student awareness
- Increase academic success
- Predict career choices and specialty affiliations
- Design continuing education programs for practicing professionals

SOME EXAMPLES OF LEARNING STYLE INSTRUMENTS[2,8,14,15]

Cognitive preference inventory—Tamir, Elstein, Molidor, and Krupka
Cognitive style inventory—Hill
Decision making inventory—Johnson
Embedded figures test—Witkin, Moore, Goodenough, and Cox
Inventory of learning process—Stritter and Friedman
Instructional preference questionnaire—Stritter and Friedman
Learning preference inventory—Rezler
Learning style inventory—Dunn, Dunn, and Price
Learning style inventory—Kolb
Learning styles inventory—Canfield and Lafferty
Matching familiar figures test—Kagan
Myers-Briggs type indicator—Myers and McCaulley
Personal style indicator—Cotroneo
Productivity environmental preference survey—Dunn, Dunn, and Price
Student learning style scales—Grasha-Reichmann
Style delineator—Gregoric
Teacher assessment of student learning styles—Hunt
Transaction ability inventory—Gregoric

suring learning style exist. Although some tools are superior to others, learning style instruments as a whole are criticized for their weak validity, reliability, and theoretical frameworks.[2,8] Various tools were developed by different researchers, are targeted at different audiences and ages, and reportedly measure different aspects of learning style.[3,14] The box identifies some of the many tools. Unfortunately, the literature often describes learning style as a cohesive phenomenon that can be tapped equally well by the numerous conceptually diverse tools. Consequently, generalizations are made rather than keeping the tools and their respective concepts separate. As a result, the literature can be confusing and potentially misleading. Despite conceptual concerns, the notion of learning style can still be used for staff development educators responsible for cultivating the learning environment to achieve intended outcomes. Nurse educators should be aware of the contradictory nature of learning style literature and use appropriate caution in applying learning style research to their educational practice.

KOLB'S EXPERIENTIAL LEARNING THEORY AND LEARNING STYLE INVENTORY

Kolb's learning style inventory (LSI) is a frequently cited instrument in medical and general higher education,[2] adult learning,[39] and nursing education.[10] Kolb's experiential learning theory, on which the LSI is based, asserts that adults refine their approaches to learning over time and strengthen a particular learning style that they believe helps them learn best. The LSI asks learners to rank their preferences in learning situations. For example, learners may say they learn best from personal relationships, observation, rational theories, and a chance to practice, in that order.[25]

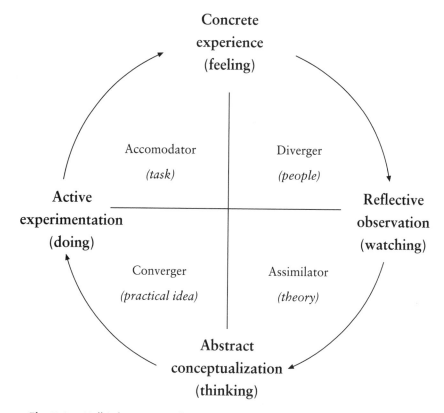

Fig. 5-1   Kolb's learning cycle. (From Kolb, DA: *Learning-style inventory: self-scoring inventory and interpretation booklet,* Boston, 1985, McBer.)

Kolb attributes learning style to various sources, including heredity, personality type, past experiences, education, career choice, and demands of the current environment. In turn, learning style enables individuals to adapt to their physical and social environments and respond to learning situations in addition to work demands and personal development opportunities.[24]

Kolb conceives of learning as both cyclical and dialectic processes (Fig. 5-1). Adults grasp and interpret reality by the following four modes of the learning process:

1. *Concrete experience*—New information is perceived through tangible reality, the senses, feelings, and intuition.
2. *Reflective observation*—Information is processed by impartially watching, listening, reflecting, and describing observations.
3. *Abstract conceptualization*—New information is gained through symbols, abstraction, and logical analysis.
4. *Active experimentation*—Information is processed by acting, experimenting, getting involved, and seeing what works.

Individuals acquire all four modes by adolescence. As adults, individuals use these modes in a clockwise, repetitive cycle of feeling (concrete), watching and listening (reflective), thinking (abstract), and doing (active) in each learning situation. The model is dialectic and cyclical, so learners must choose between polar opposite abilities in each learning situation. The vertical continuum represents the way new information is gained (concrete versus abstract); and the horizontal continuum represents the way information is processed or transformed (active versus reflective). Adults are capable of using all four modes, but flexibility among the modes is desirable. Because of the dialectic dimension, however, a learner develops particular strengths in two of the four modes (one on each axis). This results in a relatively stable but potentially adaptable repertoire of learning skills that can be categorized into one of Kolb's four learning styles (Fig. 5-2). Each style has distinct characteristics, strengths, and weaknesses.

According to Kolb's theory,[24] adults maintain and refine successful learning strategies over the years. They discard the techniques that are less preferred or that do not bring consistent success. This phenomenon of refining learning style is heightened in early adulthood during formal education and career specialization. Kolb suggests that each professional discipline or career field exhibits a characteristic learning style. An individual is drawn to a field because of its congruence with personal learning style, skills, and interests. Through the process of accentuation, the early education and experience of a well-chosen career reinforces the student's skills and learning style. At mid-career, adults become more flexible and begin to exhibit nondominant learning styles, a process Kolb calls *integration*. Most studies show that nurses and nursing students favor the concrete learning mode, which places them in the diverger and accommodator styles. However, some nurses may be found among all learning styles.[37]

IMPLICATIONS FOR STAFF DEVELOPMENT

Despite its confusion and contradiction, learning style literature conveys an important message to staff development educators—*learners learn differently*. Learning style theories or instruments are not intended to pigeonhole learners by relegating them to a particular set of characteristics or implying limits to their success with other learning strategies. Regardless of the theory or instrument an educator prefers, the professional literature advocates that learning activities offer a variety of strategies and opportunities. From these learning activities, learners can choose and be exposed to information according to their strengths, preferences, and needs. The popular notion of matching teaching strategies to learning styles is not recommended. However, recognition by educators that all learners do not learn alike paves the way for variety and creativity in each teaching-learning encounter. The process of facilitating the growth of nurses is enhanced if staff development educators recognize differences in personal styles. Staff development educators can encourage learners to explore a wide range of learning styles.

Diverger
(concrete experience + reflective observation)

Divergers have particular strengths in imagination, awareness of meaning and values. They listen with an open mind, see different perspectives to situations, and can generate many alternative ideas. They are especially interested in people and sensitive to feelings. They can organize many relationships into a meaningful whole. Divergers particularly are interested in cultural activities and the arts.

Assimilator
(reflective observation + abstract conceptualization)

Assimilators emphasize inductive reasoning, organization of information, analysis of quantitative data, creation of conceptual models, testing of theories and ideas, and synthesis of diverse observations into an integrated explanation. They are more focused on ideas and abstractions than people. They find logical, precise theory to be more important than practicality of ideas. They set goals and plan systematically.

Accomodator
(active experimentation + concrete experience)

Accomodators are particularly adept at doing things, carrying out plans, seeking opportunities, getting involved with new experiences, adapting to changing circumstances, taking risks, and influencing others. They use intuitive, trial-and-error problem solving skills. Accommodators are more oriented to facts and ideas than theory. They rely more on other people for information than on their own analytic skills. They are comfortable with people but sometimes are viewed as impatient.

Converger
(abstract conceptualization + active experimentation)

Convergers exhibit special strength in setting goals, solving problems, making decisions, experimenting with new ideas, and implementing practical applications. They utilize deductive reasoning. They are extremely focused on specific problems or best solutions. They prefer technical tasks rather than interpersonal interactions.

Fig. 5-2 Characteristics of Kolb's learning styles.[24,26,41]

Considering Various Learning Styles

Several assumptions are inherent in learning style literature in general and in Kolb's theory of learning styles in particular. These assumptions have received inconsistent research support, but their truth is accepted commonly as fact. For this reason, the following assumptions are presented as myths:

1. Professions are characterized by a particular learning style.
2. Each learning style is associated with unique preferences for learning environments and instructional strategies.
3. Educators can improve instructional outcomes by matching teaching strategies to learning styles.

Myth 1

Kolb[24] offers evidence that individuals are drawn to occupations because of congruence between the individual's learning style and that of the group. Affiliation with the correctly chosen specialty further reinforces the characteristic learning style. Smith and Kolb[41] identify favored careers of each learning style as follows:

- *Diverger*—arts/entertainment and service (including nursing)
- *Assimilator*—science and information (including education)
- *Converger*—technical and specialist
- *Accommodator*—business and organizations

Assuming that learning style and occupations are linked, it could be further assumed that educators within each specialty can capitalize on the discipline's characteristic learning style, tailor instruction for the professional group, and make learning more efficient or otherwise enhanced. However, nursing research does not support this approach. Several studies show nurses and nursing students to be predominantly concrete learners, specifically divergers and accommodators, but nursing professionals and students can be found in all four of Kolb's learning styles. Even Kolb places nursing in three of the four learning styles.[24,41] Evidence that nursing specialties lean toward one learning style over others does not exist.[37] Regardless of how persuasive isolated research evidence may appear, characterizing nursing by one dominant learning mode or style and using that research as a basis for making instructional decisions is not justified. Such an approach ignores many nurses with different learning styles.

Myth 2

According to Kolb, the relative importance learners place on each learning mode indicates the way learners learn best or believe they learn best. Kolb and Smith[24,41] offer evidence that each learning mode is linked with the following preferred teaching strategies:

- *Concrete experience*—Individuals learn from specific experiences and by relating to other people. They benefit most from discussion, games, role playing, personalized or peer feedback, application of skills to real-life problems, and sharing feelings. Teachers are seen as coaches or helpers. Self-direction and autonomy are helpful; theory readings are not.

- *Reflective observation*—Learners view things from different perspectives and precede judgments by careful observations. They prefer lectures because they can assume an observer role. They also prefer objective tests of knowledge. Learners want their work evaluated by extrinsic criteria and prefer teachers who provide expert interpretations and serve as guides or taskmasters. They are not helped by task or outcome-oriented applications of information.
- *Abstract conceptualization*—Learners make logical analyses and like systematic planning. They prefer theory readings; case studies; thinking and studying alone; and clear, well-structured presentations. Teachers are seen as communicators of information. These learners are not helped by skills application, group exercises, simulations, sharing feelings, and peer feedback.
- *Active experimentation*—Individuals take risks, get things done, and attempt to influence people and events. They value practice with feedback; self-evaluation of work; small group discussions; projects; homework; individualized, self-paced learning activities; and practical application of skills to tasks and problems. Teachers are seen as professional role models. These learners are not helped by lectures.

Although it may be an attractive and reasonable assumption, a link between learning style and preferred instructional strategies is not consistently supported by research. Research in the health care professions validates,[30,46] modestly supports,[5] and does not support this link.[6,16,29] Myth 2 addresses the presumed effect of learning style on selection of instructional strategies. A subsequent assumption holds that using preferred instructional strategies affects other variables such as learner achievement, attrition, or satisfaction.[44] When learners are allowed to satisfy their personal preferences regarding learning activities, it is natural to think that learners learn best and that instructional outcomes are enhanced.

Myth 3

The concept of matching learning styles and preferred teaching styles or instructional strategies has intuitive appeal. This assumes that if an educator's instructional approaches take advantage of learners' preferred styles or strengths, learners will excel. This idea is not new and is certainly not limited to use with Kolb's LSI. Despite its attractiveness as a teaching strategy, the process is not as simple as it sounds. Bonham[3] asks several relevant, rhetorical questions that are useful to staff development educators. These questions include the following:

- What is being matched?
- Are the constructs of teaching and learning equivalent?
- Is the same instrument used to measure both constructs, or are different tools, which may have different theoretical frameworks, used?

- What other variables affect learning?
- Will matching help or hinder learners in a particular situation?
- Is there evidence that matching works?

Messick[34] identifies an array of matches designed to suit varied teaching purposes and different learner needs. These are corrective, compensatory, capitalization, and challenge matches, as well as various combinations of matches and mismatches. Capitalization matching encourages learners to use their dominant or preferred skills, which is the usual intent of matching. In contrast, challenge matching actually is a mismatch because it deliberately challenges learners to use unfamiliar or less preferred skills to encourage flexibility.

The notion of matching assumes that deliberate matching of teaching strategy to learning style directly and positively affects learning outcomes as evidenced by increased achievement, efficiency, satisfaction, comfort, attitude, and decreased attrition or anxiety.[44] However persuasive this reasoning might appear or how popular the practice might be, professional literature does not particularly support matching.[13,43] In addition to the lack of clear research support, a number of reasons exist for educators to resist deliberate matching. These reasons include instruments, resources, variables, teaching style, flexibility, and learner needs.

Instruments. Matching assumes that the instrument used to determine learning styles was appropriately selected for the current purpose and target audience and that it is a valid and reliable measure of the concept of interest. This assumption is questionable considering the conceptual confusion in the learning/cognitive style literature, the criticism of various tools, and the general weakness of research. Given the proliferation of different theories and instruments, a teaching style may be difficult to accurately match with a learning style. In some cases, companion instruments exist to measure teacher and learner characteristics on the same dimensions. This is certainly the preferable approach. In the absence of these specially developed tools, it is risky to use one measure for learning style and another for teaching style with the intent of comparing the two.[3] For example, McCarthy's 4MAT system is identified as a companion instrument to Kolb's LSI. This measures teaching style against Kolb's learning styles.[41] Other instruments, such as the Teaching Style Q-Sort, do not clearly relate to the LSI.[4]

Resources. Copyrighted style instruments are often costly. Teacher time to develop style matches on a large scale may be prohibitive. If matching is done for each individual in a large group, the potential for classroom chaos is high. Without clear evidence that matching improves instructional outcomes, such investments are hard to justify.

Variables. Learning style is only one learning variable. Matching only emphasizes a relatively narrow aspect of the complex teaching-learning interaction. Other important factors that affect learner achievement are shown in the box.

Although one study[42] showed a modest relationship between learning style and achievement, the author acknowledged that other variables within the learning environment could have been operational. Another study[27] found learning style and environment to be significantly interactive, but neither variable can predict achievement. The teaching-learning environment is characterized by complex, interacting variables that are not easily isolated, yet the practice of matching focuses on only one narrow aspect. Until matching is validated by further research, it is a simplistic approach to teaching.

Teacher Style. Teachers probably cannot and should not change their teaching styles to accommodate students with different styles. All teachers have characteristic styles that directly influence the way they teach.[4,35] They tend to select teaching methods based on their own learning styles, not necessarily the styles of their students.[9] A teacher may be less comfortable and therefore less effective teaching in a substantially different style from the familiar and more natural one. This does not mean educators should not try new strategies or use unfamiliar techniques that learners with different styles may prefer. Indeed, offering a variety of strategies within the teaching-learning environment is recommended. However, the deliberate manipulation or change of an educator's style specifically to match a learner's style is not warranted.

Flexibility. The idea of matching teaching styles with learner styles implies that a learner's style, once measured, remains fixed. This also implies that the learner consistently uses only certain techniques in all situations.[20] Adults are capable of changing their approaches over time and in different teaching-learning environments. Learning style theory emphasizes the potential adaptability of learning style as opposed to more stable aspects of the personality. Kolb's theory of experiential learning describes a learner who becomes increasingly flexible in

---

VARIABLES IN THE TEACHING-LEARNING PROCESS[34,35,38]

- Purposes and goals of learning
- Subject matter
- Outcomes to be accomplished
- Levels of the program and learner
- Physical environment
- Context of learning
- Student characteristics
- Facilities and resources
- Time
- Relationship between student and teacher
- Teaching strategies
- Teacher style

learning strategies with age and experience. Classification stability of the LSI has been criticized.[40,45] This criticism represents a limitation of the tool or actual change in learning styles over time. Matching offers a limited, static focus in a dynamic learning environment that responds to multiple variables and with learners who may be quite capable of style flexibility. The goal of adult instruction should be to encourage learners to explore a variety of styles and strategies in all instructional settings rather than narrowly focusing on the strengths and weaknesses of their particular learning styles.

Learner Needs. Although a learner's preferences are probably familiar and comfortable to them, these preferred styles may not always be what the learners need. Self-matching allows the learners to select learning strategies. This notion is limited by learner abilities to distinguish between their preferences and their needs.[34] Educators who only match teaching strategies to learner preferences may be ignoring real needs, including the need to grow as learners. Learners who habitually only use familiar styles may be at a disadvantage when pressed to use unfamiliar skills. Parallel to Messick's challenge match,[34] Joyce[21] maintains that discomfort in the learning environment is essential for growth. He makes a case for deliberately mismatching learners and environments in order to create "dynamic disequilibrium." The goal is to force learners to feel uncomfortable with the unfamiliar. This challenges learners without overwhelming their conceptual systems, thereby encouraging them to move to greater levels of sophistication and complexity. Smith and Kolb[41] echo the prevalent professional thought by stating that "real education lies in helping learners grow in all four learning modes: in their favored ones to be comfortable and successful part of the time; and in their nonfavored ones to stretch their other learning abilities."

Teachers often advocate diagnosis of learning style as a preliminary step in prescribing instructional strategies that notably match but educators must exercise care regarding what is done with this learning style information. Consistent matching of teaching modes to an individual's preferred learning style is a reductionistic approach to teaching and limits the learner. Conversely, consistent mismatching to stimulate growth is also not the best approach. Encouraging students to rely on their own, possibly limited, preferred styles is not helpful either. The cumulatively negative research currently provides less than enthusiastic support for matching. However, many potentially valuable research questions are suggested in this field of study.[3,13,35] Until matching is more clearly defined and better supported, the teaching approach most consistently advocated in the literature is simply to increase learner awareness of differences in learning styles, offer diverse teaching strategies that allow students to develop flexibility in their learning styles, and assist learners to make more informed choices for themselves. Several authors provide especially useful advice about the general use of learning style information.[3,9,11,20]

HOW TO USE LEARNING STYLE INFORMATION
Select and Use Learning Style Instruments Carefully

Dozens of learning style and cognitive style instruments exist. They represent a broad, contradictory field of theory and research. Because style instruments do not have a particularly good reputation for validity, reliability, and theoretical framework,[3] the options should be studied before selecting a tool. Several authors[3,14,36] provide useful comparisons of many instruments and characteristics of these instruments. Educators should critically evaluate proposed tools and the purpose for using these tools. The box suggests questions to ask when selecting a tool. After an instrument is selected, more should be read about the instrument and it should be used as the author intended. Educators should plan in advance ways to use the information.[3] Inferences drawn from one instrument should be reviewed carefully to avoid making generalizations between and among different instruments. Educators should share validity, reliability, and other information about the tool with learners to help learners understand the applicability and limitations of the tool.

Kolb's LSI is one of the most frequently cited learning style tools. As with any other tool Kolb's LSI should be used cautiously. The LSI, like all style instruments, has received criticism primarily directed at the original 1976 version (LSI-I) rather than the revised 1985 version (LSI-II). The reliability, validity, and utility of the LSI-II have not been widely reported,[1,10] and the lack of differentiation between the two versions is another source of confusion. Numerous authors give clear support to the validity of the LSI-I[15,31,33] and the LSI-II.[19,22] Others acknowledge LSI weakness but cautiously support continued improvement of the tool and validation of the theory.[18,45] A few critics recommend cessation of research and normative use of the LSI based on its questionable psychometric properties,[10,17] which is probably a prudent approach. However, even critics of the LSI state that this tool does not categorize learners randomly. These critics say that the LSI classifies at a level beyond chance[45] and may be a useful descriptive mea-

QUESTIONS TO ASK WHEN SELECTING A LEARNING STYLE TOOL

- Whose theory or model is preferred?
- What aspect of learning style will be measured?
- With what age group will the tool be used?
- Is the selected instrument valid and reliable?
- How much time is required to complete the tool?
- How difficult is the tool to complete?
- How difficult is the tool to score and interpret?
- How much does the tool cost?
- Are resources available to cover this expense or has permission to use the tool been granted by the publisher?

sure.[28] Several authors recognize that although learning style research in general is conflicting and quite possibly weak, the concept of learning style *is* useful to educators, and practical applications can be derived.[9,11]

Share Learning Style Information with Learners

Information about the learning style should be shared with learners primarily for *their* use rather than for instructional prescriptions. Before being taught about style instruments, learners may be egocentric and assume everyone learns the same way.[9] Until learners become aware that different styles and strategies exist, they may only use familiar approaches because they do not know of any others.[11] Learners may be unaware or intolerant of learning approaches of others. Some learners may think of themselves as poor learners when they are simply *different* learners.[11]

Educators need to become familiar with the underlying theory and interpretation of the tool. They should point out the characteristics, strengths, and weaknesses of each style and encourage their own tolerance and appreciation of all styles. Faculty learning styles should be shared with learners.[3] Educators should convey the fact that pigeonholing learners into stereotypical learning behaviors is not the purpose of any learning style instrument. Learners should be advised that flexibility among modes and styles is desirable and that the use of only their learning style deprives them of potential success with other strategies possibly helpful to them. Learners should be cautioned that they may experience content or learning situations in which adaptability is necessary.[3] Many different learning options and approaches can be explored through discussion with learners. These discussions can identify incremental steps for learners, particularly learners who have strong preferences or extreme scores in their own style who want to try new approaches.[3] Style should be treated as actions of the learner, which are amenable to change, rather than as a measure of aptitude or general ability to learn which are beyond a learner's control.[3,20] Interpretation and discussion of various learning styles gives learners insight into their own and others' learning styles, acknowledges the important fact that people learn differently, and enables learners to more fully appreciate and better use various strategies and methods offered by educators.

The most important aspect of using these tools is possibly the discussion of results with learners. Dixon[11] advocates using learning style information to shift the focus from the educator's attempts to improve instruction to learners' opportunities to improve learning.[11] Similarly, Hyman and Rosoff[20] implore teachers to abandon their traditional, unilateral, approach to diagnosing and controlling the learning environment. These authors advocate cultivating a mutual planning approach between the educator and learners by using learning style information as one source of collaboration to empower learners and encourage them to take more responsibility for their own learning and behavior. Smith and Kolb[41] assert that the LSI is of particular benefit when used by educators and learners to understand the contributions of both parties to the educational process. Bonham[3] advocates a novel reason to use learning style information—the creation of the Hawthorne effect in the educational setting. Teachers and learners who are aware of and excited about learning style differences improve the instructional environment and outcomes. Instead of just emphasizing content, educators focus deliberate and creative attention on the *process* of learning. Identifying learning styles is the first step in creating a teaching-learning climate that recognizes and encourages individual differences, in addition to offering an environment in which learners can experiment with different learning styles with little or no risk.

In selected situations, it may be appropriate to share the learning style of employees with managers. Some style instruments are particularly well-suited to work settings and management applications. Managers may also find the information helpful. Before sharing this information, educators should be sure to have employee permission. Also, managers should understand the proper ways to use the style information.

Create a Flexible Learning Environment with a Variety of Teaching Strategies

A flexible learning environment that represents all learning styles is advocated even by researchers whose studies found a predominant learning style within a professional group.[37] This approach satisfies and stimulates the most learners, regardless of whether learning style instruments are used. Learners should be given opportunities to experience different strategies and not just discuss them abstractly. This takes thoughtful planning because identifying different perspectives of a subject and varied ways to study that subject is more resource intensive than simply delivering a well-rehearsed lecture.[11] Educators may find it helpful to start with Kolb's preferred strategies for each learning style to get ideas. Doing a literature search on teaching strategies is also recommended because the professional literature is so rich in this area. Brainstorming with learners to identify multiple ways to accomplish selected projects may also be helpful. Information gained by brainstorming may be used to develop and maintain a departmental list or file of teaching-learning strategies for general use or specific topics. Educators should refer to this list often. The box on p. 78 offers a short list of teaching strategies to get educators started. Whenever possible, a variety of ways to meet the same instructional objective should be offered. Learners should be allowed to choose activities. This is possible even in mandatory requirements. For example, accredited cardiopulmonary resuscitation (CPR) training generally requires standardized written and performance tests. Beyond these usually nonnegotiable aspects, the way learners prepare for the tests may be discretionary, particularly for recertification.

Different approaches available for learner selection might include manuals, programmed instruction, or other written materials for self-study outside of class; computer-assisted instruction or simulation; lecture and discussion; movies or videotapes; demonstration of skills; and supervised practice with feedback. Participants may feel comfortable enough with the content to simply take (challenge) the tests without special preparation.

Educators need to create a collaborative environment in which learners recog-

TEACHING STRATEGIES

Audiotape	Journal club
Brainstorming	Lecture
Cartoons	Movie
Case study	Newsletter
Competency-based education	Observation
Computer (for example, CAI,	Panel discussion
bulletin boards, networks)	Poster
Contract	Practical exercise
Critical incident	Printed materials
Debate	Programmed instruction
Demonstration or return	Puppets
demonstration	Puzzles
Discovery learning	Question and answer
Discussion	Report or presentation
Drama, skit	Role modeling
Fact sheet	Role playing
Fair or carnival	Seminar
Field trip	Simulation
Film or filmstrip	Skills practice
Games	Television
Grand rounds	Transparencies or slides
Humanities (that is, arts,	Values clarification
music, literature)	Videotape
Humor	Video teleconference
Independent study or project	Workgroups
Interview	

nize and use each other as resources, in addition to capitalizing on the unique strengths of each learning style. Educators can identify ways in which learners with different styles can help and complement each other. Learners should discuss their less preferred strategies and consider the reasons this is so. Educators may help learners select specific ways to use their nondominant styles with minimal or no risk in group process or to meet a learning objective. A reputation for fun and diversity in the staff development department can be cultivated by varying the instructional approaches to educational activities. The following lists some ideas:

- Serve popcorn during educational films.
- Sponsor a skills carnival with balloons, booths, music, and prizes.
- During orientation, send new employees on a scavenger hunt around the facility to search for answers to specific questions.
- Host an interdisciplinary panel discussion with respected experts on a topic of current interest in the organization.
- Publish staff development crosswords or other puzzles in the employee newsletter.
- Use small groups to do reality-based problem-solving exercises.
- Offer learners a variety of teaching strategies to acknowledge the importance of individual differences and demonstrate commitment to the principles of learner-centered adult education.

SUMMARY

There are many questions relating to the appropriate use of learning styles in staff development. Learning style, cognitive style, and personality type always need to be distinguished. According to his theory, Kolb's four distinctive learning styles include: concrete experience, reflective observation, abstract conceptualization, and active experimentation. Most learners can be flexible within these styles. Staff development educators can dispel the three myths of learning styles and create flexible learning environments.

REFERENCES

1. Bonham LA: Learning style instruments: let the buyer beware, *Lifelong Learn* 11(6):12, 1988.
2. Bonham LA: Learning style use: in need of perspective, *Lifelong Learn* 11(5):14, 1988.
3. Bonham LA: Using learning style information, too. In Hayes ER, editor: *Effective teaching styles: new directions for continuing education*, No 43, San Francisco, 1989, Jossey-Bass.
4. Carrier C, Melvin K: *Linking teacher theories to teacher practice*. Paper presented at the Annual Meeting of the Association for Educational Communications and Technology, Research and Theory Division, Dallas, May 1982.
5. Carrier CA, Newell KJ, Lange AL: Relationship of learning styles to preferences for instructional activities, *J Dent Educ* 46:652, 1982.
6. Christensen LM et al: Learner preferences of primary care physicians in continuing medical education, *Mobius* 5(2):13, 1985.
7. Claxton CS, Ralston Y: *Learning styles: their impact on teaching and administration*, Washington, DC, 1978, American Association for Higher Education and ERIC Clearinghouse on Higher Education Research Report No 10.
8. Curry L: *An organization of learning styles theory and constructs*. Paper presented at the annual meeting of the American Educational Research Association, Montreal, Apr 11-15, 1983.
9. Davidson GV: Matching learning styles with teaching styles: is it a useful concept in instruction? *Performance Instruction* 29(4): 36, 1990.
10. DeCoux VM: Kolb's learning style inventory: a review of its applications in nursing research, *J Nurs Educ*, 29:202, 1990.
11. Dixon NM: The implementation of learning style information, *Lifelong Learn* 9(3):16, 1985.
12. Dixon NM: Incorporating learning style into training design, *Train Dev J* 36(7):62, 1982.
13. Doyle W, Rutherford B: Classroom research on matching teaching and learning styles, *Theory Pract* 23:20, 1984.
14. Dunn R et al: Learning style researchers define learning differently, *Educ Leadership* 38:372, 1981.
15. Ferrell BG: A factor analytic comparison of four learning-styles instruments, *J Educ Psychol* 75:33, 1983.
16. Fox RD: Learning styles and instructional preferences in continuing education for health professionals: a validity study of the LSI, *Adult Educ* 35(2):72, 1984.
17. Freedman RD, Stumpf SA: Learning style theory: less than meets the eye, *Acad Manage Rev* 5:445, 1980.
18. Gregg N: Learning style inventory. In Conoley JC, Kramer JJ, editors: *The tenth mental measurements yearbook*, 1989, Omaha, University of Nebraska Press.
19. Highhouse S, Doverspike D: The validity of the learning style inventory 1985 as a predictor of cognitive style and occupational preference, *Educ Psychol Measurement* 47:749, 1987.
20. Hyman R, Rosoff B: Matching learning and teaching styles: the jug and what's in it, *Theory Practice* 23:35, 1984.
21. Joyce BR: Dynamic disequilibrium: the intelligence of growth, *Theory Practice* 23:26, 1984.
22. Katz N: Construct validity of Kolb's learning style inventory, using factor analysis and Guttman's smallest space analysis, *Percept Mot Skills* 63:1323, 1986.

23. Keefe JW: Learning style: an overview. In *Student learning styles: diagnosing and prescribing programs*, Reston, Va, 1979, National Association of Secondary School Principals.
24. Kolb DA: *Experiential learning: experience as the source of learning and development*. Englewood Cliffs, NJ, 1984, Prentice-Hall.
25. Kolb DA: Learning style inventory: self-scoring inventory and interpretation booklet, Boston, 1985, McBer.
26. Kolb DA, Plovnick MS: The experiential learning theory of career development. In Van Maanen J, editor: *Organizational careers: some new perspectives*, New York, 1977, Wiley & Sons.
27. Korhonen LJ, McCall RJ: The interaction of learning style and learning environment on adult achievement, *Lifelong Learn* 10(2):21, 1986.
28. Kruzich JM, Friesen BJ, Van Soest D: Assessment of student and faculty learning styles: research and application, *J Soc Work Educ* 22(3):22, 1986.
29. Laschinger HK, Boss MK: Learning styles of baccalaureate nursing students and attitudes toward theory-based nursing, *J Prof Nurs* 5:215, 1989.
30. Leonard A, Harris I: Learning style in a primary care internal medicine residency program, *Arch Intern Med* 139:872, 1979.
31. Lewis R, Margerison C: Working and learning—identifying your preferred ways of doing things, *Personnel Rev* 8(2):25, 1979.
32. McCaulley MH: The Myers-Briggs type indicator: a measure for individuals and groups, *Measurement Eval Counsel Dev* 22:181, 1990.
33. Merritt SL, Marshall JC: Reliability and construct validity of ipsative and normative forms of the learning style inventory, *Educ Psychol Measurement* 44:463, 1984.
34. Messick S: Personal styles and educational options. In Messick et al, editors: *Individuality in learning*, San Francisco, 1978, Jossey-Bass.
35. Ostmoe PM et al: Learning style preferences and selection of learning strategies: consideration and implications for nurse educators, *J Nurs Educ* 23:27, 1984.
36. Partridge R: Learning styles: a review of selected models, *J Nurs Educ* 22:243, 1983.
37. Penn BK: *Correlations among learning styles, clinical specialties, and personality types of U.S. Army nurses*, doctoral dissertation, Austin, 1991, The University of Texas at Austin.
38. Reichmann-Hruska S: Learning styles and individual differences in learning, *Equity Excellence* 24(3):25, 1989.
39. Rule DL, Grippin PC: *A critical comparison of learning style instruments frequently used with adult learners*. Paper presented at the annual conference of the Eastern Educational Research Association, Miami Beach, Fla, Feb 25, 1988.
40. Sims RR et al: The reliability and classification stability of the learning style inventory, *Educ Psychol Measurement* 46(3):753, 1986.
41. Smith D, Kolb DA: *User's guide for the learning style inventory: a manual for teachers and trainers*, Boston, 1986, McBer.
42. Sparks BI III: The Kolb learning style inventory: predicting academic potential among optometry students, *J Optometric Educ* 15(2):52, 1990.
43. Thompson C, Crutchlow E: Learning style research: a critical review of the literature and implications for nursing education, *J Prof Nurs* 9(1):34, 1993.
44. Underwood SM: Application of learning style theory to nursing education and nursing practice. ERIC No ED 287 415, 1987.
45. Veres JG III, Sims RR, Shake LG: The reliability and classification stability of the learning style inventory in corporate settings, *Educ Psychol Measurement* 47(4):1127, 1987.
46. Whitney MA, Caplan RM: Learning styles and instructional preferences of family practice physicians, *J Med Educ* 53:684, 1978.
47. Witkin HA et al: *Manual: embedded figures test, children's embedded figures test, and group embedded figures test*, Palo Alto, Calif, 1971, Consulting Psychologist Press.

Managing Nursing Staff Development

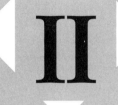

II

Organization of Staff Development Activities

6

The placement of a staff development department within an organization plays a major role in shaping employee education and the way education can be accomplished. The centralized staff development department within the nursing service department provides the greatest opportunity to influence decision making at the executive level of nursing service. The staff development division within a hospital-wide education department provides the greatest opportunity to influence other departments within the organization. Decentralized staff development activities on each patient care unit provide the best opportunities to influence care at the bedside.

The organization of staff development activities also reflects an organization's commitment to the development of its employees. If the director of staff development reports to an executive, this demonstrates a higher value for education activities than if the director is placed at a lower level in the organization. Reporting relationships and resources allocated to staff development are influenced by many factors that should be considered before investigating the types of organizational structure.

INFLUENTIAL FACTORS
Philosophy and Mission

In addition to the organization's philosophy and mission, the associated implementations affect all activities and therefore influence the organization of staff development. The nursing or patient care service's philosophy should flow directly from and be consistent with the organization's philosophy and mission statement. A hospital mission statement provides the initial impetus for identification of educational beliefs within a department philosophy. Many organizations today are embracing Peter Senge's premises[14] related to a learning organization. Belief in this viewpoint prominently positions staff development within the organizational structure.

Another example of a philosophic tenet that affects staff development structure is a professional practice model ascribing to shared governance concepts. This model may dictate that the practicing staff member has authority, control, and autonomy for staff development. As such, an organizational model must exist in which staff members play an integral role in staff development activities.

Philosophic beliefs and goals related to education must be reflected in formal department policies and procedures. The organization of staff development must then facilitate implementation of these policies and procedures. For example, if a department is committed to competency-based education (CBE) and principles of adult education, the staff development structure must support these ideas.

Structural Organization

The organizational structure of the organization directly reflects the way that staff development is organized. As hospitals become involved in reengineering and begin focusing on patient and family needs (patient-focused care) rather than on staff needs or environmental limitations, the workflow and practice patterns change dramatically.[11] In turn, traditional organizational structures may be dismantled. In organizations involved in these efforts, staff development must be organized to respond to this new paradigm.

In organizations that retain a distinct nursing or patient care service department with dedicated staff development personnel, the structure of staff development usually reflects the department's structure. For example, if the nursing department favors centralization, so will the staff development department. Likewise, a decentralized nursing department will probably spawn a similarly organized staff development department.

The roles and responsibilities of educators within a nursing staff development department are affected by the way staff development is accomplished for personnel in other departments. Some departments, such as the laboratory, physical therapy, radiology, and respiratory therapy, may have their own staff development personnel. They provide education for their own staff and serve as valuable resources for educational activities for nursing staff. As long as these other disciplines do not address issues and responsibilities within nursing care, their participation as a resource is appropriate.

On the other hand, nursing or patient care services and staff development personnel may be required to help provide staff development for employees throughout the organization. Their responsibilities may include ensuring that all regulatory agency educational requirements such as cardiopulmonary resuscitation (CPR), fire safety, and infection control reviews are met by *all* hospital personnel. In-service classes or continuing education courses related to an individual educator's expertise may also be requested.

Regardless of staff development structure, staff development educators must be given a position of status in the organization to achieve educational goals and perform their roles successfully. The director of staff development should have a direct reporting relationship to a hospital executive. For example, the staff development director within a nursing or patient care services department should report to the chief nursing executive. If the staff development department is more global, perhaps hospital wide, the director should reprot to a senior hospital executive such as the vice president for human resources or even the chief operating officer.

Staff development personnel must be recognized within the formal organizational structure. Coye[4] writes, "It is imperative that evidence of support for staff development become an identified component within the organizational structure. If staff development has no existing formal structure and is accorded neither identity nor visibility, it is difficult for staff development educators to achieve the goals and purposes of their efforts."

In most instances the formal staff development structure reflects a staff relationship rather than a line relationship to colleagues throughout the organization. According to del Bueno,[7] educators not only provide education but also promote the organization's service mission. Educators must work with managers to solve unit or department problems by using their educational expertise in the problem-solving process. Thus the organizational structure must foster formal and informal meetings and relationships between educators and managers at the administrative level and between educators and staff; the specific association depends on the organizational structure. In a decentralized environment, educators may regularly plan with the department manager and attend unit meetings to communicate with staff members.

Roles and Responsibilities

The roles and responsibilities of educators also influence the department's organizational structure. Roles are shaped by the beliefs and desires of the educators, expectations of people outside the department, and hospital and nursing department philosophies related to education. As del Bueno[7] states, "It is important that staff development personnel be perceived as proactive rather than reactive. They should not wait to be told what the organization wants from them, but rather be prepared with proposals and plans to meet anticipated organizational needs." This proactive stance helps establish the roles and responsibilities most appropriate and desired by staff development personnel.

First, educators can define and expand their roles by becoming involved in all facets of the organization. Staff development personnel should volunteer to serve on hospital and nursing department councils, committees, and task forces. They should communicate the importance of their involvement persuasively. Wide-ranging involvement within the organization assists in creating a politically strong staff development organizational structure.

Second, expectations of personnel outside the staff development department help define the role of educator. For example, an organization with a commitment to community outreach programming may create special role expectations for the staff development department. In addition, patient care unit managers may desire educational programming specific to their patient population; this may lead to the creation of a decentralized organizational structure.

Third, the roles and responsibilities for educators are conceived in philosophies and associated policies and procedures. A clinical advancement system with standards for in-service and continuing education stimulates the development of this programming by staff development personnel. An organization with a belief in and commitment to a preceptor model may need staff development educators to devise educational programming for the preceptors and serve as facilitators to the preceptors.

As mentioned, an organization's belief in CBE and adult learning principles may affect the staff development structure by creating certain roles for educators. For example, the use of learning contracts to improve or maintain performance requires an educator's expertise in developing teaching strategies, creating conditions for learning, and evaluating employee performance. The many self-directed learning resources required by a CBE system also require staff development educators who are proficient in adult learning strategies.

Educational Preparation

Formal educational preparation of staff development personnel must be considered in determining department structure and associated roles and responsibilities. As previously stated, staff development directors should be at the same hierarchical level as clinical directors or administrators. As such, directors should be members of the nursing executive team. For this role to be effectively carried out, a master's degree should be the minimum requirement. Staff development directors must be knowledgeable in clinical nursing practice and educational and administrative theory.

Educators should also be prepared at the graduate level to assume the roles and responsibilities outlined. Their expertise should be in clinical nursing practice and educational theory. In addition, educators must be able to successfully facilitate change within the organization; this requires knowledge related to systems and change theory, program evaluation, and group processes. These proficiencies and formal education should be recognized through appropriate positions for staff development educators in the organizational structure.

The educational level of other personnel within the hospital, patient care, or nursing services must be considered in structuring staff development. This becomes especially important in determining reporting relationships. For example, organizations may have unit-based educators with master's degrees who report to the unit managers. In this instance, managers should also have graduate degrees.

A hospital with a staff nurse clinical advancement system may require a baccalaureate or graduate degree for advancement. If staff development personnel are to evaluate or assist these advanced practitioners in skill or other developments, staff educators should have achieved an equivalent level of education at the least.

Availability and Use of Clinical Nurse Specialists

The use of clinical nurse specialists (CNSs) within an organization affects the roles and responsibilities of staff development personnel and the organization of the department. If CNSs are employed within a hospital, their roles and responsibilities must be clearly defined. The degree to which CNSs may be involved in staff development varies.

First, CNSs may function as staff development educators. In this case the job description is the same as that of a traditional staff development role and includes few or no aspects of a traditional CNS role. A concern with this practice is that the CNS, although prepared at the graduate level, may have little formal preparation in educational theory and methods.

Second, CNSs may function as CNSs *and* staff educators. The title for this role varies according to the organization and the department's organizational structure. The rationale for this dual role is cost containment and the belief that the appropriate role may be implemented based on demonstrated need. In reality, however, one role is typically carried out more frequently than the other. The role selected to be carried out may result from the individual's preferences or proficiencies, patient care needs, or the expectations of others.

Third, CNSs and staff educators may have distinct and clearly defined roles and responsibilities. Boyer[3] describes the collaboration and cooperation between the CNS-"the expert in clinical knowledge and skill"-and the staff development educator-"the expert in educational processes"-as a means to provide "ongoing cost-effective programs to insure nursing excellence."

Wolf[18] speaks of first- and second-generation CNSs. She believes that first-generation CNSs initially focus on the patient and then on the patient and nurse. Wolf asserts second-generation CNSs need to focus on systems-wide factors such as problematic patient care outcomes, inefficient and ineffective nursing practices, and innovative approaches to care delivery. If this happens, the roles between staff development educators and CNSs can be further differentiated and keep staff education responsibilities in the role of educator.

Two trends seem to support this prediction of a role differentiation between CNSs and educators. The first trend relates to the expanding managed care environment, in which the role of case manager is increasingly being assumed by CNSs. A second trend involves the educational preparation of CNSs, in that several colleges and universities throughout the United States are designing a role that combines the CNS and nurse practitioner tracts. Both examples point to the evolution of the CNS away from a staff development focus.

Diversification of Patient Care Services

The diversification of patient care services should also be considered in organizing staff development activities. A highly diversified organization that has numerous goals and purposes tends to assume a more decentralized structure.[7] For example, an organization that has been approved by the state as a trauma center must provide designated types and amounts of trauma-related continuing education activities for its staff. This same organization may also provide different services such as maternal-child or cardiology services and may also need to provide continuing education in these areas. On the other hand, smaller or single-service organizations may benefit from a centralized structure for staff development.

Physical Layout of the Hospital

According to del Bueno,[7] the physical layout of the hospital may affect staff development organization. An organization that has multiple buildings spread over a large geographic area may favor a decentralized staff development department. As mergers result in organizations that have several sites or campuses, decentralization is important to meet the specific educational needs of the staff at each site. Organizations with only one building may be better served by a centralized staff development department.

Financial Status

Despite a philosophic commitment to education, monies budgeted for staff development directly relate to the financial status of an organization. As the financial picture for a hospital becomes bleaker, dollars budgeted for staff development are frequently the first to be reduced or eliminated. Therefore an organization's financial status and future plans must be considered when designing the staff development department.

Organizational structures of staff development departments should not only consider the philosophy, mission, and organizational structure of the organization but other factors as well (box). Only after considering these factors can an effective organization of staff development activities be decided. The three most prevalent designs are (1) a hospital-wide education department, (2) a centralized staff development department within nursing services, and (3) a decentralized staff development department within the nursing service department. The remainder of this chapter discusses these three designs and other considerations and innovative methods for organizing staff development.

FACTORS INFLUENCING THE ORGANIZATION OF STAFF DEVELOPMENT ACTIVITIES

Philosophy and mission of the organization
Organization of the nursing department
Scope of staff development roles and responsibilities
Educational preparation of the staff development director and educators
Educational preparation of executives, managers, and staff nurses
Availability and use of clinical nurse specialists
Diversification of patient care services
Physical layout of the hospital
Financial status of the organization

HOSPITAL-WIDE EDUCATION DEPARTMENT
Organizational Structure

Some organizations have an education department that is responsible for the staff development of all hospital personnel. The manager of such a department may report directly to the hospital administrator or associate administrator and, within the organization's hierarchy, may be on the same level as the chief nursing executive and other executives. This person may also report to a vice president (Fig. 6-1). The specific structure is largely related to the organization's mission statement and philosophy concerning education.

Because the staff members of nursing services comprise the most employees in the organization, nurses are and should be members of a hospital-wide education department. Nurses who have graduate degrees are increasingly becoming managers of hospital-wide education departments. In addition to nurses, education department staff members are usually formally prepared as educators and often have degrees specifically in health education. In hospitals with large ancillary departments or hospitals that are focused on singular or specialty services, clinical practitioners who are specific to these services may also be members of the education department.

The Education Department in Relation to Nursing Services

The relationship of a hospital-wide education department to nursing services varies. The hospital-wide education department may be responsible for all nursing service staff development or only certain aspects of it. Regardless of the scope of the responsibilities, methods must be designed to ensure satisfactory communication between the hospital-wide education department and the nursing department. The nursing department must be actively involved in all phases of the educational process, especially in the assessment of learning needs, formulation of the action plan to meet those needs, and the evaluation process.

Jernigan[9] describes a centralized, hospital-wide education department with nursing unit or department consultants who form a multidisciplinary committee. This committee may answer to the director for hospital-wide education and the

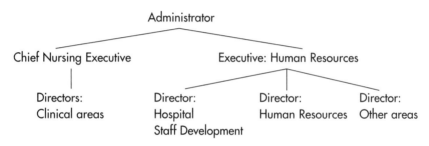

Fig. 6-1   Organization of a hospital-wide education department.

chief nursing executive. The unit or department consultants assist unit managers and personnel by facilitating educational activities.

Jernigan[9] also describes a committee exclusively made up of representatives from nursing units rather than hospital-wide departments. The multidisciplinary committee oversees hospital-wide educational activities, whereas the nursing consultant group is a decision-making committee that focuses on educational activities for nursing.

Many hospitals have a staff development department within the nursing ser-vices department *and* a hospital-wide education department. Clearly, effective com-munication between the two departments is essential. Simple strategies to achieve this communication include having a representative from each group attend the other group's staff meetings and exchanging minutes of these meetings. Organization with a shared governance model probably have a nursing education council. If so, these council meetings are ideal for hospital-wide education depart-ment representatives to attend to facilitate communication between the two groups.

Department Responsibilities

Management Training. A common responsibility of a hospital-wide education department is to develop and implement management training. A structure that allows for the inclusion of nurse managers in this training has many advantages. Because the target audience is larger (that is, all hospital managers), the pro-gramming budget may be larger than the budget for nursing alone. Therefore the training itself may be significantly broader in scope and depth than nursing ser-vices could support independently.

Another advantage of involving nurse managers in education with other managers from throughout the hospital is to provide an opportunity for man-agers to become acquainted. This fosters communication and collaborative prob-lem solving. Finally, having nurse managers attend management development sessions conveys the message throughout the organization that nurse managers are indeed department heads who possess the power and decision-making authority associated with that hierarchical level.

Orientation. Hospital-wide education departments customarily provide em-ployee orientation programs. Increased cost effectiveness related to reduced dupli-cation of effort and expenses is an important advantage to assigning responsibili-ty for orientation to a single department. Even when a nursing staff development department exists, it is wise for the departments to collaborate on orientation.

The hospital-wide education department typically performs all generic orien-tation necessary for all personnel. The Lehigh Valley Hospital's hospital-wide education department offers an 8-hour employee orientation program that includes the following:

- Welcome by hospital-wide education department representative
- Welcome by president or chief operating officer
- Benefit overview and paperwork

- Tax shelter annuity availability
- Safety, hazard communication, back safety
- Infection control
- Employee health
- Employee wellness program
- Employee assistance program
- Welcome by senior vice president for human resources
- Risk management
- Patient representatives
- Employee ombudsman
- Pastoral care
- Organ donation
- Fire safety
- Potential for violence alert
- Parking
- Security identification badges
- Hospital tours

Regulatory and Agency-Required Programming. A hospital-wide education department can also cost-effectively coordinate all regulatory and agency-required programming throughout the organization. If there is a nursing staff development department, educators and unit staff members can assist as requested. As with orientation programming, reduced duplication of effort and decreased expenses are achieved by designating an individual or a department to coordinate all regulatory and agency-required programming. For example, a hospital-wide education department could coordinate and hold monthly CPR certifications and recertifications for a designated time. Any hospital employee could attend. The hospital-wide education department would be responsible for all coordinating functions, including communicating information about the program to all personnel, obtaining supplies and audiovisuals, completing paperwork, and scheduling faculty. The faculty could include representatives from individual hospital departments.

Benefits to Nursing

If nurses are staff members within a hospital-wide education department or if means exist to secure nursing input, programs initiated by a hospital-wide education department will be more likely to incorporate a nursing perspective. This benefits the nursing department by providing more programming for nurses than a nursing staff development department alone could provide. Multidisciplinary programs are also likely to result, thereby stimulating a collaborative practice environment.

One farsighted RN, who was the director of continuing education for a nursing department, transferred within the same organization to become the hospital-wide education department's director. Under her leadership, the hospital's medical symposium series began to incorporate content appropriate to nurses and involved nurses as faculty members. Attendance and revenue significantly improved as a result of the larger target audience. Also, physicians and nurses reported an opportunity to network and enhance collaborative efforts.

This same organization conducts management development training for all managers and nurses. This training is coordinated by the hospital-wide education department. Specially trained and certified hospital managers serve as faculty members. Before the arrival of the new director, few nurses served as faculty members. This changed because the new director made special efforts to recruit nurses. Certainly this strategy helped gain nursing management's commitment to the program. It also made a statement throughout the organization that nursing managers work at the same hierarchical level as other department managers and have the exceptional managerial skills required to serve as faculty. In summary, nursing's involvement in and cooperation with a hospital-wide education department can prove extremely beneficial to the nursing department.

CENTRALIZED STAFF DEVELOPMENT WITHIN NURSING SERVICES

Coye[4] defines a *centralized staff development* as "an organizational approach in which a central nursing administrative authority is assigned the major responsibility to meet the learning needs of the nursing staff. In this approach, all staff education activities are assumed by a central staff."

The Director's Role and Reporting Structure

In practice, centralized nursing staff development educators report to one of many individuals, including the following people:
- Hospital-wide staff development administrator
- Performance improvement administrator
- Nursing research administrator
- Clinical director or administrator
- Affiliated dean or school of nursing director
- Chief nursing executive

Ideally, educators in a centralized department should report to a staff development director or administrator (Fig. 6-2). If the staff development department director has many different assignments in addition to staff development (for examples, clinical units, performance improvement, research, or school of nursing responsibilities), educators may not receive sufficient attention. Also, the staff development director may have been selected for expertise in assigned areas other than staff development and may not be qualified to lead or direct the entire department.

The staff development director may have the opportunity to report to the most senior nursing executive, whereas colleagues who are clinical directors report to an associate administrator. Although this may appear favorable and

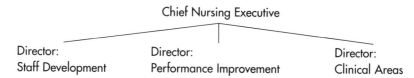

Fig. 6-2   Organization of centralized staff development within nursing services.

prestigious for the staff development department, it may not be advantageous. The other clinical directors or the associate administrator may resent the staff development director's "special" reporting relationship. This can thwart a collaborative, collegial relationship between the nursing service and nursing education departments. Even without resentment or intentional sabotage, this type of structure may prohibit effective communication between the staff development director and clinical peers, make attainment of staff education goals difficult, and hinder achievement of service goals.

The staff development director must participate as a regular member at operational meetings of the clinical directors and must have a similar workload to maintain a comparable status. Examples of a similar workload might include sharing in administrative house-call responsibilities and being responsible for the budgets of staff development and other services such as product departments. The director should volunteer for and request these additional activities.

During management decision-making meetings and activities, Tobin and Beeler[16] suggest that "the role of listening with an 'educational' ear can not be emphasized enough." Nursing service administrators expect the staff development director "to focus on and speak to the educational components of planned organizational changes."[16] As such, the director becomes a valued member of the management team and gains important early information that affects staff development.

Centralized Organizational Structure

Centralized staff development departments may be organized in several ways. Key factors in the design are the organization's and staff development department's sizes. In larger departments in which the director has multiple administrative responsibilities, one or more coordinators may manage and direct the operations of the department.

One method for organizing the educators themselves is to identify certain functional areas (Fig. 6-3). Educators are then assigned to one or more functions. These functional areas include the following:

- Orientation
- Product-related issues and in-service classes
- Regulatory agency and organizational requirements

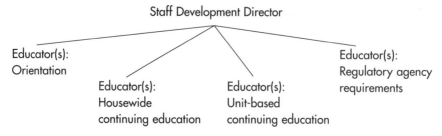

Fig. 6-3   Functional organization of educators.

- Hospital-wide continuing education programs
- Unit-based continuing education programs
- Management development

The number of educators assigned to each function varies depending on the requirements and associated goals. For example, an organization committed to community continuing education has more people dedicated to that function. If unit-based preceptors are used for orientation, fewer centralized personnel are devoted to orientation.

If a coordinator is assigned to any or all of these functional areas, the roles of this person and the staff educators must be clearly defined. For example, it should be determined whether the coordinator is in a purely managerial position or expected to participate in staff functions such as implementing programs.

In another design for a centralized staff development department, educators are organized according to patient types or services. These services may include medical-surgical, critical care, maternal-child, psychiatry, and outpatient services or neuroscience, cardiology, psychiatry, orthopedics, and burns. If two or more educators are working within the same functional or service group, they can function independently or as a team. For example, if two people are assigned to the orientation group, one may be responsible for RN and LPN/LVN orientation and the other may be in charge of unit clerk and nursing assistant orientation, or they may work together.

Yet another way to centralize the organization of staff development is to combine the functional and patient types or services approach. For example, an educator may be assigned to a particular patient type or service in addition to being responsible for coordinating hospital-wide and centralized orientation activities. Another educator may have maternal-child service responsibilities and be accountable for all educational programs related to regulatory agencies.

Advantages of a Centralized Structure

There are many advantages to a centralized staff development department. One of the most obvious advantages is that secretarial and support services are more extensive. Clerical and support personnel can be organized and used in several ways. In a large department with several clerical staff members, they may be assigned to support designated functions, thereby enhancing their proficiency in assigned areas. In contrast, all support staff may share responsibilities. This latter approach is best used when workloads related to different functional areas are unevenly distributed or vary in intensity at different times of year.

The responsibilities that clerical and support staff assume can and should be varied. Staff development educators must be creative in using personnel to control expenses and save valuable RN time. For example, having a former unit clerk train other clerks is more cost effective than employing an RN for this activity. Also, clerical personnel may effectively conduct all classes related to the hospital information system.

Clerical and support staff can also be used to assume other nonteaching activities within the department. In an effort to control costs, one acute care hospital with a large staff development department eliminated the department's coordinator positions. These staff members had coordinated orientation and continuing education programs. Many of their responsibilities, which included scheduling, distributing and summarizing evaluations, registering participants, writing confirmation and thank-you letters, and keeping records, are now effectively handled by clerical personnel.

Another advantage to having a centralized staff development department is the availability of volunteers. Volunteers can do many tasks, including taking inventory and stocking an educational resource center or learning laboratory, designing and making posters, completing literature searches, obtaining references for educators, and performing clerical functions. Volunteer RNs can implement educational programming that primarily focuses on teaching or validating the skills of nursing assistants.

Another advantage of a centralized department is the opportunity for collegial support among educators. One way to heighten this benefit is to provide centralized offices and other opportunities that facilitate group or one-on-one interactions. Another strategy to facilitate informal networking is to organize a breakfast or brunch before monthly staff meetings. The staff development director can also foster collegial sharing by referring individual staff members to consult with peers as appropriate.

A centralized department also has the opportunity to provide continuing education for its members. The staff may take turns presenting topics of interest to peers. If budgeted monies are available, outside speakers may be brought in for discussions. For maximum cost-effectiveness, educators from other hospital departments may be invited to speak.

Another advantage of a centralized department is the ability to conduct team teaching with more experienced educators. This provides opportunities for individual growth by sharing lesson plans, strategies for teaching, and evaluation methods. Integrating adult learning principles into teaching strategies is enhanced when less-experienced teachers can observe expert educators.

ADVANTAGES OF A CENTRALIZED STRUCTURE

More extensive secretarial and support services available.
Opportunity exists for collegial support among educators.
Opportunity exists for continuing education for staff members.
More experienced educators are able to team teach.
Library and audiovisual resources are more plentiful and accessible.

Library and audiovisual resources are more plentiful and accessible in a centralized department. Projectors and films are easier to share with a centralized reservation system. Also, books and magazines specific to staff development can be ordered and shared. Many educational resources specific to adult educators are discussed during peer dialogues. When educators are decentralized in the patient care areas, dialogue tends to focus on clinical problems and solutions rather than on educational problems and solutions. The advantages of a centralized structure are listed in the box.

Strategies to Minimize Disadvantages

One major disadvantage to centralized staff development is that educators may be unaware of, unresponsive to, or incapable of implementing unit-based programming. The following lists several strategies to help minimize this potential problem:

- Regular meetings should take place between the staff development director and clinical directors. During these meetings, educational needs and priorities need to be communicated. The staff development director must then communicate these needs to the educators and hold them accountable for meeting these needs.
- Formal and informal meetings should be conducted between staff development educators and head nurses to communicate the educational requests of individual units.
- Staff development educators need to attend regularly scheduled meetings of the management staff. This provides a prime opportunity for the educators to use their problem-solving skills to recognize educational needs that may go unnoticed by the managers.
- Staff development educators should attend unit staff meetings. This gives educators another opportunity to learn staff perceptions of educational needs. It also gives the staff a chance to directly communicate their desires regarding education to the educators.
- Formal needs assessments of the entire nursing staff should be conducted annually, if not more often. This assessment should include educational content needs and preferences related to scheduling. Each assessment

---

STRATEGIES TO MINIMIZE DISADVANTAGES OF A CENTRALIZED ORGANIZATION

Conduct regular meetings between the staff development director and clinical directors.

Ensure that regular meetings occur between staff development educators and head nurses.

Require staff development educators to attend management meetings.

Direct staff development educators to attend individual unit meetings.

Conduct a formal needs assessment of nursing staff annually.

Ensure that staff development educators maintain clinical competence in the skills they teach.

Form an education committee or council composed of managers and staff to participate in educational decisions.

---

should contain a summary of the previous assessment's results and a list of any educational programming done to meet the identified needs. This serves to communicate to nursing service staff the ways in which staff development has responded to their requests.

- Staff development personnel need to maintain clinical competence, particularly in skill areas for which they are responsible. For example, it may not be necessary for medical-surgical educators to remain competent in primary nursing; rather they should attain or maintain clinical expertise in working with a patient-controlled analgesia pump and other equipment for which in-service education is routinely required.

- An education committee or council should participate in recommendations or decisions related to education. This group can include representatives from management and the nursing staff who meet regularly with all or designated members of the centralized education staff.

The strategies to minimize the disadvantages of a centralized organization are summarized in the box.

DECENTRALIZED STAFF DEVELOPMENT

Decentralized staff development is defined by Coye[4] as "an approach in which nursing leadership personnel in a designated clinical area are vested with the major responsibility to identify and seek ways to meet the learning needs of the nursing staff within the designated clinical area."

Examples of Decentralized Organization

The first consideration in organizing decentralized staff development is to identify the individuals or leadership personnel who will be responsible for over-

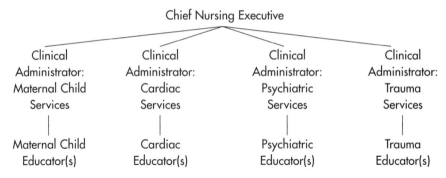

Fig. 6-4   Organization of decentralized staff development.

seeing educational activities in the designated clinical areas.[4] These individuals may be administrators or directors of various clinical services or individual unit managers.

If an individual service administrator has this responsibility, one or more decentralized educators could be assigned to educational activities within that service division. These educators may work independently to cover designated units or work as a team within the service as a whole. They typically report to the service administrator (Fig. 6-4).

If the department manager is responsible for ensuring educational activities for the unit staff, multiple organizational designs are possible. One method is to assign certain individuals to be responsible for particular aspects of staff development. For example, the associate head nurse might facilitate orientation activities and enlist staff nurses as preceptors. Other unit staff may be responsible for additional designated functions such as product-related in-service classes, patient care conferences, or continuing education. The unit staff member accountable for each area may be a volunteer or a more advanced practitioner in organizations with a clinical ladder.

Another method used to organize decentralized staff development at an individual unit level is to identify one staff member per unit as an educator. The ideal but seldom realized candidate should have clinical expertise, a master's degree, and theoretical knowledge of and practical experience in implementing adult education techniques. This person usually reports to the unit manager. As stated, however, the educational levels of the staff development educator and staff development manager should be considered in determining the reporting relationship.

Yet another method is to establish an individual unit education committee. Committee members representing all shifts determine the educational needs and methods and the people responsible for implementing particular educational efforts. Unit education committees can also be used in conjunction with the other decentralized structures presented.

Involvement of Decentralized Educators in Nursing Service Delivery

Determining the amount of involvement educators should have in delivering nursing care is a frequent dilemma for managers, staff nurses, and decentralized educators. The advantages of educators providing direct patient care include (1) maintaining educators' skills, (2) developing and preserving educators' credibility with the staff, (3) providing an opportunity to display role model behaviors, and (4) identifying staff educational needs firsthand.

Because of the limited staff available to perform a unit's patient care or budget constraints that require staff development educators to perform dual responsibilities, educators have sometimes been required to serve as direct patient caregivers. Often, a designated number of hours is set aside for that purpose. If an educator is requested to perform in a staff nurse capacity, that educator may not have enough time to perform necessary and assigned educational activities. Another dilemma occurs when educators are prescheduled to work as staff nurses and an unexpected educational need develops.

The key to successfully assigning educators who are required to work patient caregiving hours is a trusting, respectful relationship between educators and unit managers. Managers must give the educator options when prescheduling staffing hours. Educators cannot be expected to perform patient care duties only on weekends and hours other than during the day shift. On the other hand, educators should volunteer to do some patient caregiving hours during these less desirable times. If the educator is prescheduled to perform direct patient care and an unexpected educational need arises, the manager and educator must be flexible and able to communicate openly to mutually set priorities. Communication and priority setting should also occur if an educator is responsible for more than one patient care unit.

Many educators who want or are required to deliver nursing care do not preschedule staff hours. Rather, they assist on the unit in times of crisis, in times of unanticipated decreased staffing, during staff meals and breaks, during a preceptor's day off, or at times when an orientee is having difficulty. Another strategy is for the educator to assist staff in a particular aspect of patient care when two or more nurses are required.

Prescheduling staff hours or assisting only in times of need, taking a full patient assignment or assisting staff with their assignments, requiring a set amount of direct caregiving hours in educators' job descriptions, and having an informal nursing care requirement of educators are all possibilities. The system that works best depends on the needs and philosophies of the organization and the personalities of the personnel involved. However, a formal requirement for staff development educators to perform direct patient care often sets up an adversarial relationship between nursing service and education.

Proactive educators, who voluntarily and at their own discretion assist staff at times of true need, schedule themselves as staff during off hours, weekends, and holidays. They also participate in aspects of care that dictate their involvement in nursing service delivery without being required to do so. In such instances, nursing service and educators truly work together to ensure optimal patient care.

Advantages

The obvious advantages of decentralized staff development are that educational needs may be more readily acknowledged and appropriate programming is often more timely. Decentralization is becoming more necessary as individual unit or service staff needs become increasingly diverse and specialized.

Decentralized educators and the leaders responsible for overseeing the education process are usually more aware of their specific unit or service educational requirements than centralized educators. Working as a team, these individuals can set priority needs and decide on and implement educational programming. In a centralized system, prioritization of needs is typically accomplished among all units and services throughout the organization. Usually, needs that are shared by the majority of staff members or a need to meet a specific hospital goal takes priority over individual needs.

Timeliness is another advantage of a decentralized structure. Decentralized educators can often respond more promptly to a recognizable deficiency, and in some cases, they can respond immediately.

Another advantage is that decentralized educators and managers responsible for education are clinical experts in the associated area. This facilitates effective needs assessment and associated problem solving to identify educational strategies. This can also reduce the time spent by educators to gain the expertise needed to provide appropriate education.

Flexibility in providing education is yet another advantage. The decentralized educator can make presentations at times that best accommodate the staff. For example, one unit's staff may prefer in-service classes during their on-duty hours and at a particular time. Another staff may voluntarily choose to come in for presentations during off-duty time or may prefer programming at a different time. Different units and staffs often work varying shift lengths, and stagger their hours differently. Therefore a good time for programming for an 8-hour shift may not be ideal for the 12-hour shift or a unit with staggered hours. Clearly, decentralization can best accommodate these differences.

A final advantage of decentralized staff development involves evaluation. Trainor, Robinson, and Parlor[17] relate four levels of outcome criteria described by Dixon that can be used to evaluate nursing continuing education.[17] The higher third and fourth levels relate to changes in clinical performance and a positive impact on patient care outcomes, respectively. Decentralized educators are more able than centralized staff to evaluate these higher outcome levels. These advantages are summarized in the box.

Disadvantages

Duplication of Services. As decentralized educators focus on individual unit and service programming, it is "tragically easy for each to lose contact with the

---

ADVANTAGES OF A DECENTRALIZED STRUCTURE

Educational needs are more readily acknowledged.
Programming is implemented in a timely manner.
Educators and managers are clinical experts.
Ability to deliver education is more flexible.
Evaluating clinical outcomes of education is possible.

---

other."[8] This results in a needless duplication of services and efforts. Many educational sessions are provided for one or two staff nurses when the same material could be cost effectively presented to many staff nurses.

Inappropriate Use of Resources. Haggard[8] cites the inappropriate use of resources as another frustrating problem in a decentralized system. As educational personnel work independently on programming, multiple resources, which could have been shared, may be ordered or purchased by several individuals. These resources include audiovisual equipment, computer software, reference books, magazine subscriptions, literature searches, anatomic models, and technical demonstration equipment.

Inadequate Record Keeping. In a decentralized system, record keeping tends to be decentralized as well. This may make it difficult to gather and present data clearly and uniformly for review by regulatory agencies. In addition, the specific requirements related to record keeping for different regulatory agencies change constantly and are often quite extensive. Therefore decentralized educators may have difficulty remaining current in all requirements.

Limited Clerical, Audiovisual, and Reference Support. Decentralized systems usually do not have clerical support specifically for education. Educators share secretaries and support personnel with other nursing service peers. As a result, educators tend to perform many clerical functions themselves, thereby increasing their workload and decreasing efficiency. Also, audiovisual resources and other reference materials may be limited or nonexistent because decentralized systems usually do not have an education budget.

Difficulty Remaining Focused on Education. Educators in a decentralized system are frequently asked to perform duties outside of education. They often serve as committee chairpeople or become active members of unit or service committees. They tend to become involved in special projects such as patient and family support groups and reward and recognition programs. The tendency to help provide direct patient health care services is greater for decentralized educators. These demands make remaining focused on educational processes difficult for staff development educators.

Lack of Collegial Support. Decentralized educators may suffer from lack of collegial support. They have no one with whom to discuss problems related to education. This is especially difficult for new educators who benefit and learn from more experienced educators.

Limited Support for Education. Oftentimes managers to whom educators report have not had formal preparation in education. As a result, these managers may not value educational theory and practice, so staff development activities become secondary to other responsibilities. This causes limited support for educationally sound practices and education itself.

Strategies to Minimize Disadvantages

Regular Opportunity to Communicate Education Activities. Educators should meet monthly (every 3 months minimally) to communicate and mutually plan their activities. At this time, resources that need to be purchased should be discussed and mutually agreed on to prevent duplication and inappropriate use.

Methods should also be developed to communicate outside the planning meetings to share unanticipated programming. Strategies include using electronic mail bulletin boards or a designated communication book or bulletin board located in a central area. Educators should use these methods to announce planning of previously communicated education and completed literature searches.

Central Programming Schedule. A centralized schedule listing all educational programming is a necessity in a decentralized system. This schedule of listings can be generated via electronic mail, if available, or assigned to a clerical person to type and distribute a weekly or monthly calendar to all units. Educators should be responsible for submitting the required information. Another idea is to post a large wipe-off board in a central location so that educators can list programs occurring that day, week, or month.

Centralized Record Keeping. A process describing the minimal requirements for record keeping should be developed. Haggard[8] suggests that any program given within the agency should centrally file an outline, behavioral objectives, and an attendance record. This not only serves as evidence of what has been done but "promotes quality improvement by requiring well-planned classes of all educators."[8] At the least, evidence of education required by regulatory agencies must be retained and readily available in a consistent and organized format.

Clerical and Support Personnel. Clerical and support personnel must be assigned to help educators become most effective. These people are usually employed within the nursing service administration, but unit-based personnel should not be overlooked. For example, unit secretaries or clerks, especially during evening and night shifts, may perform educational clerical tasks. Even nursing assistants or unit volunteers may help with various projects such as copying and collating handouts or making posters.

Collegial Support for Educators. Methods to enhance collegial support among staff development educators are especially important in a decentralized system. The planning meetings mentioned earlier are one way to enhance personnel relationship.

Another strategy is to have a formal performance improvement standard requiring all educators to be critiqued by peer educators during "dry runs" of any new formal programs. Critiques should be done at least once a year for each educator while teaching a session. A standardized check list can be developed and used for this evaluation. This serves to enhance networking, develop educators' presentation skills, and promote high-quality programming.

Another strategy is to centralize office space. Although it is unlikely that all decentralized educators can have offices together, those in the same or related service areas could share an office or have offices close to one another.

Educators themselves must seek and take the initiative to network with their colleagues. Taking breaks and eating meals together, consulting more experienced people, or acting as mentors for new staff members are all keys to survival. Educators who receive staff development journals can share these by copying and posting the indexes in a central location. If any article is of particular interest, copies may be requested.

OTHER ORGANIZATIONAL STRUCTURES

As the health care delivery system undergoes significant changes, the more traditional methods used to organize staff development activities may not be the most advantageous. Administrators and staff development personnel must creatively design a staff development organizational structure to meet the organization's unique needs and achieve the desired outcomes.

Combining Centralized and Decentralized Structures

Combining centralized and decentralized structures maximizes the advantages and minimizes the disadvantages of both. Combinations may be achieved in a number of ways. One method is to assign centralized and decentralized functions within a designated staff development department. For example, one or more staff members can be assigned general centralized functions related to orientation, continuing education, and in-service education; other department staff members may be responsible for the decentralized activities related to these same areas. Centralized staff can plan and conduct orientation activities that are the same for all nursing staff. Decentralized personnel can implement the more specific unit-based aspects of orientation. If a preceptor model method is used, the decentralized educator facilitates the preceptor's work.

For continuing education, centralized personnel perform tasks such as scheduling rooms, registrations, faculty confirmations and evaluations, contact hour applications, and evaluation summaries. Decentralized staff serve as faculty for programs related to their areas of expertise.

In-service classes are implemented by both centralized and decentralized personnel. Hospital-wide in-service classes are coordinated and conducted by centralized educators, whereas unit-specific in-service classes are implemented by the appropriate decentralized staff.

Clearly, this type of structure may require many dedicated staff development educators, particularly in large organizations. An alternative is to use centralized staff development educators in conjunction with staff nurses who have been groomed as educators in their own units. Haggard describes a structure that uses three staff nurses per unit (that is, one for each shift) as the decentralized educators. These nurses are responsible for providing "the follow-up for orientees, in-service classes for new equipment and forms on the unit, update the staff on new developments in their area of practice, and conduct patient care conferences and unit classes."[8] The centralized staff development educators conduct the classroom portion of the orientation.

One model that successfully combines centralized and decentralized structures is in place at the National Institutes of Health Clinical Center Nursing Department. The Division of Professional Development, which is made up of a director and four centralized educators, meets generalized learning needs and provides universal nursing department orientation. Decentralized educators are responsible for addressing specialized learning needs and coordinating specialty orientation for their designated clinical areas. These educators report directly to the nursing administrator of their respective clinical areas and do not have a formal line relationship with the centralized nursing educator or their administrator.[5]

Spalt and Moellering[15] describe a structure called the *staff development educator/facilitator concept*. Head nurses select professional nurses from each patient care unit to be responsible for staff development. Instructors from the centralized department of education act as facilitators, or "coaches," to the designated staff nurses in all aspects of unit-based teaching activities.

McElroy[12] offers another example that pairs a centralized staff development department with decentralized unit-based nurses for staff nurse orientation. The staff development division conducts a 2-week centralized orientation for new nursing staff. Assistant head nurses within one nursing division then implement a decentralized unit-based orientation plan. One staff development educator serves as a liaison or coordinator to help the assistant head nurses with such things as obtaining and organizing course materials, designing appropriate teaching strategies, and evaluating their performance as teachers.

All examples of combining centralized and decentralized structures offer the following advantages:
- Identification of individual unit needs
- Timely responsiveness to individual unit needs
- Use of clinical experts to implement unit-based programming

- Flexibility in delivering unit-based education
- Availability of clerical and support services within the centralized department
- Coordination by the centralized department to reduce duplication of services and inappropriate use of resources and to ensure accurate and necessary record keeping
- Support for education by having an administrator or director of staff development
- Collegial support within the centralized staff development department and support for decentralized educators through a liaison relationship

Matrix Structure

Another method that may facilitate staff development effectiveness is to organize activities through a matrix structure. Anders[1] asserts that "the matrix organization is not a replacement for the traditional pyramidal organizational structure. It simply allows the existing organizational structure to be more flexible in accomplishing specific goals which call for a unique blend of specialists." Matrix organizations are characterized by a team of "diverse specialists working on a specific task," each with equal power and responsibilities.[1]

Mintzberg[13] points out that matrices can be either permanent or shifting. The shifting form is geared to project work and could last from several hours to several years.[1] A dual authority structure is inherent in a matrix organization. As a result, "matrix structure sacrifices the principles of unity of command."[13] Personnel report to different supervisors depending on the assignment or task. Matrix structure appears to be most useful to develop new activities and to coordinate complex, multiple interdependencies.[13]

Many examples for using the matrix system to structure and organize staff development activities are available. Staff development personnel are often appointed to chair or be members of committees or task forces. These work groups benefit from the expertise and responsibilities of each member and the direction provided by the designated manager. As a committee or task force chairperson or project manager, the staff development educator has the "authority and accountability to solve specific problems. This provides the sanction to move horizontally across the organization to obtain personnel and other support necessary to accomplish the mission, thus bringing interdepartmental resources to bear on a problem."[1]

When staff development educators have both centralized and decentralized functions, a frequently expressed frustration of the staff development director and clinical directors is a lack of control or knowledge. For example, a centralized staff development educator reporting to a staff development director may have centralized responsibilities and may also be assigned to provide educational needs within a particular specialty division. The staff development director can guide the educator in centralized responsibilities but may be unaware of the specialty division's specific education needs. In this case a matrix reporting structure may be the most viable organizational structure. However, authority-responsibility relationships must be defined for the educator and *both* directors. This structure will only succeed in organizations in which open communication and trusting, collegial relationships exist among service and education staff members.

Relationships with Schools of Nursing

Relationships involving organizations and local schools of nursing offer many unique and creative opportunities for staff development. Shared or joint appointments for organizations and affiliated schools of nursing are successful in university and non–university-affiliated hospitals. In a joint appointment, faculty from a local or affiliated college or university and hospital personnel have responsibilities at the academic organization and the health care agency. For example, the Lehigh Valley Hospital and the Allentown College of St. Francis de Sales have two joint appointees. Both are employed as 60% of a full-time equivalent at the hospital and 40% at the college. Their salaries and benefits are proportionally contributed by the college and hospital.

One appointee teaches in the undergraduate nursing program and is responsible for developing and maintaining the computer-assisted instruction program at the hospital. The other also teaches in the undergraduate nursing program and is a diabetes patient education specialist at the hospital.

A clinical educator role implemented at Georgetown University offers another example of a joint appointment. Nurses in this role assume dual responsibilities for nursing staff development and clinical supervision of undergraduate nursing students. The clinical educators have joint appointments in the Department of Nursing and the School of Nursing.[10]

In a shared appointment a college or university faculty member shares the same position with a hospital staff member. An exchange of hours is negotiated between the two individuals. In one instance a hospital nursing staff development educator had the opportunity to share an appointment with a sophomore-level faculty member at a local college. An exchange of roles occurred for 12 hours a week during a designated semester. The staff development educator supervised students in a 6-hour clinical experience and participated in didactic presentations for the remaining 6 hours. The college faculty member assumed designated staff development functions for the staff development educator. An obvious advantage of having joint or shared appointments is the establishment of collegial working relationships between the college or university and the organization. Many other advantages exist, including the following:

- Academic faculty and nursing students become aware of the trends and realities in hospital nursing practice through exposure to expert clinicians.
- Theory-based practice is reinforced within the hospital setting by academic personnel.
- Educational resources are communicated and shared, preventing duplication and creating cost effectiveness. Shared resources may include self-

learning packets, audiovisual materials, and even a computer or learning laboratory.

■ Personnel salaries may be reduced and recruitment aided. For example, a hospital may not be able to afford to employ a full-time nurse researcher or recruit such a person for a part-time position. The shared or joint appointment solves this dilemma. In another instance, the organization may need an additional staff development educator only during the summer for assistance with orientation and vacation coverage. Again, recruitment may be difficult, but a joint appointment in which the staff member spends the academic year at the college or university and the summer in the hospital could prove successful.

Curran[6] offers another example of the way colleges and organizations can collaborate staff development activities. She specifically describes the way that the continuing education department of a college of nursing and the staff development department of a hospital can work together to provide continuing education for professional nurses. Curran[6] believes that "without coordination, efforts are duplicated and resources wasted, and educational gaps occur." She recommends that a joint committee, with equal representation, equal respect, and equal workloads be formed from the hospital and college to plan, implement, and evaluate continuing education programs.

Consortium among Hospitals

Cooperation to provide staff development activities can be carried out among not only colleges and hospitals but also two or more hospitals. Cooperative ventures can be related to almost any aspect of staff development activities, including orientation, in-service, and continuing education.

For example, several hospitals in mideastern Pennsylvania formed a consortium to implement competency-based education in each organization. Costs were shared to hire an outside consultant to develop resources. After the initial implementation, consortium members continued to meet to network and address associated issues and concerns. As a result, development expenses were cost effective, and networking and mutual problem solving occurred.

The Houston Area Collaborative Critical Care Program illustrates another model for a consortium among hospitals. This alliance of 10 competing hospitals and a local school of nursing has resulted in a successful critical care program comprised of 15 modules. Support services contributed by each participating organization provide the required foundation for operation of the venture. No exchange of money takes place; only services necessary for program functions are offered. Beyond providing high-quality critical care education, this venture has promoted a professional network for educators and participants, increased educator effectiveness because of less duplication of lectures or programs, opportunities for expert peer consultation, and the exchange of clinical experiences and knowledge by participants.[2]

SUMMARY

Many factors influence the organization of staff development activities and the outcomes of specific organizational structures. Whether a hospital-wide, centralized, decentralized, or matrix organizational structure is chosen, many activities can be adapted to ensure the greatest benefits for educational endeavors. As health care delivery changes, successful staff development organizations will be flexible enough to quickly recognize and respond to educational requirements prompted by system changes and associated learning needs, performance improvement studies, professional review organizations, and changing regulatory agency requirements.

Jernigan and del Bueno offer interesting perspectives on the organizational structure that they believe leads to staff development effectiveness. Jernigan[9] states that "effective staff development depends on the proper climate and conditions, not upon specific organizational structure." del Bueno[7] concludes that "in the final analysis it is usually the individuals involved who make a system work regardless of the formal structure portrayed on paper."

REFERENCES

1. Anders RL: Matrix organization: an alternative for clinical specialists, *J Nurs Adm* 5(5):11, 1975.
2. Aulbach RK, et al: Collaborative critical care education: the educator link, *J Nurs Staff Dev* 9(2):63, 1993.
3. Boyer VM: The clinical nurse specialist: an underdeveloped staff development resource, *J Nurs Staff Dev* 2(1):23, 1986.
4. Coye D: Organizational structures: considerations which facilitate effectiveness, *J Contin Educ Nurs* 8(3):42, 1977.
5. Cummings C, McCaskey R: A model combining centralized and decentralized staff development, *J Nurs Staff Dev* 8(1):22, 1992.
6. Curran C: Collaboration not competition: a model for nursing continuing education, *J Nurs Educ* 20(6):24, 1981.
7. del Bueno DJ: Nursing staff development: critical times, critical issues, *J Nurs Staff Dev* 2(3):94, 1986.
8. Haggard A: Decentralized staff development, *J Contin Educ Nurs* 15(3):90, 1984.
9. Jernigan DK: *Human resource management in nursing*, Norwalk, Conn, 1988, Appleton & Lange.
10. Lachat MF, Zerbe MB, Scott CA: A new clinical educator role: bridging the education-practice gap, *J Nurs Staff Dev* 8(2):55, 1992.
11. Kerfoot K, Green S: Redesign vs. "fix-it-up": the case for reengineering, *Capsules Comments Nurs Leadership Manage* 1(4):1, 1993.
12. McElroy MJ: Decentralized orientation: a model for professional practice, *J Nurs Staff Dev* 5(2):84, 1989.
13. Mintzberg H: *The structuring of organizations*, Englewood Cliffs, NJ, 1979, Prentice-Hall.
14. Senge P: *The fifth discipline*, New York, 1990, Doubleday.
15. Spalt SM, Moellering JA: The education connection: a staff development concept, *J Nurs Staff Dev* 5(3):116, 1989.
16. Tobin HM, Beeler JL: Roles and relationships of staff development educators: a critical component of impact, *J Nurs Staff Dev* 4(3):91, 1988.
17. Trainor S, Robinson EM, Parlon D: Utilization of a staff development department to promote the philosophy and goals of nursing management, *J Nurs Staff Dev* 5(2):97, 1989.
18. Wolf GA: Clinical nurse specialists: the second generation, *J Nurs Adm* 20(5):7, 1990.

LORI RODRIGUEZ ◆ ROBERTA S. ABRUZZESE

Enhancing Human Resources for Staff Development

Staff development departments focus on assessing and developing the abilities of nursing service employees. This is an important focus because the abilities of employees directly affect the quality of patient care provided. Ultimately, the quality of patient care depends on the quality of the educational programs designed to maintain and increase employee competency. Too little attention, however, is focused on developing the capabilities of educators in staff development, even though their abilities directly affect the quality and quantity of the teaching and learning activities structured for employees. It is wise to permit only well-qualified educators to hold positions in staff development.

An examination of the major functions of staff educators, standards for staff development departments, and position descriptions leads to an understanding of the necessary qualifications for staff development educators. The assumption is that no one possesses all the necessary qualifications of this position.

Miller suggests that the minimum requirements for a staff development educator may include the following[15]:

- A desire to instruct
- The knowledge of what to instruct
- The knowledge of the way to instruct
- An understanding of the way people learn
- The "right" personality
- The ability to communicate
- Flexibility

After a candidate satisfactorily demonstrates all competencies of the position, other items also influence the candidate's success or failure. For example, the right personality and flexibility are requisites or indicators of qualified candidates. Characteristics of people who have the right personality for this job involve caring about others; being sensitive to the feelings and family problems that may influence a person's work performance; and understanding people's foibles. Another personality trait needed by staff development educators is flexibility. Educators should expect things to go wrong and be mentally prepared for alternatives. David Hartl, an adult educator, said Murphy was an optimist when he stated, "If anything can go wrong, it will go wrong at the worst possible moment." Hartl amended Murphy's statement by saying "Something will always go wrong; be ready to fix it."

According to Miller,[15] staff development educators should be skilled questioners, listeners, counselors, and reinforcers. As questioners, educators must question routine ways of teaching, learner interactions, outcome evaluations, and more effective ways to achieve the same outcome. As listeners, educators need to really hear what learners are saying and then respond respectfully. As counselors, educators should guide individuals regarding present dilemmas and future career development. As reinforcers, educators periodically work in the clinical areas to reinforce learning and provide explanations for difficult situations.

Jacobs and Jones[10] suggest that a willingness to share is another valuable attribute for educators. This characteristic is important because learners need to hear about personal solutions to problems—successes and failures. If educators only share their success stories, learners may be unable to share their own problems and uncertainties.

When a new educator is hired, the ideal is to assess their qualifications and deficiencies and then hire the person with the most potential to learn and grow. A tip for all educators is to construct a self-development plan to assist them as they acquire or enhance needed competencies. Performing this assessment requires an analysis of the functions and standards of staff development educators.

FUNCTIONS

The functions of staff development educators arise from the philosophies, goals, objectives, and mission statements of the nursing service department and the organization. These functions reflect national standards for staff development departments and the specific needs of nursing service departments. The organizational structure of each staff development department influences these functions as well, causing centralized and decentralized departments to differ.

The American Nurses Association (ANA), the American Society for Healthcare Education and Training (ASHET),[5] and the American Society of Training and Development (ASTD) are all especially interested in the functions of staff development educators. Each organization has analyzed the activities of staff development educators and grouped these activities into function categories. In 1966 the nursing service administrators section of the ANA[4] proposed 15 functions for staff development educators (box). The major roles of staff development educators were reiterated in 1978 as "those of facilitator, teacher, and resource person. Expectations of this role include the responsibility of assessing needs, planning, organizing, implementing, and evaluating the staff development pro-

FUNCTIONS FOR IN-SERVICE EDUCATORS

The responsibilities of the in-service educator are to plan, organize, direct, coordinate, and evaluate the in-service program of the nursing department.

1. Provides leadership in formulating the philosophy and objectives of the in-service education program in accordance with the philosophy and objectives of the nursing service department.
2. Determines the educational needs of the employees necessary to accomplish the objectives of the nursing service through collaboration with line and staff personnel.
3. Plans and implements the program of instruction designed to meet the nursing service needs.
4. Communicates the plan for the program in such a way as to encourage and foster participation, involvement, and cooperation.
5. Participates in counseling and guidance of personnel in relation to their educational needs.
6. Recommends a budget to meet the objectives of the in-service education program.
7. Plans and organizes the resources and facilities needed to accomplish the objectives of the program.
8. Contributes in the development of philosophy, objectives, policies, procedures, and job descriptions for the nursing service department.
9. Develops, maintains, and utilizes records and reports pertinent to the in-service program.
10. Supervises the in-service staff and teaches in the program.
11. Evaluates study and research findings for application to in-service education programs.
12. Initiates and/or participates in studies and research activities related to in-service education.
13. Participates in activities which further his/her professional growth and development.
14. Prepares an annual report of the in-service program, including evaluation and recommendations for future programming.
15. Participates in and promotes membership, interest, and participation in the activities of the professional nursing association, in allied health organizations, and in supportive community activities.

Courtesy American Nurses Association, Kansas City, Mo, 1966.

gram."[1] These responsibilities were further described as the following[1]:

- Collaborating with nursing service personnel to provide educational activities
- Stating philosophy and goals of staff development congruent with those of nursing service
- Implementing a cost-effective budget
- Identifying learning needs
- Planning learning activities to achieve desired outcomes
- Communicating the plan for learning activities to foster participation
- Implementing the plan to meet learning needs
- Evaluating educational outcomes
- Counseling nursing service personnel about their learning needs

- Initiating and participating in research activities
- Implementing record-keeping systems
- Engaging in activities to promote personal professional growth and development

Current functions and responsibilities were first developed by the ANA in 1990. These provided criteria for 11 standards related to organization and administration, human resources, learners, program planning, educational design, material resources and facilities, records and reports, evaluation, consultation, climate setting, and systematic inquiry.[2] In 1994 these standards were modified further by the combining of continuing education and staff development standards. The 11 standards were grouped into 6 professional standards related to administration, human resources, material resources and facilities, educational design, records and reports, and professional practice.[3] A comparison of these standards to the standards and functions described by ASHET and ASTD shows similarities and differences. This is expected because educator activities are similar even if target learners and settings are different.

ASHET focuses on hospital-wide education and training personnel, whereas ASTD is concerned with trainers in business and industry. In 1990, ASHET published standards in the areas of philosophy and mission, organization and structure, functions, facilities and equipment, financial management, policy and procedure, productivity measurement, clinical affiliations and contracts, record keeping, professional development, research, quality improvement, and the educational process. Three standards fall under the heading "functions." These standards describe the responsibilities of adult educators in education services departments in various settings, with different audiences, and with activities in human resource development, internal consultation, and change agents.[6]

Many staff development functions and responsibilities identified by the ANA and ASHET have previously been delineated by ASTD in their 1983 competency study.[7] In the 1983 study, key functions were listed under the following headings:

- Evaluator
- Group facilitator
- Individual development counselor
- Instructional writer
- Instructor
- Manager of training and development
- Marketer
- Media specialist
- Needs analyst
- Program administrator
- Program designer
- Strategist
- Task analyst
- Theoretician
- Transfer agent

This extensive study by the ASTD was intended to answer questions about the competencies required to practice in human resource development currently and in the future. The ASTD estimated that the human resource development field (called *staff development* in nursing) would cost approximately $100 billion annually by 1990. This expense continues to give human resource and staff development departments additional motivation for striving to enhance the competencies of their educators.

POSITION DESCRIPTIONS

Each organization with a staff development department has its own position descriptions for staff development educators. Each position description, however, contains the title, general description, functions, and qualifications of the position. These elements reflect the philosophy, goals, and organization of that department. For example, one organization may describe the position as a competent clinical nurse who performs educational activities, whereas another organization may describe the position as a competent adult educator who occasionally teaches in clinical areas. These divergent views of staff development educators indicate a need to write position descriptions only after thorough analysis of the position expectations.[11] First, the title to best define the position, the tasks and decision making involved, and the requirements necessary to implement the tasks and decisions must be determined.

Before writing the position description, the terms *competencies, functions, tasks, skills,* and *knowledge* must be clarified. Competency, as defined by Benner,[8] means a defined area of skilled performance, identified and described by its intent, function, and meanings. Functions refer to a person's characteristic activities. Skill means a person's present, observable competence. Knowledge refers to a body of learned information.[9]

One of the first steps in writing position descriptions is to specify the specific functions of the position. These functions must be congruent with the mission and objectives of the nursing service department and the organization. One way to accurately specify the position functions is to ask the person who previously held the position or someone who holds a similar position to list the functions. Another way is to ask consumers who interact with the person holding that position the major activities they see in that position. For example, for the position of emergency department educator, the nursing staff in that department could be asked to describe the activities carried out by an educator in that position. Careful attention should be focused on the priorities and importance of various activities so someone new to the position would have an accurate understanding of the expectations. The activities described can then be grouped into major categories or functions. The box shows an example.

Congruence with Missions and Objectives

After generating a long list of possible functions for staff development educators, the functions that are congruent with the organization's mission and objectives should be determined. These functions must be chosen for their ability to support the goals and further the objectives of the organization. As new responsibilities are added to the position, such as quality improvement or marketing, the position's functions also change. Some factors that influence the responsibilities of the staff development department include the following:

- Overall future needs of the organization
- Incremental needs of each department
- Current resources for the nursing department
- Turnover trends
- Allocation of current and future resources
- Strategic plans of the organization

FUNCTIONS OF STAFF DEVELOPMENT EDUCATORS

Instructional design
Assessment and planning activities
Teaching in-service classes and workshops
Orientation
Evaluation of activities or the impact of an activity
coordinating workshops
Educational problem solving

Clinical support
Bedside clinical consultation
Skill training
Product review
Troubleshooting equipment problems

Administration
Meetings
Communications such as memos and fliers
Writing policies
Community liaison: student placement

Instructional materials preparation
Producing self-study learning modules and packages
Serving as a resource to the staff for obtaining educational materials

Consultation
Coaching and assisting staff in handling specific performance problems

Professional development
Participating in continuous self-development by reading professional journals, attending workshops and seminars, and setting goals for growth.

Courtesy El Camino Hospital, Mountain View, Calif.

Examples of Position Descriptions

A position description provides a general description of a position's responsibilities and areas of accountability. The position description usually outlines the levels of authority; the immediate supervisor; other reporting relationships; supervisory responsibilities; working conditions; and required knowledge, skills, and abilities (box). The description does not state the factors that may be necessary for success or failure. These descriptions tend to be general

---

EXAMPLES OF POSITION DESCRIPTIONS

Example 1: medical, surgical, orthopedic educator
El Camino Hospital, Mountain View, California
Position summary:
Provides high-quality education programs and activities that promote individual development of medical, surgical, orthopedic (MSO) staff nurses according to learning needs identified jointly by department directors, staff development educators, and unit staff nurses to facilitate patient care at El Camino Hospital.
Responsibilities:
1. Uses a variety of sources to identify learning needs of staff of five MSO units and plans either formal or informal learning activities in response.
2. Plans and conducts preceptor training program and ongoing preceptor training and support on MSO units.
3. Presents and coordinates educational activities on MSO units.
4. Assists directors, assistant head nurses, and staff nurses with complex clinical situations and acts an an internal consultant to MSO staff, staff development instructors, and coordinators.
5. Develops and evaluates learning materials for preceptors, in support of Medical Information Systems (MIS) training, clinical practice committee, and learning materials to be placed in the learning center.
6. Maintains liaison between El Camino Hospital and community learning sources.
7. Enhances self development on a continual basis by participating in Management and Organizational Development (MOD), setting goals and objectives, reading professional literature, providing direct patient care, preparing manuscripts for journal publications, and attending conferences.
8. Coordinates and develops procedures and protocols for nursing service resource manuals for clinical units.
Education:
Masters degree in nursing or education
Previous experience:
Minimum of 2 years in direct patient care roles
Judgment, planning, initiative required:
High degree of initiative, planning, and judgment required to prepare, implement, and evaluate educational experiences
Skills required:
One-to-one and small group communication, use of adult learning principles, program planning, and experience with coaching and validation

Courtesy El Camino Hospital, Mountain View, Calif.   *Continued.*

---

statements of the position's role within an organization. Educational and experiential requirements for a position should be listed, and a general role description should be given. The person writing the position statement needs to use the most appropriate and self-explanatory statements to describe the role.

EXAMPLES OF POSITION DESCRIPTIONS—cont'd

Example 2: critical care instructor, evening/night shifts
El Camino Hospital, Mountain View, California
Position summary:
Evening and night staff development instructors are responsible for assessing the learning needs of the critical care units on the 3 PM to 11 PM or 11 PM to 7 AM shifts and for providing education opportunities that will meet those needs. These instructors act as an education resource for all evening or night staff, including assistant head nurses and nursing coordinators.
Responsibilities:
1. Supports the philosophy of education at El Camino Hospital to promote individual responsibility for self-directed growth and development.
2. Works closely with other critical care instructors to provide follow through and continuity of educational programs on a 24-hour basis.
3. Uses a variety of sources to identify learning needs of staff on the critical care units, and plans either formal or informal learning activities in response to these needs.
4. Helps nurses problem solve complex clinical situations.
5. Participates in patient care as vehicle for coaching staff.
6. Educational resource for staff regarding continuing education opportunities in the community as well as in hospital activities.
7. Coaches and supports preceptors in orientation of new employees.
8. Acts as a resource for new graduate RNs and for new employees.
9. Responds to all emergency or "stat" pages to give staff support and guidance as appropriate.
10. Provides support to nursing coordinators and leadership in emergency situations, such as fire, disaster, CPR, etc.
11. Assists in the updating of learning center materials for critical care.
12. Involved in special projects as designated by the director of nursing staff development.
13. Participates in continued self-development by reading professional journals, attending workshops and seminars, and setting goals for continued growth.
Requirements:
Bachelor of science in nursing
Three years of critical care clinical experience
Evidence of continuing education
Desirable:
Knowledge of adult learning principles
Evidence of good communication skills and ability to work well one-to-one or in groups.

INTERVIEWING AND HIRING

Interviewing is a skill that most people need to improve. Inexperienced interviewers tend to do most of the talking, whereas the person being interviewed should ideally talk about 70% of the time. The formulation of interview questions that elicit long answers from the applicant can achieve this. Some interviewing guidelines can make the process more efficient for the interviewer and applicant. For example, the interviewer should thoroughly review the application, and note previous positions and indications of teaching ability. Often, the cover letter provides clues about the reasons that the person wants to be involved in staff development.

Interview questions should clearly relate to the job and must meet equal employment guidelines. For example, questions related to marital status, spouse's work, number of children, age, religion, and ethnic background are not permitted. The purpose of the interview is to establish a relationship with the applicant and determine if there is a fit between the "corporate culture" of the staff development department and the applicant. Questions should be clear and unambiguous; they should proceed from simple to complex. All questions should relate to the functions of educators. For example, questions should be worded to elicit information about lesson plans, preferred teaching techniques, use of audiovisual equipment, familiarity with adult education principles, and expertise in areas of clinical interest. Other questions should relate to previous positions held, such as the following:

- Why did you leave your most recent position?
- What did you like best about your most recent position?
- What did you like least about your previous position?
- What is one project that you were especially proud of?

More complex questions that reveal the applicant's attitudes and abilities are as follows:

- What are your career goals in relation to the educator role?
- How does this position match your goals?
- Describe one accomplishment in the last 6 months that you are most proud of.
- What teaching and learning experiences have you most enjoyed?
- What was a difficult problem that you have recently faced and solved?
- What was an instance in which you persuaded others to take actions you wanted?
- What is the toughest decision you have had to make recently? What options did you need to consider?
- What has been your biggest disappointment in the work setting? How did you handle it?
- Describe an instance when you had to make plans for yourself and others to achieve a goal. How did you set priorities?
- Describe an instance in which you worked well with others to achieve a goal.

Although the final decision to hire someone as a new educator belongs to the director of the staff development department, other people are also important in the hiring process. Other instructors, managers of the units on which the person will provide educational services, and a select group of staff nurses from those units can be involved in the interviewing process. The hope is that the interview process provides an accurate assessment of the candidate's congruence with the staff development department's values and goals. The ideal outcome is to find a person whose goals, teaching style, communication abilities, and educational philosophy match those of the department.

DETERMINING COMPETENCIES OF EDUCATORS

Nurses who are new to staff development usually come from one of two backgrounds—clinical nursing or education. Their educational preparation also may vary from a graduate degree in a clinical specialty or nursing service administration to a graduate degree in education. Some graduate degrees in education relate to undergraduate education, whereas others relate to adult education. The educational preparation and experiential background of each new educator has implications for the staff development functions and activities. Each new educator will be competent in some areas and require enhanced skills in other areas. The abilities of educators may be as varied as their educational and experiential background and may indicate the need for greater facility in clinical practice skills or in learning facilitation skills.

New staff development educators should be involved in identifying gaps in their own knowledge and skills as required by the position. Knowles,[12] the Ontario Society for Training and Development,[16] and ASHET[6] suggest that a rating scale be used to identify the functions and activities of staff development educators (Fig. 7-1).

After identifying the function requiring more proficiency, Knowles suggests that the activities of that function be identified. For example, if consultation is the function needing improvement, the elements of consultation could be specified as the following abilities[12]:

- Establish rapport
- Present oneself authentically
- Help others define problems
- Help identify and collect needed data for problem solving
- Help specify and test options
- Help others devise strategies for implementing options
- Help others evaluate results
- Maintain objective relationships
- Terminate consultant relationship constructively

After specifying the abilities needed for effective consultation, a plan can be constructed to attain an improved level of proficiency. The plan should state objectives for learning; resources used to develop knowledge, skills, and attitudes; and strategies for attainment.[12] The time for completion and the criteria for judging improvement in the area of proficiency should also be included. This

Competency Area									Proficiency Rating Scale	
	Beginning								Proficient	
1. Instructional design	1	2	3	4	5	6	7	8	9	10
2. Clinical support	1	2	3	4	5	6	7	8	9	10
3. Administrative activities	1	2	3	4	5	6	7	8	9	10
4. Instructional materials	1	2	3	4	5	6	7	8	9	10
5. Consultation	1	2	3	4	5	6	7	8	9	10
6. Professional development	1	2	3	4	5	6	7	8	9	10

Now draw a line to connect each of the numbers you selected.
What is your most proficient area? Which is your least proficient area?
Develop a plan to enhance your competency.

Fig. 7-1   Competency self-rating scale for staff development educators. (Modified from Knowles M: *Self-directed learning: a guide for learners and teachers,* Chicago, 1975, Follett Press.)

plan should be discussed with the director of the staff development department and perhaps with a colleague who can act as a mentor.

ORIENTATION OF NEW STAFF DEVELOPMENT EDUCATORS

In addition to identifying and planning strategies for increasing competency, new staff development educators should receive a general orientation to the organization and department. New educators should be introduced to the entire staff development program through experiences with other educators and reading the department's annual reports. They should become familiar with the functions required for their position through hands-on experiences, simulated situations, and practice teaching with a mentor. New educators need an opportunity to design a teaching and learning activity, evaluate outcomes, and use audiovisual equipment. Special attention may be needed to make audiovisual teaching aids, use the computer, and locate learning resources. Review of departmental fiscal constraints on previewing new books, films, or videotapes and opportunities for personal growth is important. Becoming familiar with the staff development monthly and annual cycle of learning activities, meeting key people in the organization, and becoming oriented to secretarial services are all important for new educators. Evaluating the speaking abilities of new educators and helping them increase their skills can be accomplished by videotaping a mini-teaching session. Resources should be available to review teaching strategies such as questioning techniques, use of humor, self-study modules, games and role playing, and construction of simulations. Just as most staff development departments are always changing and updating their orientation program for new nursing service employees, so should the orientation for new educators continuously be updated and improved.

It is helpful to negotiate the orientation schedule with the new educator to adapt it for experienced and inexperienced learners. This is time-efficient and therefore cost-effective. Many new educators can plan their own objectives, resources for learning, and time frame for completion. This is more satisfactory for the new educator because it allows progress at the learner's own pace and remains in keeping with the learner's negotiated outcomes.[13]

EVALUATION

The primary evaluation of staff development educators should be done with a review of their self-designed plans to increase areas of competency. Their progress should be compared with their stated objectives and the criteria for judging attainment of those objectives. The strengths and weaknesses of educators should be discussed in terms of performance standards, productivity standards, and values of the department and organization. The evaluation should include evaluations of the programs for which they are responsible in terms of cost-benefit and cost-effectiveness so determinations can be made about the value of the time and money spent in proportion to the positive outcomes achieved.

In addition to self-evaluation and evaluation by the director, educators are often critiqued by the learner and peer evaluation of their classroom and clinical teaching effectiveness. Some questions that might be used in educator evaluations are provided in the box.

EXAMPLES OF EDUCATOR EVALUATION QUESTIONS

1. Was the time adequate for covering the content?
2. Did the content have relevance for the group?
3. Was the teaching pace too fast, too slow, or adequate?
4. Were the methods of presentation appropriate?
5. Were the audiovisual materials appropriate and interesting?
6. Did the handouts aid in learning?
7. Was group discussion included in the learning activity?
8. How were the participants motivated to learn?
9. Was there adequate time for questions and answers?
10. Were questions handled in a respectful manner?
11. Did the instructor demonstrate an in-depth grasp of the contents?
12. Were the educator's voice, gestures, and manner effective?
13. Were the classroom facilities conducive to learning?
14. Was feedback used to determine if class objectives were met?

Modified from Magner M: *Inservice education manual for the nursing department,* St Louis, 1980, The Catholic Health Association.[14]

Instructional materials used in learning may also be evaluated as a measure of teaching effectiveness. Some staff development departments evaluate learner outcomes as a measure of teaching effectiveness. Such departments believe educators have not successfully taught unless learners have integrated the learning into clinical practice. The goal of all evaluations should be to increase the professional growth and proficiency of staff development educators.

SUMMARY

The functions, standards, and qualifications of staff development educators have been matters of concern for the ANA, ASHET, and ASTD for many years. These concerns have resulted in statements of functions and standards for the practice of staff development in nursing service, hospital-wide education departments, and business and industry. These statements have formed the basis for position descriptions, interviewing, hiring, orientation, and evaluation of educators. The delineation of standards, functions and roles, and activities currently sets the stage for an emphasis on the results and outcomes of staff development departments.

REFERENCES

1. American Nurses Association: *Guidelines for staff development*, Kansas City, Mo, 1978, The Association.
2. American Nurses Association: *Standards for nursing professional development: continuing education and staff development*, Washington, DC, 1994, The Association.
3. American Nurses Association: *Standards for nursing staff development*, Kansas City, Mo, 1990, The Association.
4. American Nurses Association: *Statement of functions and qualifications for inservice educators*, Kansas City, Mo, 1966, The Association.
5. American Society for Healthcare Education and Training: *Pursuing mastery: professional development tools and techniques*, Chicago, 1990, American Hospital Association.
6. American Society for Healthcare Education and Training: *Standards for health care education and training*, Chicago, 1990, American Hospital Association.
7. American Society for Training and Development: *Models for excellence: the conclusions and recommendations of the ASTD training and development competency study*, Washington, DC, 1983, The Society.
8. Benner P: *From novice to expert: excellence and power in clinical nursing practice*, Menlo Park, Calif, 1984, Addison-Wesley.
9. Gales KL: The recruitment process. In Lewis EM, Spicer JG, editors: *Human resource management handbook*, Rockville, Md, 1987, Aspen.
10. Jacobs RL, Jones MJ: *Structured on-the-job training*, San Francisco, 1994, Berrett-Koehler.
11. Knowles M: *The adult learner: a neglected species*, ed 2, Houston, 1978, Gulf Publishing.
12. Knowles M: *Self-directed learning: a guide for learners and teachers*, Chicago, 1975, Follett Press.
13. Kotecki CN, Eddy JR: Developing an orientation program for a nurse educator, *J Nurs Staff Dev* 10(6):301, 1994.
14. Magner M: *Inservice education manual for the nursing department*, St Louis, 1980, The Catholic Health Association.
15. Miller VA: Selecting, developing, and evaluating trainers. In Miller VA, editor: *The guidebook for global trainers*, Alexandria, Va, 1994, Human Resource Development Press.
16. Ontario Society for Training and Development: *Competency analysis for trainers: a personal planning guide*, Toronto, 1979, The Society

DONNA RICHARDS SHERIDAN ◆ PATRICIA FROST-HARTZER

Documenting Effectiveness: Budget and Cost Considerations

Health care economics has radically changed the way health care agencies allocate their financial resources. Limited reimbursement has meant fewer dollars for nonpatient health care activities. Budgets for essential and support services are closely scrutinized with cost-containment and cost-reduction strategies as the norm. In this environment, staff development departments have been directly affected by a loss of fiscal resources.[13,25,26]

Staff development departments must be financially responsible and have creative programming to remain viable. Sophisticated fiscal management and shrewd financial planning are needed to justify current resource allocation and prevent further shrinkage of these departments. Staff development managers and educators need to work closely to demonstrate that the financial resources provided by the organization are being used effectively and efficiently in response to the organization's needs and goals.[7] Program evaluation and cost analysis must be integrated with all activities to generate essential data to measure departmental productivity. Staff development departments justify their existence based on the organization's needs that they meet; that is, education must be congruent with the organization's goals.[17] Awareness of the organization's goals and priorities is essential to successful budget planning. The staff development setting, organization's structure, and philosophy and goals of the organization influence the scope and components of a staff development department's budget.[28] The resources of the department also influence budget preparation. High-quality data collection throughout the year facilitates the preparation and accuracy of the statistical budget, which drives the operating budget by predicting volume in the units defined by the department. Staff development departments use such units of volume as number of continuing education hours, number of in-service classes, and number of orientees. Departmental computerization of data is a must for current education departments.

BASIC BUDGETARY CONCEPTS

The budgetary process is built on some common principles that are relevant to all staff development settings. To effectively understand, prepare, and manage a staff development budget, knowledge of budget terminology is essential.

Fiscal Year

All budgets are administered on the organization's fiscal year. The organization's fiscal year often differs from the calendar year and may vary among organizations. Many organizations begin their fiscal years on July 1 of the present calendar year and run to the end of June of the next calendar year. September 1 through August 31 or January 1 through December 31 are other common fiscal years.

Data Collection

The budget preparation process requires a significant amount of time. Preparation usually begins 4 to 6 months before the end of the current fiscal year. Although the trend is to increase the overall process period, some hospitals now have an almost year-long process with various stages of planning throughout the year.

Budget preparation requires substantial data collection. The data collection comes from a number of sources including staffing data bases, turnover, and staff development department figures such as orientation, in-service, and continuing education records. Data from the human resource department, nurse managers, and advanced practice clinicians may also be useful. These data provide the statistics necessary for generation of the financial budget.

Data collection is time consuming and should begin well in advance of the budget preparation process if it is not maintained on an on-going basis. Staff development departments that monitor data on an on-going basis will find it much easier to prepare their budgets. Automation provides substantial time savings in data management. Investing in computer software that can quickly compute numbers and readjust calculations when individual data items are changed can greatly enhance the data collection process.[5]

Budget Preparation

Budget preparation is a negotiated process. A strong financial base depends on the department's ability to produce a budget document that is comprehensive, well-substantiated, clearly supportive of the organization's goals, and stands alone when reviewed by those unfamiliar with staff development services. After a preliminary budget is drafted, it is submitted by the staff development manager to the next administrative level for feedback and revision. Variance in line items and new program proposals require carefully written justifications. The budget travels up administrative hierarchy until it reaches the board of directors for final approval. Throughout this process, the budget is reviewed by many individuals who make recommendations to support, revise, or reject specific aspects.

The budget preparation process is participatory. To generate an accurate database to formulate sound staff development budgets, all members of the staff development department should be involved. Without this level of cooperation and participation, valuable data and insights for creative programming, cost-effective outcomes, and overall justification may be lost. Conversely, "buy in" and accountability for the budget by educators begin with their involvement during planning. As a service department, the staff development department budget must reflect programming that is responsive to the "buyers of educational services," that is, the nursing staff and nursing managers.

The budget preparation process is influenced by internal and external factors of the organization.[18] The process itself may be complicated by the organization's politics, reimbursement patterns, and changes in structure and culture of the organization such as corporate downsizing, merger, consolidation, buy out, or takeover. No departmental budget is immune to cuts and reprioritization, even if the budget is a well-prepared document. However, staff development departments that base their programming and expenses on supporting the organization's goals of cost-effective, high-quality patient health care are less likely to suffer budgetary cuts. Educational programs that support state licensure or Joint Commission on Accreditation of Healthcare Organizations (JCAHO) accreditation requirements are defensible but should be tied to quality patient care goals.

Operational Budget

The operational budget translates the operational plans for the department into its financial requirements for one fiscal year. The staff development department's operating budget reflects the day-to-day costs of operating a staff development department. Components of an operational budget may vary from organization to organization; however, the basic elements include the projected revenue (if applicable) and the expenses such as the personnel budget and the materials and supplies budget, which includes purchased service expenses.

The personnel budget consists of personnel or staff salary expenses, including benefits. Expected salary increases resulting from tenure or advancement are added to these calculations. The cost of adding new staff positions must also be included along with appropriate proposals and justification. The personnel budget also reflects salary or honoraria costs for per diem or contracted instructors. To calculate the latter, the projected number of hours needs to be determined and multiplied by the per diem instructor's hourly rate of pay, adding benefits, if appropriate.

The material and supplies budget, also known as the M & S budget, consists of expendable items such as instructional materials; reference and course textbooks; audiovisual material; office supplies; postage, printing and duplication; dietary expenses for class participants; small medical supplies and equipment for training; repairs and maintenance of education equipment; advertising and promotion costs; facility fees for space and equipment rental and setup; and departmental telephones. These M & S items vary depending on the organization's generic operational expense categories. The organization's finance department defines each expense category. In some organizations, dollars cannot be shifted from one line-item category to another. For example, if the "office supplies" allocation is used up, extra money cannot be taken from an under-used line such as postage. This makes careful estimation of monies for each line-item critical to smooth budgetary management. In other organizations, a lump sum of money is designated for the M & S category. The department manager can allocate the money to various line-items as needed.

Capital Budget

Capital budgets supplement the department's operational budget. The purpose of a capital budget is to provide for the acquisition of major equipment that typically costs more than $500 per item. Each organization defines its capital budget minimum. The capital budget may vary from as low as $300 to as high as $3000. Capital items for a staff development department may include TV monitors, videocameras, teaching manikins, classroom furniture, and computer monitors or programs. Renovation of existing facilities within the staff development department may also be considered capital expenditures.

In contrast to the operational budget, capital budget items are projected to last longer than 1 year or have a function lifetime of 3 to 7 years. Purchase of these budget items may be planned for anywhere from 1 year to as many as 10 years, although few organizations plan beyond 5 years because of rapid economic and technologic changes. Most organizations ask departments to project capital expenditures for 2 to 3 years. Requests for capital items are reviewed and priorities are set by the organization in terms of the facility's total capital allowance. Funds available for capital expenditures are characteristically less than those for operations. These funds are derived from "profit" or "retained" earnings from previous operating years. The process of developing a capital budget includes brainstorming and analyzing the items needed; exploring alternatives with cost comparisons; and preparing proposals to purchase the best alternative with justification of need. Factors considered in capital budget purchases include expected contribution to revenue (for example, a new scanner will produce a chargeable service); expected decrease in expenses (for example, a copy machine may allow a substantial decrease in outside printing costs); equipment to meet a patient safety or regulatory requirement; and needed replacement of equipment.

Hoffman[11] and McAlvanah[21] also recommend developing an evaluation plan and timetable for the acquisition once capital equipment approval has been obtained. Well-prepared capital budgets that are linked to increasing efficiency, cost-effectiveness, and nursing service department-wide needs are most likely to be given a higher priority within the organization. In times of financial instability, an organization may freeze even approved capital budgets.

Congruence with Organizational Goals

Staff development activities must be translated into budget formats that are congruent with the norms set by the organization's finance department. The congruence is necessary for hospital-wide bookkeeping. Both materials and salaries must be budgeted and controlled according to the organization's financial policies and procedures. Because the staff development budget reflects the costs of departmental activities and the relative values of these activities within the department, it is essential that all activities emanate from the goals and objectives of the organization as a whole.[2,4,13,26,30]

The staff development department must not be viewed as idealistic or impractical in its assessment of the organization priorities and educational needs for the nursing staff.[30] Effective collaboration among staff development educators, managers, and the nursing staff results in the efficient use and justification of all fiscal resources for educational activities. Staff development budgets that are planned and developed in isolation of nursing service considerations threaten the staff development department's credibility and survival.

To increase the success of appropriate budgetary allocations for staff development activities, it is important to prepare a budget that is in line with nursing division and the organization's goals, using figures based on accurate data collection and showing a track record of maintaining departmental operations within allocated fiscal resources. The staff development department must strengthen budget justifications to show both quantitative and qualitative benefits and must demonstrate that "every dollar counts" by evaluating programs for effective educational outcomes and cost-efficiency. Being prepared to "put a price tag" on educational services by documenting the costs and benefits of staff development services is an expectation in current health care organizations.

Preparing a staff development budget with these considerations reflects a "systems view" strategy in which nursing educational goals and management goals are compatible with each other. This strategy is highly valued within the organization and is significantly more effective in gaining budget approval.[8]

CALCULATING COSTS OF EDUCATIONAL ACTIVITIES

A basic component of fiscal management within a staff development department is the ability to accurately calculate costs of educational programs and activities.[10] Quantifying these costs assists staff development educators in responsibly projecting costs for new programs and assessing costs of current educational activities.[20] Individual elements of cost accounting vary depending on line items listed on the department's operational budget, data monitored for departmental reports and record keeping, fiscal priorities of the organization and department, and information needed for program justification and future strategic planning.[29]

Monitoring the costs for an educational activity may be done in a variety of ways. Two approaches frequently used can be characterized as a traditional system, consisting of labor, costs, materials, and overhead expenses,[22] and as a more comprehensive system, including planning, implementing, and evaluating costs.[4]

Traditional System of Cost Accounting

In the traditional revenue and expense monitoring system, revenue includes participant fees and sponsor donations and expenses include labor, materials, and overhead. Labor encompasses contracted or subsidized faculty and "outside" speaker costs, in addition to "in-house" salaries and benefits of staff development department personnel. Labor costs of coordinators, instructors, and secretaries are based on the amount of time spent on planning, implementing, and evaluating the educational activity. In-house labor costs are usually calculated by multiplying the number of hours involved by the individual's hourly salary plus benefits. Honoraria and fees of outside speakers are added for the total labor costs.

Material costs include audiovisual charges, printing and duplication, postage, telephone charges, advertising, and dietary expenses for participants. Learner materials, such as name tags, folders, and handouts, are included, as are costs of materials used in skill teaching such as small medical equipment, intravenous (IV) catheters and tubing, or emergency medications. Some staff development departments also build in depreciation costs for capital equipment such as computers, manikins, and videotapes. Overhead costs for space, maintenance of facilities, and utilities may also need to be calculated as part of educational activity costs. In some organizations, overhead costs are not included in departmental budgets. If overhead costs are included, this information can be obtained from the financial department within the organization. Adding overhead charges ensures a more accurate accounting of expenditures. An example of an educational activity cost worksheet based on the traditional system of cost accounting is presented in Fig. 8-1. This method is essentially a costing-per-program approach. Revenue recoveries are also included.

Comprehensive System of Cost Accounting

A more comprehensive system for the cost accounting of an educational activity is recommended by del Bueno and Kelly.[4] Their model is based on total costs of the three phases of program development—planning, implementation, and evaluation.

Planning costs represent all expenses associated with planning the educational activity. This includes salaries and benefits for all people involved in planning activities such as planning committee members, costs of marketing and promotion, brochure preparation, postage, and travel and meal expenses for the planning group. Implementation costs include such expense items as faculty salaries and benefits or honoraria. Secretarial salary costs based on hours of typing, record keeping, and other tasks performed while involved in program implementation are also included. All costs associated with preparation of handouts, course registration, and coordination activities are also considered. Materials for

REVENUE AND EXPENSE MONITORING

Program title: _____ Date: _____ Time: _____

Location: _____ Fee: $ _____ (Inhouse) $ _____ (Outside)

Coordinator: _____ Speakers: _____ , _____

Enrollment maximum: _____ Actual enrollment: _____ (Inhouse) _____ (Outside)

Number of contact hours: _____ Approval for C.E. credit: ☐ yes ☐ no

---

Expenses
  Labor
    Instructor/speaker expenses:
    hrs x (salary/hr + benefits)
    Coordinator expenses:
    Secretarial expenses:
    Other labor expenses:

  Subtotal of labor expenses:

  Materials/fees
    Supplies:
      Printing/duplication:
      Promotion:
      Food:
      Postage:
      Telephone:
      Small medical equipment:

  Subtotal of materials expenses:

  Overhead
    Rental fees/room charges:
    Utilities:
    A-V rental:
    Maintenance:
    Other general overhead:

  Subtotal overhead expenses:

TOTAL EXPENSES:

Revenue
  Income in-house participants
  (number x fee)
  Income outside participants
  (number x fee)
  Sponsor contributions:

TOTAL REVENUE:

PROFIT (LOSS):
Total revenue - total expenses =
Adjusted program balance or profit (loss)

Cost analysis: Total expenses/total number of participants = Total cost/participant

Adjusted program cost balance (profit or loss)/total number of participants = Profit/participant or uncompensated cost/participant

Cost per participant/program contact hours = Cost per contact hour for participant

Fig. 8-1 Courtesy Patricia Frost-Hartzer and Donna Richards Sheridan, Palo Alto and San Francisco, Calif, 1991.

the program, including duplication costs, teaching materials, and office supplies, are in this category, as are costs for refreshments and overhead. What is unique about this approach is that learner salaries and their replacement costs are also calculated as part of program cost. These learner costs are calculated only if the employer is paying for the learner to attend.

Evaluation costs are limited to the department's staff salaries based on hours spent in evaluation activities and the actual cost of evaluation materials and secretarial support for program evaluation. A comparison of two systems of educational activity cost accounting is summarized in Table 8-1. Fig. 8-2 shows an example of an educational activity cost worksheet based on a comprehensive costing system. In general, the comprehensive costing system is better for documenting educational costs than the traditional revenue and expense monitoring system because it includes learner costs. However, if learner costs are included, the costs of all educational activities are considerably higher and must be justified by greater documentation that the learner's information makes a positive difference in the work setting (impact evaluation). Learner costs may also be added to the calculations done in a traditional expense monitoring system. The selection of a system to monitor educational activity costs and individual line items should be based on the organization's needs. Some items are included primarily to facilitate data collection during the budget preparation process. Other items are included because of specific departmental needs or concerns. For instance, a department may want to monitor the amount of hours instructors spend on planning programs to develop a standard or evaluate productivity.

Table 8-1   Comparison of traditional and comprehensive cost accounting

Traditional expense system	Comprehensive expense system
Includes all direct and some indirect program costs	Includes all direct and all indirect program costs
Does not include learner costs as part of cost accounting	Includes learner costs as part of cost accounting
Calculates cost per participant hour based on direct expenses only	Produces higher cost per participant hour figures because calculations are based on direct and indirect costs
Monitors cost data as traditional budget line items, facilitating line item cost monitoring from program to program	Requires additional calculations to monitor traditional operational budget line items such as salaries and duplicating costs that involve more than one phase of program development
Limits view of full educational cost within the organization	Captures many hidden costs of educational activities (e.g., learner costs and planning costs)
Less time consuming to complete for staff development department	Requires additional cost-benefit and cost-effectiveness analysis to support additional educational activity baseline costs

COMPREHENSIVE COSTING SYSTEM

Program title: _____ Date:_____ Time: _____

Location: _____ Fee: $_____ (Inhouse) $_____(Outside)

Coordinator: _____ Speakers: _____ , _____

Enrollment maximum: _____ Actual enrollment: _____ (Inhouse) _____ (Outside)

Number of contact hours: _____ Approval for C.E. credit: ☐ yes ☐ no

---

Expenses
  Planning Costs
    Instructor expenses:
    hrs x (salary/hr + benefits)
    Coordinator expenses:
    Secretarial expenses:
    Other labor expenses:
    Supplies:
  Promotion
    Food:
    Travel:
    Postage:
  Subtotal of planning/promotion expenses:

  Implementation costs
    Instructor expenses:
    Coordinator expenses:
    Secretarial expense:
    Learner expenses:
      (cost of lost work time)
    Supplies:
    Printing/duplication:
    Food:
    Telephone:
    Small medical equipment:
    Overhead:
  Subtotal of implementation expenses:

  Evaluation costs
    Instructor expenses:
    Coordinator expenses:
    Secretarial expenses:
    Supplies and materials:
  Subtotal evaluation expenses:

TOTAL EXPENSES:

Revenue
  Income outside participants
    (number x fee)
  Income in-house participants
    (number x fee)
  Total income from course fees:

  Sponsor contributions:
  Other revenue:

TOTAL REVENUE:

PROFIT (LOSS):
Revenue − Expenses =
Total profit (loss)

Cost analysis: Program cost (expense)/total number of participants = Program cost/participant

Cost per participant/number contact hours = Cost per participant hour

Fig. 8-2 Courtesy Patricia Frost-Hartzer and Donna Richards Sheridan, Palo Alto and San Francisco, Calif, 1991.

Some organizations set up a standard such as ½:1 preparation for a repeat course (½ hour preparation allowed for 1 hour presentation for a repeat program) and 4:1 for a new program. Preparation requiring greater than 4:1 needs to be closely scrutinized in terms of need, and outside speakers should be considered for cost-effectiveness.

There may be other line items that are included or excluded as part of a departmental procedure. It is essential to keep the process consistent for accurate comparison. If changes are adopted that will significantly increase the costs of educational services, the staff development department should fully inform administrators involved in the budget approval process of the rationale for and the benefits of including specific costs. For example, if a staff development department elects to change from a cost accounting system that does not include learner costs to one that does, the costs per participant hour will rise significantly. If the staff development department neglects to justify these increased costs, educational costs may appear unacceptably high to administrators and may raise unjustified concerns. This can place the staff development department in jeopardy and threaten its credibility.

Once educational activity costs are quantified, they then can be analyzed. Cost analysis is an important part of the staff development department's fiscal management. It is tied closely to program evaluation and subsequent revision and may be accomplished by using cost-benefit or cost-effectiveness measurements. Cost analysis raises two questions for staff development—can the same educational benefits be obtained at a lower cost, and can greater educational benefits be obtained at the same cost?

Cost-Effectiveness Models

Descriptions of staff development cost-effectiveness models vary; however, most authors agree that the purpose of a cost-effectiveness analysis is to measure the efficiency in achieving outcomes in relation to costs.[4,24] The purpose of cost-effectiveness is to achieve objectives with minimum costs. An analysis of cost-effectiveness enhances a staff development department's ability to use resources efficiently because costs are related to outcomes.

Cost-effectiveness analysis has been described as a three-step process: (1) determining program objectives, (2) computing program costs, and (3) defining learner outcomes.[22] In the first step, realistic, measurable objectives are defined. In the second step, the program's costs are delineated as accurately as possible. Step 3 requires that the program's learner outcomes are defined and measured to evaluate success.

For example, a program on IV certification may have the following objective: by the end of 1 year, 50% of all RNs attending the course will be effectively using IV skills on a regular basis ("regular" is defined as at least once per week). The total IV certification program costs are estimated at $25,000 per year. The desired learner outcomes are described as 100 RNs attending the program at a cost of $250 per participant and 50 RNs using IV skills once a week (that is,

50% of the attendees who complete the class use the skill). If only 80 RNs complete the requirements for IV certification, program costs increase to $312 per participant and only 40 participants (50% of attendees) are expected to use IV skills weekly. If staff are surveyed 1 year later and if it is found that 42 of the 80 participants are starting IVs at least once per week, 35 are starting IVs less often, and 3 participants are no longer working at the hospital, the final program cost (based on 77 nurses who attended and are still starting IVs) is $325 per participant. The analysis reveals that of the 80 RNs who completed the program, over 50% of them are using those skills weekly; another 44% are using those skills less often. These data indicate that the program at 1 year was successful at meeting one of its learner outcomes, percent of skill use, but the cost was $325 per participant instead of the original projected cost of $250 per person. This indicates that the cost objective was not met at 1 year.

One comprehensive cost-effectiveness model is recommended by del Bueno and Kelly.[4] The model has been frequently cited in the literature and adapted many times.[14,16,19] The key elements of measuring cost-effectiveness include the following:

- Accurate assessment of program costs, including learner costs
- Measurable learner outcomes and the value to the organization
- Cost-efficiency criteria based on program cost per participant hour
- Program costs and learner outcomes that can be measured and justified

Determining the cost-effectiveness of each course begins with an accounting of program costs and calculating the cost per participant hour as shown in Fig. 8-2. In addition to the costs per participant hour, del Bueno's original cost-effectiveness model[3] also established cost-efficiency criteria in the following areas:

- Learner costs based on replacement and salary costs to the employer
- Job performance criteria demonstrating levels of ability in applying learning
- Cost of manager time required for reinforcement of learning
- Travel and lodging cost per participant

Adapted models most frequently use only two cost-efficiency criteria—salary and replacement costs for learners and cost per participant hour.[14,16,26] A typical example of a modified cost-effectiveness model based on all four criteria follows.

A 4-hour CPR recertification class has a cost per participant hour of $12.50. A staff development department assigned the following cost-efficiency values for all educational programs based on cost per participant hour.

- Less than $10 per hour = 1
- $10 to $15 per hour = 2
- $16 to $20 per hour = 3
- More than $20 per hour = 4

Under this system, the program would be assigned a cost-efficiency value of 2 on a scale of 1 to 4. Specific evaluative criteria measuring course-effectiveness were also established by the staff development department, as follows:

- Attendance only; no other documentation of learning = 1
- Passed written examination documenting evidence of acquired knowledge and skills = 2

- Return demonstration; ability to apply knowledge and skills in classroom setting = 3
- Work performance; documented evidence that learners can apply knowledge and skills in the workplace (that is, real or mock codes) = 4

Using the department's course-effectiveness criteria, the CPR recertification course receives a minimum course-effectiveness value of *3* on a scale of *1* to *4*. This could be raised to an effectiveness value of *4* at a later time, based on educator and manager feedback or code review data from the quality improvement program.

In analyzing the effectiveness, a course-effectiveness and cost-efficiency rate of 3:2 can be assigned to the program. This gives the staff development department a representative value of the relationship of this program's outcomes (level 3) to the program's costs (level 2). This indicates that the outcomes were of a higher level than the cost of the program. The course effectiveness to cost-efficiency ratio of 1:4 would be an undesirable finding because the interpretation is that attendance is associated with a very high cost. A ratio of 2:2 is a reasonable finding, showing a moderate cost and acquired knowledge or skill. A ratio of 4:1 is an extraordinary outcome, demonstrating that the work performance of learners is associated with a very low cost.

This method of analyzing effectiveness may be too complex to be useful beyond the staff development department. If it is used in budget justification, the assumptions behind the ratios must be explained. Numbers should never be used without explaining the somewhat subjective assumptions that underlie them.

Cost-Benefit Model

Cost-benefit analysis is also a complex method of cost analysis. Rossi and Freeman[24] define cost-benefit analysis as a process that expresses the economic efficiency of a program in terms of the relationship between program benefits (expressed in monetary terms) and program costs. Because a cost-benefit analysis is based on comparing dollar benefits with program costs, the strategy is most useful when the benefits are tangible and easily translated into monetary units.[22,26]

Cost-benefit analysis allows staff development educators to determine if the monetary benefits of an educational activity are appropriate to the costs of that activity. The process involves three steps: (1) cost itemization, (2) benefits itemization, and (3) translation of benefits and costs into monetary units.

Cost itemization involves the complete accounting of all educational activity costs. This process was described in detail in the previous section on calculating costs for educational activities. Benefit itemization is the more difficult and subjective part of the process. It requires that decisions be made about which benefits can be monetarily measured and therefore included. In the hospital setting, Kelly[16] recommends using three perspectives when attempting to quantify program benefits. They are benefits received by the hospital, the learner, and the patient. Examples of benefits that can be identified as part of a cost-benefit analysis are the following:

- Increased retention
- Increased productivity in patient health care activities
- Decreased patient health care incidents
- Decreased Worker's Compensation claims
- Increased service availability for patients
- Decreased hospital pay
- Decreased overtime costs
- Improved reimbursement[16,23,27]
- Improved quality of care
- Improved patient safety
- Increased compliance with regulatory agencies

The translation of costs and benefits into monetary units is the last step in the cost-benefit analysis process. Translating program costs into monetary units is a relatively simple process when compared with assigning monetary costs to benefits. The examples of benefits listed above show that some benefits are easier to measure in dollars than others. For example, the benefit of decreased overtime costs is much easier to translate into dollars than is the benefit of increased nurse retention. Accurate measurement of dollars associated with benefits requires important judgments and assumptions about the value of educational outcomes.

An example of a cost-benefit analysis is a program designed to prevent medication errors. In cost itemization and monetary translation, the total program costs per year are estimated at $5750, based on learner and educator salaries and educational program costs for a 1-hour, self-study module administered to 200 nurses. The cost per participant is $25 plus $600 for educator development time, $50 for typing costs, and $100 for copying costs.

The benefit itemization shows increased reimbursement as a result of improved documentation of medications on program completion at an estimated cost benefit of $250 per month × 12 months, or $3000. The potential for decreased hospital litigation related to medication errors was another benefit estimated as one case per year at an organization's value of $10,000. In summary, the cost-benefit analysis shows benefits at $10,000 + $3000, or $13,000 per year compared with the costs of $5750. Net benefits are $13,000 − $5750, or $7250 per year. The cost-benefit ratio is 5750:13,000. This means that for every dollar invested in this program, there was a $2.26 return on that investment to the hospital. The net benefit for the hospital is $7250 for 1 year.

The cost-benefit analysis has some limitations. Whatever method is used, it is a difficult, time-consuming, and complex process to measure educational outcomes quantitatively or qualitatively.[6,9,12] Measured learner outcomes may be valued by the organization differently than they are by the staff development department. Also, it may be difficult to compare the cost-benefit analysis of one program with that of another. All data for calculations may not be available, and cost assumptions not based on quantifiable data may be open to criticism, such as the $10,000 litigation cost savings. Finally, the time involved in producing a cost-benefit analysis may be prohibitive in staff development departments that already have limited human resources.

Despite these problems, the use of a cost-benefit analysis can help the staff development department identify many benefits that might otherwise go unidentified.[9] It is a tool that can strengthen justifications for fiscal resources and that can provide valuable information for strategic planning.

METHODS OF CALCULATING INSTRUCTIONAL COSTS

Calculating instructional costs is a simple process, provided that mechanisms are in place to identify and monitor individual program costs. Staff development educators must first decide how to define instructional costs. The definition of instructional costs is based on the department's rationale for determining the costs. Does the staff development department want to evaluate aspects of departmental productivity or individual educator productivity? Does the department need instructional cost data to complete internal or external reports? Does the department need to use the data to determine tuition rates for continuing education programs?

Once the department determines the use of instructional costs, pertinent expenses can be isolated from the education activity cost worksheets and evaluated. Common methods for calculating instructional costs include the following:
- Dividing the total expenses for an educational activity by the number of participants (program costs per number of participants) gives the total cost per participant
- Dividing the total program costs less the program's revenue by the number of participants (program costs minus revenue per number of participants) shows the profit or loss per participant
- Dividing the total program costs plus learner costs minus the revenue by the number of participants (program costs plus learner costs minus revenue per number of participants). This formula demonstrates the real cost to the organization per participant, including the opportunity cost—the cost of the learner learning in lieu of working.

Each of these methods represents instructional cost in terms of the cost per participant. This information can be used to project fiscal requirements for future programs so that appropriate tuition charges can be established, program-to-program costs can be evaluated, and departmental averages or standards can be determined.

Sometimes staff development departments wish to monitor a particular element of instructional costs, such as program preparation or number of classroom instructional hours. Determining these costs usually requires additional data collection by the instructor or program coordinator. Various tools can facilitate this data collection. Basically, all that is required is a tool that allows the instructor to record the hours involved in the activity (that is, library time, A-V time, class time). Costs can then be determined by multiplying total class hours by the instructor's hourly salary plus benefits. If many instructors at different pay scales are involved, an average hourly salary with benefits should be used.

An example of calculating costs for actual instructional hours follows: Four instructors are used for a 2-day, 12-hour continuing education program with breakout sessions. The average hourly salary plus benefits among the four instructors is $20 per hour. Instructor A teaches 3 hours, B teaches 6 hours, C teaches 4 hours, and D teaches 5 hours for a total of 18 hours. Eighteen hours times $20 per hour equals a $360 cost of instructors for the program.

In addition to class time, some staff development departments also include preparation time for the class. Standards exist in some institutions regarding preparation time. For example, 4 hours of "prep time" is budgeted for the *repetition* of a 6 contact hour class, whereas 18 to 24 hours of preparation may be allotted for a *new* 6 contact hour class. This assumes some relevant expertise exists on the part of the instructor.

Costs per Contact Hour

Calculating the cost per contact hour (time actually spent in contact with the learner) begins with determining the educational activity's cost per participant. Having determined this figure, the staff development educator divides it by the number of contact hours to establish a cost per participant hour. For example, if the program cost is $100 per participant and the program contains 10 contact hours, then $100 for 10 contact hours is $10 per participant contact hour.

Another way to calculate the cost per contact hour is to divide the total program costs by the number of contact hours. For example, a 6-hour program with a total cost of $3000 has a cost per contact hour of $500, or $3000 divided by 6.

Each method helps the staff development department evaluate program costs from a different perspective. The method chosen should meet the organization's needs and should be used consistently to provide comparability from course to course. Also, the methodology should be explained to those who have access to the data.

Educator Productivity Worksheets

In an effort to demonstrate the optimal use of both financial and personnel resources, many staff development departments monitor educational activities using productivity worksheets.[13,14] The term *productivity* has many meanings. Simply defined, productivity is the relationship between input and output. Productivity measures in staff development are generally used to analyze the amount of time being spent on various types of departmental activities. The information generated from productivity reports is useful in monitoring individual workloads and in setting realistic workloads or outcome expectations. It also allows for the evaluation of individual and departmental performance and justifies educator time. Johnson[14] sees a value in evaluating work distribution.

In addition, educator productivity reports demonstrate outcomes such as total learner contact hours per activity or per year. Productivity reports provide a data base for setting departmental standards, for example, time standards for program planning or for analyzing operational changes such as time impact of new program activities. These reports also assist with identifying departmental patterns.[13] Productivity reports facilitate program decision making, allowing for an analysis of whether the time spent in an activity justifies its outcomes. Productivity measurements also provide information on how efficiently the staff development department contributes to the organization's goals.

When measuring educator productivity the staff development department determines the following:

- Activities to measure
- The frequency and duration of data collection
- Method of collecting and reporting the productivity
- Use of the productivity data

For example, if a staff development department evaluates faculty workload distribution, a productivity worksheet must include a list of educator activities (for example, program preparation), a unit to log educator time (that is, hours), and a method to summarize the data at the end of a designated period of time (for example, weekly or quarterly totals).

A variety of ratios may be used to measure productivity. One example of a common productivity measure involves measuring educator hours in relation to contact hours produced. This involves a productivity worksheet that allows the educator to document actual time (in hours) spent on a learning activity in relation to the number of total contact hours provided to learners. For example, an educator may spend 18 hours preparing a learning experience, 6 hours teaching, and 24 hours evaluating the learner outcomes in clinical practice. For 24 learners, 6 contact hours would be multiplied by 24 for a total of 144 contact hours. Adding the 24 hours of evaluation of learners in the clinical areas yields a grand total of 168 contact hours. For 48 hours of the educator's time, there were 168 learner contact hours. Based on this information, many additional questions can be answered. Is this an appropriate educator output? What is the ratio of cost per learner? Could the same outcome be achieved by a self-study format? Would the self-study format cost less? How the data are used depends on the needs of the staff development department and the organization. Regardless of how educator productivity tools are used, they provide valuable data to evaluate departmental effectiveness and efficiency.

Allocation of Learner Costs

Educational activities are carried out in a variety of ways, but generally, they can be categorized as decentralized or centralized educational efforts. Decentralized educational activities may be assigned to unit-based staff educators, advanced practice clinicians, or a combination of these individuals. Monies for these decentralized educational activities may be allocated to the budgets of the individual areas in which these services take place. In contrast, centralized

Table 8-2   Comparison of centralized and decentralized education

	Advantages	Disadvantages
Centralized	Most data for budget preparation tracking and analysis centrally located	Individual unit data possibly difficult to extract
	Improved efficiency of fiscal resources and FTEs[2]	May jeopardize unit manager accountability for proper use of staff development resources
	Enhanced ability to formulate viable justification because of the ability to comprehensively collect data on staff development activities and benefits	May limit unit manager knowledge of staff use of education services, which can threaten ability to justify services provided
Decentralized	Unit manager is directly accountable for use of staff development services provided to unit	Justification of staff development fiscal requirements may possibly be seen as a unit priority
	Education services highly visible when linked to day-to-day unit activities	Budget for educational activities may be combined with other noneducation line items
	Unit manager knowledgeable and involved in planning and justification of staff development monies for unit	Decreased ability to access necessary data for staff development budget preparation and to look at staff development for the entire nursing division

educational efforts are organized under a department with sole responsibility for education and usually include centralized and decentralized educational activities. Monies for centralized educational services within the hospital are more likely to be allocated to a cost center aligned with the administrative or support components of the organization. The budgetary advantages and disadvantages of each system are reviewed in Table 8-2.

Currently, most staff development departments and their budgets are organized using both centralized and decentralized systems. The way that the department is structured is reflected in its budget components. For example, some staff development departments have all staff orientation hours charged to their budget. In this case extensive data on the previous year's orientation hours and costs need to be obtained for each job category. These data are used for projections for the coming fiscal year, taking into account the average orientation costs per job category and staff turnover trends. Data must also include anticipated new positions, the percentage of positions currently not filled, and changes in hiring and orientation practices, such as a decrease in new graduate hiring.

Assigning total orientation costs to one cost center, such as the staff development department, can reveal trends that may be missed with decentralized allocation. These trends provide important information for planning cost-efficient staff development activities and evaluating outcomes. Decentralization also loses the economies of scale and invites dissolution of educator positions during downsizing, "right-sizing," or other major efficiency drives of the organization.

PROGRAM PROPOSALS WITH FINANCIAL IMPLICATIONS

As new programs are planned, the development of a proposal offers a clear direction or points of discussion to determine a direction. The proposal should include a needs assessment with a clear connection to the organization's goals, a purpose statement, an implementation plan, a timeline, a target market, details of the program, and a budget. The budget is the core of the proposal, delineating expected revenue and expenses for labor, materials, and marketing. The budget format may be similar to Fig. 8-1 or Fig. 8-2, or with proposed numbers rather than actual numbers. Several scenarios may be necessary, with differing assumptions about the number of participants or other selected variables. Cost-benefit analyses may be included with the proposal and should be based on statistical records of the department.

Statistical Records as a Base

Statistical records can provide valuable information for all levels of departmental planning and are especially useful in new program proposals. A departmental proposal analysis is impossible without statistical records on work produced and services used. According to Dombro,[5] Holzemer,[12] and others,[1] staff development departments receive higher levels of administrative support when departmental activities can be measured by quantifiable data. These data are essential in formulating departmental statistics on costs, revenue, effectiveness, outcomes, productivity, and contribution to organizational and nursing goals.

Statistical records are especially useful in evaluating departmental patterns and trends. This information is essential to budget planning, justification of departmental resource use, and explaining the feasibility of new programs. Statistical data are highly valued by administration and should be used to share departmental outcomes.

Compiling statistical records can be a laborious and frustrating process if appropriate resources are not available to facilitate data collection and analysis. It is worth the staff development department's time to carefully plan the statistical records necessary for budget planning and for activity justification. Once this is determined, policies, measurement tools, and maintenance systems can be implemented to effectively manage the data collection. Personal computers and educational data base management programs contained within integrated medical information systems facilitate the process of data collection. The key is to make sure that statistical records for projecting staff development program needs are accurate, current, and accessible. Staff development departments that review statistical records on an on-going basis will be more successful in ensuring the department's financial support within the organization.

Documenting Cost-Effectiveness

Statistical records should include documentation of cost-effectiveness. All these statistical records are extremely time consuming to document.[5,9] However, documentation is essential because staff development activities, similar to patient health care services, are impossible to verify and justify if they are not documented.

Staff development departments that have established comprehensive cost-effectiveness documentation systems still need to reevaluate the priority of their activities.[12] Some departments spend large amounts of time to document the cost-effectiveness and cost-benefit of activities. To justify the time and expense of these activities, managers have to consider them an essential part of the program evaluation and to demonstrate that the benefits of cost-effectiveness documentation outweigh the costs.[5,15] However, for most staff development departments, this is not a realistic allocation of time. All departments should carefully consider documentation that is essential, realistic, and relevant in their setting. Methods of documentation using computer programs take considerably less time than the allocated 25% to 50% of total hours estimated by del Bueno and Kelly.[4]

The theme of cost-effectiveness in staff development was prevalent during the 1980s and continues today. Pressures for staff development departments to demonstrate efficiency, productivity, and value to the organization will only increase in the future. Staff development departments that document qualitative and quantitative outcomes are positioned for success.

SUMMARY

This chapter presented the concepts of budgeting with an emphasis on cost-benefit and cost-effectiveness. Basic budgetary concepts were reviewed in terms of fiscal year, data collection, preparation of operational and capital budgets, and congruency with the organization's goals. In the calculation of the costs of educational activities, examples were provided of both traditional and comprehensive systems for cost accounting, cost-effectiveness models, and cost-benefit models. To facilitate the budgetary process, examples of calculating instructional costs, contact hour costs, educator productivity, and learner costs were explored. Statistical records of activities throughout the year are important for justifying budget requests and documenting that the staff development department can respond to change quickly, can proactively plan for the future, and can continuously respond to the organization's needs for nursing service personnel who can provide high-quality patient health care.

REFERENCES

1. Bethel PL: Inservice education: calculating the cost, *J Contin Educ Nurs* 23(4):184, 1992.
2. Boston C: Justifying costs for continuing nursing education departments, *Nurs Econ* 4(2):83, 1986.
3. del Bueno D: Nursing staff development: critical times, critical issues, *J Nurs Staff Dev* 2(3):94, 1986.
4. del Bueno D, Kelly K: How cost-effective is your staff development program? *J Nurs Adm* 10(4):31, 1980.
5. Dombro M: Using a computer data management system to measure hospital staff development productivity, *J Nurs Staff Dev* 1(2):52, 1985.
6. Farley J: Does continuing nursing education make a difference? *J Contin Educ Nurs* 18(6):184, 1987.
7. Filipczak B: Training budgets boom, *Training* 30(10):37, 1993.
8. Franks-Joiner G: Perspective used for gaining approval of budgets, *J Nurs Adm* 20(1):34, 1990.
9. Haggard A: *Hospital orientation handbook for nurses and allied health professionals*, Rockville, Md, 1984, Aspen.
10. Hassett J: Predicting the costs of training, *Train Dev* 46(11):40, 1992.
11. Hoffman FM: Developing capital expenditure proposals, *J Nurs Adm* 15(9):32, 1985.
12. Holzemer W: Evaluation methods in continuing education, *J Contin Educ Nurs* 19(4):148, 1988.
13. Jazwiec R: Economics, productivity and effectiveness, *J Contin Educ Nurs* 18(1):8, 1987.
14. Johnson JA: Cost, value, and productivity: the bottom line in education, *J Nurs Staff Dev* 2(1):28, 1986.
15. Kelly K: A productivity measure for nursing staff development, *J Nurs Staff Dev* 6(2):65, 1990.
16. Kelly K: Cost-benefit and cost-effectiveness analysis: tools for the staff development manager, *J Nurs Staff Dev* 1(1):9, 1985.
17. Kramlinger T: A trainer's guide to business problems, *Training* 30(3):47, 1993.
18. Lee C: The budget blahs, *Training* 29(10):31, 1992.
19. Lewis EM, Gygax-Spicer J: *Contemporary strategies for nursing managers*, Rockville, Md, 1987, Aspen.
20. Marcelli AF: Determining training costs, benefits, and results, *Tech & Skills Training*, Nov/Dec:8, 1993.
21. McAlvanah M: Fiscal planning: the capital budget, *Pediatr Nurs* 15(1):70, 1989.
22. Puetz BE: *Evaluation in nursing staff development: methods and models*, Rockville, Md, 1985, Aspen.
23. Redman BK, Bednash G, Amos LK: Policy perspectives on economic investment in professional nursing education, *Nurs Econ* 8(1):27, 1990.
24. Rossi P, Freeman H: *Evaluation: a systematic approach*, ed 2, Beverly Hills, Calif, 1982, Sage Publications.
25. Rowe E: Providing effective inservice training, *J Contin Educ Nurs* 15(4):119, 1985.
26. Sanger M: Overcoming the dilemma of continuing education, *J Nurs Staff Dev* 3(4):169, 1987.
27. Slate E et al: An urban consortium: a low cost quality approach to critical care education, *J Contin Educ Nurs* 16(6):193, 1986.
28. Sparks P: A systematic budget process for CE programs. In Adelson R, Watkins FS, Caplan RM, editors: *Continuing education for the health professional: educational and administrative methods*, Rockville, Md, 1985, Aspen.
29. Spencer LM: Calculating costs & benefits. In Tracy WR, editor: *Human resources management and development handbook*, New York, 1985, American Management Assoc.
30. Weeks L, Spor K: Hospital nursing education dispelling the doomsday prophesies, *J Nurs Adm* 17(3):34, 1987.

In-House Marketing of Staff Development Programs

9

Not long ago, marketing was considered an unprofessional activity in health care. This opinion has changed with time and out of necessity. Competition for patients and staff has resulted in a shift toward market-driven hospitals. A new appreciation for creative marketing plans exist, whether in the selling of health care services, physician services, or educational programs.

MARKETING

Marketing is the activity that brings products or services to the attention of consumers. As consumers for goods and services sold by the media, everyone has been on the receiving end of marketing. Survival in the competitive health care environment has necessitated that many people with no marketing background understand marketing within their organization.

The marketing of staff development is service marketing. Service marketing requires a different focus from product marketing because of certain unique characteristics. Services are distinguished from products in that they are intangible, inconsistent, inseparable, and cannot be inventoried.[2] Unlike a product, which can be looked at, tried out, and sampled, staff development services are purchased without being seen. This intangible quality becomes a marketing challenge for the staff development department. The goal of the staff development educator is to convince the customer of the benefit that may be received from the service, thereby making the intangible seem tangible. The perceived goal needs to be marketed. The notion that "You will be able to perform better" is an obvious benefit for most educational offerings.

Another characteristic to consider is that marketing services are inconsistent. In comparison to an assembly line product or a fast-food hamburger, the delivery of the service of education, training, and development is inconsistent because people are not receiving a fixed product.[3] Even when adhering to an outline or

142

lesson plan, serial orientations occur differently. An excellent educator may have an off day, thereby producing an inconsistent result. Another example of the inconsistency of services is the delivery of patient care. Given the same patient situation, an experienced nurse delivers different care than a beginner does. Hospitals attempt to reduce the inconsistency of patient care by providing training. Trainers attempt to limit inconsistencies by using outlines and lesson plans. Written educational materials help eliminate inconsistencies.

Another distinction of service marketing is its inseparability of content and delivery. For instance, although the content of a workshop is important, at the time participants attend a class, they also comment on the chairs, lighting, room, temperature, and parking. Often, instructors receive glowing evaluations about a class, only to read a comment such as "I would have preferred donuts to muffins." The delivery and content of educational services is viewed as an inseparable combination. Instructors are not only required to be content experts but also project managers and experts in logistics.

Finally, services need to be inventoried differently than products. A product can be kept in central stores and requested when needed. On-the-job training is only available when trainers are available. The use of preceptors is one way to make on-the-job training available to more people, thereby increasing training inventory. Often, training is inventoried in a procedure manual, which allows for a consistent set of instructions to be delivered to nurses at any time. Other methods of increasing training inventory include written learning modules and other media. Providing around-the-clock access to training materials and resources can be a challenge.[10]

The terms *marketing* and *selling* are often used interchangeably although they are distinct concepts. Sales is the finding of customers for goods and services. Marketing is the creation of services or products to meet customers' needs. In staff development, the needs and wants of the customer must be understood before programs are created. If this does not occur, staff development educators are placed in the uncomfortable position of selling an unwanted program. This results in dissatisfied customers.

THE CUSTOMER

No conversation about marketing can be complete without a clear understanding and recognition of the customer. Customers are individuals who buy services from staff development. They include the hospital organization and the hospital staff. Staff development can be responsible for the entire hospital staff or given distinct areas of responsibility, such as for the nursing staff.

By paying the instructors' salaries, the hospital is purchasing the services of staff development to meet the training needs of the hospital's employees. In turn, the staff development department has a responsibility to help the hospital meet its strategic goals by providing education consistent with those goals. The staff development department must be founded on the goals and values of the organization that it serves. Failure to do so can lead to department cutbacks. As a customer, the hospital must have a sense of customer satisfaction, or the hospital will not remain interested in continuing the service.[11]

The hospital staff, although not always the "paying customers," are consumers of education, training, and development provided by the staff development department. Often, the hospital employees pay for classes in valuable time. Therefore the staff development department has a responsibility to the consumer to provide a useful service. With a strong internal marketing plan, the staff development department can provide a service of value to all consumers and worthy of the time and money invested.

MARKET ANALYSIS

To determine the goods and services needed, a market analysis should be performed. Included in this market analysis for staff development are an educational needs assessment, assessment of the patient care environment for inconsistencies, understanding of health care trends, and understanding of the strategic goals and objectives of the hospital. A successful marketing analysis includes all of these; a successful marketing program satisfies the identified needs.[5]

A magic formula for the internal marketing of a staff development department does not exist. A successful program is one that considers a number of variables assessed in the market analysis. Such a program balances the wants of the consumer with the goals of the organization. The Pillsbury marketing concept summarizes this idea, "We are in the business of satisfying the needs and the wants of customers."

The Foundation of Successful Marketing

For internal marketing to be effective, a staff development department must direct its efforts toward the hospital's strategic goals and values. Just like large companies, staff development departments must focus on their business. Some departments are in the business of producing revenue or showing large attendance figures. Others increase competence or promote retention and development. Still others have a confusing combination of competing goals.

One difficulty occurs when the goals of the hospital, the accrediting body for hospitals, and the hospital staff conflict. The goal of the hospital may be to provide cost-effective, efficient education. The Joint Commission on Accreditation of Healthcare Organizations (JCAHO) may strive to adhere to certain criteria in the area of safety and competence. The staff may desire to master the latest piece of equipment or know more about certain drug interactions. In successful programs, staff development balances these conflicting needs to produce programs that satisfy all customer goals.

DEPARTMENT RELATIONSHIPS

The next step toward the success of an internal marketing program requires a positive relationship between the staff development department and the rest of the hospital. The department head of staff development should be on the same hierarchical level as other department heads. This promotes communication. In some hospitals the department head is also responsible for research, quality assurance, or marketing. These varied responsibilities can help keep the staff development department in contact with other concerns of the hospital. However, this can also result in spreading the human resources of these areas so thinly that education is neglected. Staff dedicated to the delivery of education, training, and development are needed in today's rapidly changing health care environment. When hiring educators for the department, the director should pay special attention to the goals that candidates want to achieve and the talents that they can bring to the department. The personal power and ability of the educators strengthen the department's successful marketing ability. Effective instructors build relationships with the staff that allow them to know the staff's strengths and weaknesses. Competent instructors know the staff and genuinely want to spend time with the staff and contribute to individuals' goals. By becoming acquainted with the staff, educators are more likely to produce useful educational programs at the appropriate times and for the right individuals. A successful internally marketed staff development department provides a variety of services including bedside consultation, unit in-service classes, and workshops as needed by the staff.[20]

If the educator is trusted, competent, respected, and seen as an advisor or coach, staff members will see class offerings as invitations to grow and opportunities to gain valuable information. As long as educators remain committed to contributing to others and the purpose of the class is to increase competence, this relationship between educators and staff will continue. Department offerings by individual educators will be seen as opportunities for growth and development.

By working with the staff and providing growth and development, the staff development department helps nursing department heads meet their goal of providing competent care. Staff development personnel will be valued and considered indispensable contributors to the successful attainment of staff goals. To ensure that the needs of department heads are being met, contracts can be used. A contract is an agreement between the staff development educator and manager of a department or unit to ensure that educational needs are met. The contract should clearly indicate important topics, the people responsible, and expected completion dates. A contract creates alignment between managers and educators and can reveal responsiveness. The result is a greater likelihood that what is learned will be applied to the clinical setting because the information meets that unit's unique needs. Educators who know the strengths, weaknesses, and competencies of the staff become invaluable to unit managers who need to make performance, staffing, and promotion decisions.

Program Utility

When programs meet the hospital's needs, they are said to have "program utility."[2] Programs or classes that make patient care or other tasks easier are useful to the organization and staff. Assessing newly hired employees for competence is something that staff educators can do during the orientation program. This makes the unit manager's job easier. In addition, assessment supports preceptors or clinical unit instructors by clarifying the learning needs of new employees. Staff development educators are also able to assess performance problems. A manager may ask a staff educator to identify employee learning deficits and work with the staff development department to decide the way to meet learning needs. Staff development educators can also work with staff members to identify skill deficiencies and provide programs to correct those deficiencies. By combining competency and developmental models, educational offerings can be ranked in categories to meet the needs of all hospital staff.[1] All employees must have technical skills, interpersonal skills, critical-thinking abilities, and knowledge of the organization to successfully perform their jobs.[4] Surveys and needs assessments can be built on this framework. Focus groups and advisory committees can suggest possible topics. The goal is to make people more effective in their jobs.

THE "P" FACTORS
Product

A number of factors must be considered when building a staff development program. First, the product or products offered must be considered. The product can be a class, workshop, in-service program, learning package, video, or module. Whatever the product, it must be desired by decision makers or it's use will be limited. Having decision-maker "buy-in" lends needed support to a program and will help increase attendance or usage of the program. The program's content should be high quality and consistent with the staff needs. Experts may work with instructional designers to achieve this. High-frequency, high-risk learning needs, such as using a crash cart, instituting patient-controlled analgesia, or using a bag-valve-mask device correctly, should be addressed in reusable learning formats such as modules or videotapes. Well-designed programs on high-use tasks can save instructors hours of time.[8]

Some topics, such as diagnostic-related groups and burnout, are trendy. If trendy topics are timely, attendance and interest for these programs is high. However, these same programs may not generate much interest among the staff later. A well-marketed program addresses fads advantageously and presents useful, new programs on a timely basis. For instance, courses about "renewal" currently have replaced courses about "burnout." This program title emphasizes the desired outcome rather than the problem. The most current fads in staff development are measurable outcomes and programs on quality improvement.[18]

Basic classes, such as classes about the use of chest tubes or 12-lead electrocardiograms, are needed by all staff members at some time. Practical classes that deliver basic information to the staff are usually well attended if presented well. The content must be clear, consistent, and concise. These courses should be scheduled at convenient times for the staff. Subject practicality suggests that these programs combine on-the-job training with short periods of classroom time. Well-designed classes with clear objectives can often be converted to learning modules. This may allow for more exposure of new concepts to a larger audience.

Obtaining high attendance at classic programs, such as those on immobility or care of the aging adult, is often a challenge. Staff members often believe they already know about these subjects and may not be interested. Staff development educators may need to create a demand for these classes. One method that creates interest is pretesting the target audience. The pretest should be an accurate representation of the material to be taught in the class. Staff members can test their knowledge and decide whether they would benefit from attending this class. Providing a new theme for classic classes may also boost attendance. For example, a class about caring for an aging adult that was offered at Christmas time was well attended after it included the theme of normal and abnormal changes in the aging of Santa Claus. Colorful posters were easy to obtain; clever analogies were easy to draw. Topics such as "Grandma's favorite Christmas cookies" and "Christmas gifts to buy for your aging grandparents" fit easily into this theme.

Program quality remains the responsibility of the staff development department. For instance, external sources of educational programs are now marketing themselves to in-house education departments. Because the nursing staff associates any program offered in or publicized by the hospital with their own staff development department, the content and presentation quality of these programs is often transferred to the staff development department.[13] For this reason, it becomes the role of the staff development department to determine the appropriateness and the content quality of these programs before scheduling them. In every community enough programs are available to fill an education calendar at minimal monetary cost but great cost to departmental credibility. Sometimes, outside speakers are unfamiliar with the culture of an organization so the audience has a sense of cultural dissonance, that is, the audience does not know the way to apply the information presented to the work setting. Product vendors may also supply outside speakers. A good in-service program from a knowledgeable vendor can be helpful. However, product vendors who are more interested in selling their products can be frustrating to busy staff nurses.

Carefully chosen external speakers can enhance the staff development department's effort. These speakers should have good reputations and be capable of adapting to the cultural differences of the organization. The staff and department heads can also be speakers. Before attending national conferences, department heads can be asked to notice particularly strong speakers who would meet needs of the hospital or their own units. A nationally known speaker can share the latest and most up-to-date practices with staff members and can have a positive effect on practice and patient care. Other possible speakers include physicians and external content experts.

Promotion

The best promotion is one that is timely and motivating. The first step to motivation is creating a program for which a genuine need exists. Such programs promote themselves. However, even the best program will not get the attendance it deserves if it is not well publicized. Prominently posted fliers and notices in hospital newspapers and newsletters are the most common publicity methods. Other methods include notices on computer bulletin boards, announcements made in meetings or gatherings, and telephone reminders made directly to unit or department managers. The speaker's relationship to the potential audience is often overlooked but extremely important. For example, a program was recently presented by a well-liked physician on the proper use and delivery of blood products. Although this program's title was identical to a program given by an outside vendor, the physician's program was attended by eight times as many people. A charismatic speaker draws participants to an educational offering based on that speaker's relationship with participants. In addition, the speaker's enthusiasm while producing the program is often infectious; this enthusiasm often makes people excited about coming to the program.

If a program is really strong, word of mouth works to publicize it. If a class or workshop is only scheduled once, word-of-mouth publicity has no value. Classes scheduled 3 to 4 weeks apart maximize the chances of word spreading. Workshops that are routinely scheduled at least 3 weeks apart promote the program and help the department head arrange a schedule so many staff members can attend.

Word of mouth is an underestimated promotion strategy. If the staff development department gets the reputation for making learning fun, that will be the staff's expectation. No matter how dry the topic, the learners know the material will be presented in an interesting fashion.

One way to make learning interesting is to add games. Not only do games make learning fun but, most importantly, they immediately allow learners to apply theory to practice and learners will be more likely to transfer the learning principles to their work. Enjoyable, useful learning experiences become a reputation that assists in the promotion of future programs.[12]

Place

The setting for a class or topic should depend on the content and length of time it takes to teach the topic. Certain skills are best taught at the bedside with one-on-one coaching from the educator. At other times, classrooms are more suitable. For day-long workshops, seating must be comfortable with tables available for writing and taking notes. Class setting is extremely important to future marketing efforts.

The setting for programs can also be nowhere and anywhere. The program may be a roving cart of self-contained learning modules or a newspaper sent to learners. Gloe[9] has developed a learning opportunity called the paper programs, that is, a brief synthesis of an identified topic of interest within the organization. These topics are presented as a newspaper or booklet. The cover page identifies the topic and resources, the contact hours awarded on successful completion, and the name of the contact person assisting with the topic. The body of the paper program is much like a journal article and can be made attractive with clip art. The setting is limited only by the ingenuity of staff development educators.

Premiums and Incentives

Incentives are used by people selling a product or service to draw customers and encourage them to buy. Incentives are giveaways that add value to the product or service that is already being offered. Continuing education units have long been an incentive for nursing education programs. Food can also be part of an incentive program. The costs of food can be built into the registration fee so that consumers believe the food is free.

Sometimes premiums are not always considered premiums (e.g., hand-outs from the learning experience itself). For example, Modic and Harris[17] describe a workshop on "Triple O"-overwhelmed, overworked, and out-of-control. The learning experiences stressed the physiological, psychological, and sociological aspects of stress. In addition to games, songs, dance, and lecturettes, the workshop ended with the distribution of a goody bag for each participant. The goody bag contained an apple and a bottle of water to remind participants about healthful living and a pad and pencil to remind them about managing time better and communicating effectively. These premiums are exceptionally effective because they are in the affective domain.

Duty-time pay is often an incentive to attend classes. Usually hospitals are required to pay for the "mandatory" classes they request their staff to take. However, the majority of classes do not fall into this category. Some employee contracts guarantee paid time for education on a sliding scale in which hours are accrued by the amount of time worked. Nurses can then attend the class, get paid for the day, and not be expected to work an additional day. Some staff members attend classes on their days off because they need to know the material and consider the class to be part of their professional responsibility. Most nurses can be released from staffing only if the unit can operate effectively in their absence. The ratio of nurses to unlicensed assistive personnel affects this release by making fewer staff members available to cover for nurses attending educational programs. A good marketing plan considers staffing difficulties and schedules classes that do not conflict with known unit needs.

Participants

Know the participants. A successful internally marketed staff development program can not develop unless the marketer understands the needs of the participants, demands of the working environment, and skills required to get the job done.

There is an added benefit when continuing education (CE) can be designed for nurses, auxiliary personnel, and visitors. Evanoski and Henderson[6] describe a mobile cart carrying eye-catching health topics that was originally positioned in a busy corridor. This cart became so popular that it now regularly rotates throughout the hospital. This cart demonstrates ingenuity and responsiveness to participants.

Process

The learning process in a successful staff development program must take adult learning principles into account. Two principles are especially important.

Learning does *not* start and stop sporadically. Learning is an ongoing process that begins when an employee is hired. A career path for each nurse can be established based on individual, personal goals. Learning resources and opportunities must be made known to all staff members so they can take responsibility for their own ongoing learning.

Learning *must* be reinforced. Once a topic is learned, it should be applied in the worksetting as soon as possible. For staff development educators who are available at the bedside or on units for on-the-job training, this may be the easiest adult learning principle to apply. The success of preceptor programs may be attributed to the opportunity to apply new knowledge immediately, thereby reinforcing learning. If a hospital does not have staff development educators available for on-the-job training, programs can be reinforced in the worksetting.

Presentation

Even with excellent content and an understanding of the learning process, an educational program can fail if the educator does not possess solid presentation skills. By observing effective speakers and attending classes about giving presentations, educators can learn and fine tune these skills. However, nothing works as well as practice. Effective presenters are able to empathize with their audiences. They are sincere and authentic in their delivery and can be easily heard. They make their presentations clear, appropriate, and interesting by using humor and body language appropriately.[16]

In one hospital, one of the most popular classes was called "The Joy of Presentation." This class was taught by the staff development department and participants were required to bring a topic to develop into a presentation. The class content was designed so participants would have a usable product by the end of the day. Because staff development personnel often have the most experience in presentation, this was a relatively easy class to present. This class resulted in an improvement in the quality and quantity of many small, unit-based in-service programs.

Price

Price is often the most controversial component of a marketing program. Without affixing a standard price to any class, a few simple guidelines can be followed to develop a budget. Consistency in pricing is especially important. Participants often cannot understand the reason one class costs more than another. In the pricing game, "cheap" is not necessarily a winner; potential participants are sometimes leery of free programs.

MOTIVATION

Motivation can be defined as an individual's desire to do something based on need.[14] The problem with motivating people is that they are not always aware of their needs. People may not be aware that they do not know something; if people are not motivated, they will not care about the information that they do not know.

Staff development educators can inspire, motivate, and create demand. One method is to assess the information that people know and then make them aware of the information they do not know. This can be accomplished by giving a pretest or developing a clever flier that asks puzzling questions and requires people to register for a class to learn the answers. Competency-based assessments, although time consuming, are yet another method of inspiring staff member's to learn.[7]

Unfortunate incidents and horror stories also create a desire to learn. For instance, stories about the errant placement of tubes guarantee attendance at a class on enteral tube complications. "Horror story marketing" needs to be targeted only to the staff members and not be posted or shared with patients and their families. This kind of marketing effort requires discretion and good judgment. For example, a family was recently awarded damages in one of the largest court settlements after the family's elderly mother strangled in her restraints. Without emphasizing the human horror of this story, it can serve to motivate staff members to attend classes on the proper and safe application of restraints. Such stories get people's attention and arouse interest in the course content being offered.

Courses designed "especially for you" also receive attention. Promises of course benefits should be emphasized in fliers. Benefits can be for participants or their managers. For instance, decreasing the number of falls on a patient unit by introducing a fall prevention program may appeal to managers who are aware of the number of falls on their units more than to individual staff members. However, staff members are usually anxious to attend classes that simplify the use and provide an understanding of equipment. They can readily apply this to their job and immediately attain benefit from it.

A common mistake made by staff development educators is trying to get people to do what they do not want to do. "Mandatory" classes are often seen as classes no one wants to attend. By using a little ingenuity, staff development educators can create courses and programs so staff members want to attend. The most ingenious of these are theme classes. For example, at El Camino Hospital, mandatory safety training has been transformed into "Dangerous Liaisons" by using a variety of fast-paced activities tied together by movie themes. As attendees register, their names are placed on the "wall of stars." Participants receive tickets to attend. Colorful movie posters from a video store are strategically placed for all to see. A life-size cardboard cutout of Eddie Murphy asks "Coming to Safety Training?" Mandatory activities, such as disaster planning, hazardous materials, and back safety, are transformed into games. Infection control training has been turned into a game called "Dirty Dancing." For fire safety, a picture of the hospital has been enlarged, crepe paper flames are pasted to hospital's windows, and the entire picture is covered with a heavy plastic. This creates a "towering inferno" on which staff members can practice using fire extinguishers. Many other clever activities have been added to this mandatory safety training. Attendance has gone up, the staff has learned about safety, and everyone has fun.

Reasons Given for not Attending Classes

Although staff development educators may do all sorts of creative things, sometimes people still do not participate. During these times, the problem must be identified. As Henry Kaiser once said, "I always view problems as opportunities in work clothes." Some of the more common problems and hidden opportunities are listed as following:

Exhausted staff members: In this case, in-service classes must be fast, upbeat, and empowering. Most people have energy for fun things. The key is to make classes fun. Laughter is an effective method for decreasing stress. Many training departments have interpreted this to mean that classes should be taught on laughter therapy. Another interpretation is to teach regular classes in a humorous way that gives energy to the participants.

Dissatisfaction with previous classes: Staff development educators need to determine the reason people are dissatisfied. Then promise to solve the problem. Needless to say, once this promise is made, it must be kept.

Useless courses: Staff development educators should define the personal utility of courses for the staff. For instance, if a course about fire safety is offered and there has never been a fire, the staff development educator must discover personal utility for staff members. In the case of fire safety, educators can remind staff members of the loss of lives that can occur in an organization's fire and who is responsible for those lives. For example, after the October 17, 1989 earthquake in the San Francisco Bay region, staff members at El Camino Hospital found information about disaster preparedness useful. Handout materials that had previously been ignored disappeared by the hundreds after the earthquake.

Competing priorities: Classes should be identified and well publicized in advance and offered at different times. Time is a valuable commodity in the modern world, and wise staff development educators treat other people's time as valuable and precious. Classes should begin and end on time. Material that can be covered in a handout or 5-minute in-service program should not be converted to a day-long workshop. There must be a mutual respect of time.

COMMON MARKETING MISTAKES
Poor Quality Program Announcements and Promotional Pieces

Because computers are readily available and laser printers may be found at local photocopy stores, there is no excuse for unprofessional-looking promotional pieces. A number of simple desk-top publishing programs are available and even simpler programs can print professional-looking fliers. Some programs are relatively inexpensive and easy to use. Many of the latest generation of word-processing programs can produce quality promotional pieces.

Conflicts in Scheduling

Hospital schedules are usually produced 6 weeks in advance. If the education department is expecting a large attendance for a class, the class should also be publicized in advance. Some organizations distribute class schedules a year in advance. Staff development educators should make fliers available to managers before scheduling so staff members will be available to attend.

Once the class is scheduled and publicized, educators should continue announcing the course at meetings and other gatherings to create a demand for the course. As previously discussed, if a relationship exists between educators and staff members, it is easy for educators to be persistent in letting people know the classes they should attend.

Instructional materials may become more popular training methods during census fluctuations. In some facilities the organization is responsible for paying employees if the census drops suddenly. An alternative is to use this "down time" for self-paced training activities. At such times, small guides can be given to managers to make them aware of learning activities that are available on short notice.

Complex Programming

Some departments limit themselves to delivering in-service programs or workshops exclusively. These departments do not realize that some educational methods such as in-service posters, on-the-job training, and short learning modules may be the best and most efficient methods for delivering information. Keeping information simple and accessible increases the amount of training and development that occurs and decreases the labor required for members of the education department.

Developing Unnecessary Programs

The most effective programs are supported by management and arise from the needs of the participants. Occasionally, educators operate from their mistaken beliefs about programs that are wanted or needed. This results in poor attendance. Formal and informal surveys of program participants and nonparticipants should be performed if attendance falls or other indications that the educational program is not meeting the needs of participants are given.

COMPOSING PROMOTIONAL PIECES

Attention-getting titles can spark interest in a class. For example, "High-Impact Nursing Interventions" (now affectionately called "HINI") began as a method of delivering a potpourri of quality-improvement in-service programs that would impact a variety of care areas. In a day-long workshop format, staff members can learn to prevent falls, differentiate types of chest pain, perform critical assessments, and differentiate types of bizarre behavior. The workshop is interesting and fast-paced and the contents can be applied directly to specific jobs. Managers like the program because it meets quality-improvement requirements.

When designing promotional pieces, staff development educators must be aware of what is popular and unpopular. Some methods used to determine popularity are brainstorming and reading magazine stories, headlines, and movie titles. The key is to look for something unique and to use it in the title. Of course, a little humor never hurts either.

The most common method to advertise for classes is to develop fliers. Fliers should be complete and accurate. They should include the class name, instructor, date, time, place, cost, and number of continuing education units. Text included in the flier should be structured in short sentences. The writer should strive for a crisp, clean writing style. Fliers should be colorful and professional looking.[15] They may be the only communication about the class that potential participants will receive, therefore fliers should be widely distributed. Two mailings of the same flier may be helpful. One mailing should occur several weeks before the class; the other should be sent as a reminder about 2 weeks in advance.

If fliers are routinely posted on overcrowded bulletin boards, they must be eye-catching. Separate bulletin boards for in-house education programs help overcome this problem. Fliers may get more visibility if they are posted in elevators, near elevators, or in restrooms.

The best motivation and promotion is to provide vital and timely information in the classes or courses that are presented. Staff members want to do a good job; staff development educators can provide necessary skills and knowledge. New products, goods, and services should always be introduced by in-service programs.

EVALUATING MARKETING EFFECTIVENESS

Unlike evaluating the effectiveness of education, evaluating the effectiveness of marketing is fairly simple. Many departments currently perform this evaluation and call it a measurement of the effectiveness of education. The effectiveness can be measured by dividing the number of potential attendees for a class by the number of people who attended to show what percentage of the staff attended.[19]

Market studies can be done at the end of the year. One way to do this is to list all the classes and have staff members indicate if they did or did not attend and the reason. This allows staff development educators to form an overview of popular and unpopular courses and understand the reasons staff members did or did not attend.

SUMMARY

In-house marketing of learning experiences and programs challenges the ingenuity of staff development educators. Market analysis, determination of who the customer is, and interdepartmental relationships affect in-house marketing efforts. The "P" factors—product, promotion, place, premiums, participants, presentations, and price—shape the materials used for marketing. An analysis of reasons nursing service staff do and do not attend staff development learning experiences also assists in planning effective in-house marketing. Implementing effective in-house marketing may be time-consuming but is important to achieve maximum attendance at staff development programs.

REFERENCES

1. Benner P: *From novice to expert: excellence and power in clinical nursing,* Menlo Park, Calif, 1984, Addison-Wesley.
2. Berkowitz E, Kerin R, Rudelius W: *Marketing,* Santa Clara, Calif, 1986, Mosby.
3. Cooper PD: What is health care marketing? In Cooper PD, editor: *Health care marketing,* Germantown, Md, 1979, Aspen.
4. del Bueno D, Weeks L, Brown-Stewart P: Clinical assessment centers: a cost-effective alternative for competency development, *Nurs Econ* 5(1):21, 1987.
5. Dunham JR: Marketing continuing education for nurses, *Nurs Adm Q* 10(1):73, 1985.
6. Evanoski CA, Henderson DW: MobyEd: a mobile educator unit, *J Contin Educ Nurs* 26(2):89, 1995.
7. Falkenberry J: Marketing strategies to increase participation in continuing education, *J Nurs Staff Dev* 2(3):98, 1986.
8. Freeman L, del Bueno D, Wake M: Product development and marketing in continuing education, *Nurs Econ* 2:336, 1984.
9. Gloe D: Paper programs, *J Contin Educ Nurs* 25(4):188, 1994.
10. Johnson SH: A model for marketing continuing education in a recession, *J Contin Educ Nurs* 16(1):19, 1985.
11. Kotler P: *Marketing for non-profit organizations,* Englewood Cliffs, NJ, 1975, Prentice-Hall.
12. Kuhn MA: Gaming: a technique that adds spice to learning, *J Contin Educ Nurs* 26(1):35, 1995.
13. Kuramoto A: Defining the image of your continuing education department, *J Contin Educ Nurs* 19(6):274, 1988.
14. Lambert C: *Secrets of a successful trainer: a simplified guide for survival,* New York, 1986, John Wiley & Sons.
15. Leonard K, Shinn S: Creating an effective flyer, *J Contin Educ Nurs* 24(6):280, 1993.
16. May K: A view from the side of the provider, *J Contin Educ Nurs* 14(6):24, 1983.
17. Modic MB, Harris R: A reinforcement technique: the goody bag, *J Contin Educ Nurs* 25(3):143, 1994.
18. Puetz B: Editorial: focus on outcome, *J Nurs Staff Dev* 6(3):111, 1990.
19. Ship T: The marketing concept and adult education, *Lifelong Learning* 4(4):26, 1981.
20. Southern Regional Education Board: *Marketing continuing education for nurses,* Atlanta, 1981, Regional Action for Continuing Education in Nursing Project.

Using Computers to Manage Staff Development

The days of computer ignorance have ended. Currently, computers are as important as class plans in delivering educational services. Computers also are in greater demand to assist in organizational planning, problem solving, and decision making. Staff development educators must maximize their use of computers to achieve expected performance outcomes. With tremendous capacity for storage and retrieval of data, arithmetic computations, and drawing of comparison relations, computers have become indispensable management tools. This chapter highlights computer applications in two major functions of the staff development department—administration and instruction.

PLANNING FOR COMPUTER APPLICATIONS

An accurate needs analysis must precede the implementation of computer application. This includes attention to the organization's structure, client and department needs, and regulatory requirements.

Organizational Structure

The structure of the staff development department should be determined. For instance, it should be determined whether the staff development department is part of nursing service, working exclusively with nursing service, or a hospital-wide or system-wide department responsible for delivering education services to all employees. In addition, it should be determined whether other departments offer the same or similar services to specialized clientele within the organization. For example, the organization may include a hospital-wide education department; a nursing staff development department; a group of clinical nurse specialists; and trainers in other departments such as laboratories, housekeeping, or surgery. Finally, determining whether these departments and individuals interface in the areas of record keeping, registration, class scheduling, graphics or presentation programs, and computer-based training capabilities is also important. The answers to these questions determine the kind of capacity and flexibility needed in a computer system. Verifying that the services the staff development department wishes to implement are not already available in another department is another requirement. Needless duplication can occur if the staff development department purchases a multimedia graphics package if one is already available in the information services department.

Client and Department Needs

The type and degree of the speed and frequency of record keeping and reporting services that clients want should be determined. The staff development department might provide training reports, which only document attendance at programs, or the department may receive requests for special reports to assist managers in a decision-making process. The staff development department may draw on the computer's data base capability to request such things as mailing lists and instructor productivity reports. If clients are combating a shortage of staff and an inability to schedule people for classes, nontraditional learning approaches such as computer-based training should be considered. This flexibility allows for individual client use at times scheduled by the client. Staff development members should analyze the requests received, the data currently available, and information from key client committees. A formal survey or target interviews with key clients are additional ways to determine a specific direction for computer planning.

Regulatory Requirements

The need to comply with the requirements of regulatory bodies can be a powerful argument for implementing computerized record keeping in the staff development department. The Joint Commission on Accreditation of Healthcare Organizations (JCAHO), federal and state agencies, and the parent organization may require annual employee training documentation. This can be a burdensome task for hospital managers and the staff development department. One experience with manual record retrieval for a JCAHO survey team can convince anyone that a computerized record retrieval system is a necessity. The box shows examples of record keeping that comply with regulatory bodies.

Practical Considerations

Other issues enter into the decision-making process as well. These include budget, staff capability, volume of business, storage space, and internal resources.[12]

The budget certainly dictates the computer applications that can be purchased. Secondary factors influencing this choice are the speed with which

---

EXAMPLES OF MANDATORY PROGRAM DOCUMENTATION

JCAHO requirements
Cardiopulmonary resuscitation review
Electrical safety review
General safety review
Infection control review

Federal requirements
Occupational Safety and Health Administration's "right-to-know" program
Occupational Safety and Health Administration's bloodborne pathogen program

State requirements
Certified nursing home assistant training
Licensed practical/vocational nurses' intravenous therapy training
Trauma education

Organizational requirements
New employee orientation
Nursing orientation
Specific nursing skills training

---

requests can be addressed and the quality of output desired. A dot matrix printer can be purchased for less than $200. A laser printer, on the other hand, can cost more than $1000. Software may cost anywhere from $50 for an add-on package for an existing system to thousands of dollars for interactive-video capability. At this time, the 486 class computer is the overwhelming choice for businesses when purchasing a new personal computer (PC). Prices range from a little more than $1000 to nearly $3000. Again, this choice must be based on *need*. A good rule of thumb is to buy the fastest PC that the department can afford without neglecting other components of the system, such as a printer. Software (e.g., DOS, Windows OS/2, Macintosh, VAX) should be based on personal preference, familiarity, price, and what the information systems department supports. A cost-benefit analysis can be done to determine which project will provide the greatest productivity payoff. The costs of developing and running the proposed program should be compared with current needs to determine the cost effectiveness of the proposal.[30]

Resources are needed for researching hardware and software options, writing a proposal, and learning the basic and advanced capabilities of the system to be purchased. The staff development department personnel may choose to limit the scope of the application to data entry and generation of basic reports, such as registration processing and education record keeping. In this instance, clerical staff can be trained to handle the application with initial support from the software vendor. In the instructional arena, staff development department members may choose to purchase vendor-prepared software packages to bypass the time, expertise, and expense required to develop in-house programs.

More advanced applications require dedicated personnel with in-depth computer backgrounds. For instance, database or spreadsheet applications may be used to develop specialized management reports, such as the number of educational hours spent by staff members in different job categories during a given year (e.g., the average number of hours spent per year by RNs, LPNs, and nurse assistants in education activities). A nursing vice-president could use this data to budget educational time, salaries, and supplemental staffing hours. For instructional uses the staff developer should consider the skills needed in script writing, authoring knowledge and experience, and media production to produce in-house instructional software (whether computer-assisted instruction [CAI] or interactive video [IVD]).

The volume of business also dictates the course of action. Meeting the needs of 100 staff members is different than meeting the needs of 5000 staff members. A hardware and software package that can handle the current and anticipated volume with maximal reliability and speed is needed. One approach may be to purchase a basic system with optional add-on features for future applications. For example, a computerized record-keeping package and add-on registration, classroom scheduling, and budget-tracking capabilities can be purchased as time and funds permit.

Storage space can be a critical factor in switching to a computer application in the work area. A computer disk takes up a fraction of the space of a hard-copy file. As a result, a disk makes it possible to store 10 years of training reports, program files, and instructional manuals on the secretary's desk rather than in an off-site warehouse.

In the event there is insufficient expertise to track training activity within the department, access must be available to a mainframe system and skilled information system staff who can handle an application request. It may be more cost effective to access the mainframe rather than develop a PC application specifically for the staff development department.

External Resources and Vendors

Once needs are assessed and the practical issues are addressed, staff development department members should research and evaluate the choices and define the bottom-line requirements. This entails a careful consideration of software and hardware features. These are key decisions to make because the staff development department must live with the system for several years. A mistake here can cost considerable money, lost productivity, and dissatisfaction among clients and users in the department. The boxes outline the major software, hardware, and technical details to review.

ADMINISTRATIVE SOFTWARE SELECTION CRITERIA

Record keeping
Program tracking by individual and by program
Type and scope of data fields collected including the following:
Employee name
Employee identification number
Employee work location
Class title
Class category
Class location
Instructor's name
Class date
Class hours
Contact hours
Grade or certification code
Attendance at outside education programs

Reports
Standard report formats
Standard reports included in the software package
User generation of own reports

Correspondence generation
Correspondence to program participants
Unique correspondence
Mailing lists and labels
Limited or extensive word-processing capability

Budgeting
Tracks actual and planned expenses
Handles chargeback and tuition expenses
Downloads information to a spreadsheet

Lists
Produces class rosters, course calendars, course schedules, and course catalogs
Generates user designed and standardized lists

Human resources department information
Incorporates employee development plans, career tracking, and performance appraisals

---

Modified from March J, Bernhards J: *Train Dev J* 43(6):85, 1989.[17]

Building Support

Although staff development department members may be enthusiastic about computer application in the department, other key players may not be as pleased. Examining the relationship of this application to the organization's mission statement and goals is necessary to gain administrative approval and staff "buy-in." The technology should support organizational direction and promote the accomplishment of department objectives. This technology should increase

---

ADDITIONAL SELECTION CRITERIA FOR ADMINISTRATIVE COMPUTER APPLICATIONS

Technical requirements

Monitor, memory, storage, and printer requirements
Computer hardware requirements (has PC, network, and main frame versions)
Various program versions are compatible
Program can be customized to meet user needs
Program sold in modules or as a complete package
Provision for cleaning out unnecessary and outdated files
Length and comprehensiveness of warranty

Security requirements

Limits access to certain individuals
Limits access to selected information
Contains automatic data backup capability
Provides recovery procedures
Offers safeguards and checks to prevent error in data entry

User support and training

Installation and orientation time
Access to training and ongoing technical support
Access to documentation manual or a system tutorial
Access to an 800 number
Access to a site visit by a vendor representative
Access to a user group

Updates and new releases

New releases of the program available once or twice per year
Access to new releases at reduced cost
System in place for handling updates and bugs and communicating same to client
Opportunities for users to suggest software changes

Documentation

Written guidelines and procedures logically organized, accurate, and comprehensive
Tutorial available to acquaint users with important functions
Documentation updated when the software is updated

Modified from March J, Bernard J: *Train Dev J* 43(6):85, 1989.[17]

access to services, offer productivity improvements and cost savings, improve the transfer of learning, assist management decision making, and decrease management and instructor workload. Payoffs may need to be demonstrated to staff development personnel and the administration by tying computer solutions to the removal of work obstacles, an improved ability to meet the demands of current jobs, and the provision of new services that had not been available such as the production of customized management reports.[21]

COMPUTER APPLICATIONS IN EDUCATION ADMINISTRATION

A wide range of computer applications is available for education administration (box). These applications fall under the four categories of planning, daily operations, record keeping, and reporting. Just as hospital managers need information for decision making, education managers do too. The computer can generate needs analysis information by keeping track of employee training attendance reports according to the program, instructor, and time of year. Entering financial information from individual program files and other department operations allows for accurate budget development, tracking, and forecasting. This principle allows for educator productivity tracking. Data from daily, weekly, or monthly time-accounting sheets can be entered by clerical staff to generate periodic productivity reports by instructor or program. A spreadsheet program assists with project planning and tracking. Once project parameters and deadlines are entered into the computer, the computer can keep track of compliance with major project checkpoints.

Data entry labor for tracking functions can be significantly reduced by using bar code technology. Identifying bar codes can be created for such things as educator and employee identification badges, project folders, and equipment. A light reader scans the bar code, and the computer converts the electronic impulses to a binary code and readable characters. Systems may be purchased to generate bar codes. The project folder can be scanned when beginning and ending work on the project to track the time spent. This does require a clock in the computer or recorder. Bar codes can also be used to track equipment such as cardiopul-

---

COMPUTER APPLICATIONS IN EDUCATION ADMINISTRATION

Planning functions

Needs analysis tool
Developing, tracking, and forecasting budgets
Project planning and tracking
Tracking equipment and supply inventory
Tracking instructors from outside the department, such as unit-based educators
Productivity reporting

Daily operations

Program registration and correspondence
Classroom and instructor scheduling
Daily and monthly program calendars

Record keeping and reporting

Employee training records
Department reports (e.g., annual reports, instructor program evaluation reports, and quality-assurance reporting)
Specialized management information reports (for both department personnel and other hospital clients)

monary (CPR) manikins or audiovisual equipment. Bar codes can also track library and reference books, course curriculum, and course materials. A bar code reader can replace handwritten attendance sign-in sheets if a bar code is affixed to the back of each employee badge.

For daily operations, PC software is capable of handling all aspects of program registration. This includes the generation of class rosters, confirmation notices, mailing labels, program evaluation forms, student transcripts, and program certificates of attendance. The computer eliminates the multiple actions it would take to perform each of these functions separately. Once the initial data are entered, the push of a single key can generate the various pieces of program correspondence included in the system. When using a PC to handle program registration and record keeping, educators need access to personnel data from the human resources department. A download of data every 2 weeks can keep educators up to date on employment status, job title, and work location of each employee. A good rule of thumb is to download this information after every payday. Human resource information system departments make sure employee data are accurate so that employees are compensated correctly.

Scheduling software eliminates time-consuming paperwork and double-booking of scheduling program dates, classrooms, and educators. The software accepts a set of givens about available resources and then accommodates the schedule request made. The computer can print out a daily schedule of classroom events to be posted on the classroom door. Annual program calendars can also be printed using this same database.

The large database built by the entry of registration and program attendance records allows users to obtain special management reports. Usage patterns for services can be examined. For example, hospital departments that do or do not send employees to hospital orientations can be identified. The percentage of hospital staff who have attended fire safety training in a given year and their departments can be accessed. The list of possible reports is limited only by software, personal creativity, and the way the database is designed in the first place. It is important to think about what information is to be retrieved *before* entering it, remembering the acronym GIGO meaning "garbage in, garbage out."[12] The education department can track its own performance by entering educator evaluation, department quality-assurance, and objectives analysis data to provide the information necessary to generate specific reports in each area. A program evaluation tool that assigns a number to various aspects of instructor performance may be used (Fig. 10-1). This yields a numeric instructor evaluation average, which can be used in development efforts and instructor performance appraisal. Narrative comments can be placed on the back of the card.

Finally, a software package can be used that allows for the purging of unwanted records from the current files. These files can be deleted altogether, as in the case of an employee who leaves the system, or archived for later use. Having a historical record of department activities on diskettes allows for easy retrieval of information. This also makes it easier to create trending reports that compare activities over a period of years.

Program Title _____
Program Date _____
Instructor _____

Place an x in the box that you think is appropriate.	1 Excellent	2 Very good	3 Good	4 Fair	5 Poor
1. Instructor's manner					
2. Instructor's knowledge					
3. Content applies to my job					
4. My understanding of content					
5. Encouraged, accepted, and responded					
6. Covered stated objectives to questions					
7. Use of audiovisual aids					
8. Overall rating of the instructor					
9. Overall rating of the program					
10. Physical facilities					

Fig. 10-1   Program evaluation form.

COMPUTER APPLICATIONS IN EDUCATION INSTRUCTION

The computer is revolutionizing education instruction. From computer-assisted instruction to computerized graphics packages to interactive video, the world of instructional technology is exploding with new applications. This presents exciting learning opportunities for both students and educators. Students reap the benefits of interesting learning packages tailored to meet their specific, personal needs at a time convenient to their schedules.[5] Instructors gain freedom from repetitive tasks and time to devote to more creative teaching projects. Student and educators gain by the faster and more effective transfer of knowledge.[4] The two main application areas in computerized education instruction are instructional adjuncts and instructional technology (box).

Instructional Adjuncts

Presentation packages, such as Harvard Graphics, Lotus, Freelance, and Microsoft Powerpoint, not only save instructors time and money but also produce final products that look more professional. A PC connected to a color printer, plotter (for overhead transparencies), or camera (for 35-mm slides) allows educators to enter text in a variety of letter styles and sizes, in addition to entering graphs, charts, symbols, and picture. A full-color palette is available to add visual interest and emphasis.

Word-processing software, such as Word Perfect, Word, and Ami Pro, allow for easy production, alteration, and storage of program handouts and course

---

COMPUTER APPLICATIONS IN EDUCATION INSTRUCTION

Instructional adjuncts
Graphics production
Handout and manual production
Literature searches
Test construction and analysis

Instructional technology
CAI
IVD

---

manuals. When a laser jet printer is used, the quality of printed text is comparable with that produced by a professional typesetter. Access to electronic databases and bulletin boards shortens the length of time required for a manual literature review. This access also ensures a more comprehensive and current database. A number of health care and education databases exist. Users pay a fee to hook up to an on-line database and are charged by the number of hours the service is used. Staff development educators can contract directly with the database producer, or they can use a variety of database vendors. A database vendor can allow access to a wide array of databases through one vendor versus multiple service contracts with each database producer. The subscription fee buys a password, phone line, and training to use the system. It is currently possible to access databases through compact disk technology (CD-ROM). Users can perform their own literature searches with CD-ROM. However, two drawbacks to this approach exist—the amount of time needed to perform a personal search and the information that can be accessed not always being the most recent. For example, because compact disks are updated and reissued quarterly to subscribers, journal articles published 3 months before the search may be missed. However, subscribing to a compact disk system is less expensive. The quality of any computerized literature search also depends on the search parameters used to identify an area of interest. The computer search is only as good as the identifying word parameters used to direct it.

Electronic Networking

Another valuable tool for educators lies in electronic networking. "Electronic networks link computers of various sizes and kinds. Computers on a given network share certain common specifications, called 'protocols,' that allow them to 'talk' to each other. Individual computers, which send and receive messages on a network, are called 'nodes.' A node may serve one person or thousands. Nodes are managed by systems operators."[28] Using a computer, modem, and communication software gives users access to up-to-the-minute professional news and information services. This is the ultimate networking tool. Standard costs include telephone charges and a user fee determined by the system operator. Several worldwide systems exist that connect computers in academic and research settings. In these instances the organizations become the systems operators. The organizations pay a fixed rate for the service, and individuals are not charged for their use of the system.

In a recent article, Holtzclaw, Underman-Boggs, and Wilson outlined the ways a network may be used in the following list[13]:

1. Free long-distance communication
2. The option of writing and transmitting messages to a single operation
3. Service provided 24 hours a day
4. Message storage for recipients
5. Access to electronic newsletters and forums
6. Capability for transferring documents created on and uploaded from PCs to others on the network

Currently, three major international networks exist—Internet, FIDONET, and BITNET. Internet, with the largest worldwide coverage, is owned by the U.S. government and managed by the National Science Foundation. Users can access Internet most frequently through an organizational resource. Electronic mail (e-mail); telnet sessions (communications with a remote host computer); file transfers; and synchronous, interactive messaging are all supported by Internet.

Internet has three host computer resources of special significance to nurses. Internet access allows telnet sessions to the Virginia Henderson International Nursing Library and to E.T. NET. There is now Internet access to the National Library of Medicine MEDLARS family of databases via GRATEFUL MED. A telnet session to Sigma Theta Tau International Honor Society of Nursing's Virginia Henderson International Nursing Library furnishes access to the on-line Directory of Nurse Researchers, to abstracts of recent scientific sessions sponsored by several nursing organizations and to a database of databases of nursing research–relevant information.[28]

FIDONET is an individually owned and operated midsized network. It allows for the pursuit of individual interests and hobbies, in addition to supporting e-mail, file transfers, and asynchronous and synchronous messaging with a host operator.

BITNET is the smallest international network. It is privately owned by a consortium of colleges and universities and supports the same functions as the Internet.

In addition to these major networks, others are available to nurses. FITNET is the private network of the Fuld Institute for Technology in Nursing Education Network and consists of one computer located in Athens, Ohio. FITNET "serves several hundred members of the Fuld Institute for Technology in Nursing Education Consortium who access the system via computers and modems using two 800 (toll-free) data lines."[28]

E.T. NET (Educational Technology Network) is yet another network and is sponsored by the Educational Technology Branch of the Lister Hill National

Center for Biomedical Communications. This network focuses on interactive software and hardware resources in the health sciences.

A subset of this electronic network is the electronic bulletin board. "The user calls a central number to log onto a bulletin board account and options are selected from a menu once the connection is made. Bulletin boards are often maintained by organizations to keep their affiliates informed of such information as professional meetings, policy issues, program schedules and resources."[13] A bulletin board is not the same as a network, although some bulletin boards are offered through national networks. Bulletin boards may assess a direct charge for access, or they may have a central number that must be called. This generates a long-distance telephone charge.

Aside from access to research information, electronic networking allows distance communication between instructors and students at remote sites.[13] This may become increasingly important as single hospitals join multihospital systems and education departments are combined to offer services more efficiently.

Test Writing

Computer software can also help busy nurse educators write and analyze test items. McNeal[18] describes a software package that she developed. When this software package is combined with a word-processing package and printer, it allows a hard-copy examination to be generated. The program, called *RN Banker*, "is flexible enough to allow for the sequential numbering of test items; the alteration of stems, distractors, and options to develop new test items." The program permits the creating and saving of several hundred test items on one disk. Not only does this save time for instructors and typists, but it also allows for greater depth and variety in test-item development. Purchasing a Scantron Forms Analysis Package (SFAP) can relieve educators of manual test grading. Learners fill in a card with their answers, and then Scantron grades the cards and keeps a record of the scores. Statistical Package for the Social Sciences (SPSS) allows nurse educators to perform statistic analysis of the previously scanned test questions. Although scanning packages limit the level of knowledge that can be tested, they can be useful in administering routine tests given in high volumes.

Instruction Technology

Computer-Assisted Instruction. CAI has come of age as a teaching tool. As stand-alone applications or as an adjunct to other methods of instruction, CAI has benefited learners and educators alike. The list of applications and CAI formats available is long. Drills, practices, tutorials, and simulations can assist learners to acquire new knowledge and skills, refresh previously learned knowledge and skills, and develop clinical decision-making capabilities in a safe environment. The following describes more detailed applications.

Educators have many routine and repetitive tasks to accomplish during orientation. For example, certifying nurses in drug knowledge and calculation, specific nursing skills, and CPR must all be covered during orientation. Working in a learning laboratory with a CAI program allows learners to work through orientation material at their own pace while the computer automatically scores the results and enters them into the employee training record. Developmental needs can be identified immediately, and interventions can be made to correct only those deficits identified for each employee, thereby individualizing and shortening orientation. CAI would be beneficial for any other repetitive, high-volume program such as JCAHO in-service programs or annual skill certification. The productivity gains from CAI are enormous.

Nurses in the clinical areas can participate in continuing education activities around the clock through CAI. Programs exist in such areas as fluid and electrolyte balance, arterial blood gas interpretation, and arrhythmia recognition. Again, nurses can select programs specific to their needs. They can search for patient situations that they might not frequently encounter in their practice. Howard[14] developed a simulation program to investigate cognitive and affective gains using a computerized cardiopulmonary arrest situation. The simulation was designed to recreate the events that occur just before and immediately after the discovery of an unresponsive patient. Howard found a significant increase in knowledge, as evidenced by dramatically improved posttest scores, and perceived confidence in handling an arrest after participants completed the simulation.

CAI has great application in teaching clinical decision-making skills. Patient care simulations allow nurses to practice efficient data collection, practice cue clustering for quick interpretation of patient problems, and otherwise observe a variety of cause-and-effect relationships.[5] Because the simulation compresses time, learners can see the long-term effects of a decision. The branching capability of CAI also allows patient situations to change in response to decisions made by learners. Of course, all this can be accomplished without harm to patients or embarrassment to learners when an incorrect action is chosen.

Simulation can also be used to teach in nonclinical areas of nursing. Time management and delegation skills can be taught simulating a patient care assignment. Choices made in setting priorities and delegating work can demonstrate favorable or unfavorable outcomes for completing work within a specified time frame, such as an 8-, 10-, or 12-hour shift. Staff budget awareness can also be raised. Altering the dollar amount spent on a one-line item, such as dressing supplies, can demonstrate a dramatic difference in the final bottom line for the nursing unit's budget.

The decision to use CAI depends on cost effectiveness and suitability, that is, if the staff development educator can save significant learner and educator time by using CAI and achieve the same or improved instructional outcomes. Time away from the job is the greatest cost in any educational program. This is followed closely by educator time. The literature certainly documents that CAI can save time for learners and educators. Other questions to ask include the following[1,5]:
1. Can the program be used without significant repetition?

Table 10-1   Cost effectiveness of traditional and CAI approaches to education*

Traditional approach		CAI approach	
Development costs			
32-hour preparation		Purchase CAI program	$ 200
× $18/hour instructor salary = $ 576		Purchase PC and color monitor + $1000	
Presentation costs			
1 program/month		2 hours/month coordination	
× 8 hours × $18/hour	= $1728	time × 12 months × $18/hour	= $ 432
Total program costs	$2304		$1632

*Based on an 8-hour program.

2. Can learners gain new insight or perspective with each additional use?
3. How many learners can use the program?
4. How many different areas can use the program?

The program that can be used the most times without repetition by the largest number of learners is the most cost effective.

A useful assessment model for weighing cost effectiveness should compare the development and presentation costs of traditional classroom learning with CAI. Table 10-1 demonstrates one approach for comparing CAI costs with traditional learning costs. Because initial development costs are fixed and annual presentation costs are so low, the cost per participant decreases each year the program is used. The program becomes even more cost effective if large numbers of the staff use it.

In deciding to purchase a vendor-produced program, staff educators need to evaluate the program's quality and usefulness. Bolwell[5] outlined the major points to consider in selecting CAI software (box).

Interactive Video. IVD is the latest computerized instructional option. IVD combines the technology of a videodisc, computer, and monitor to produce a moving picture that responds to computer commands. Levin's description of the CAI experience[29] eloquently describes the power of this technology:

It enables the learner to participate actively in the unfolding of an educational television presentation that is individualized to the learner's own interest level, knowledge base, and learning rate. The learner is in control, as with a book, but the information is presented through vivid personalities, multiple sound and music tracks, and motion picture action...[yet] unlike a book...[it] spontaneously reacts differently according to the immediate decisions of the student.

In a recent article, Rizzolo[22] describes four models of videodisk players:

Level 0 plays back linear applications (such as video movies and exercise workouts). Level

---

CRITERIA FOR SELECTING CAI SOFTWARE

Ease of use
Easy to begin program
User controls pace and sequence
Instructions easy to follow

Interactive characteristics
Frequent and varied interaction
Immediate and satisfying feedback

Graphics
Includes color and animation

Rapid calculation
Tracks student scores
Totals scores and calculates percentages
Performs test analysis

Interest level
Motivates learner
Individualized by use of branching
Individualized by use of varied feedback

Content
Accurate
Logical sequence
Suited to your audience

Modified from Bolwell C: *Evaluating Computer Assisted Instruction*, New York, 1989, National League for Nursing.

I has the added capacity of allowing a person to access individual frames and view them forward or backward at any speed. Level II has a built-in, programmable microprocessor. Based on the user's response, in a decision frame, the program will branch to another section of the disk. Combining a videodisk player with a personal computer creates yet another model: a level II system allowing infinitely more complex design, branching, and record keeping. Several interactive video designers have added peripheral devices to the basic system, creating a multimedia blend of video, audio, and computer.

IVD offers the clear advantages of realism and active involvement in the learning process. "The videodisc brings to the screen clear views of the patient, the equipment or the setting, rather than relying on the printed word or computer-generated graphics to get the message across."[29] This combination of realism and active involvement improves the transfer of knowledge. Land et al[15] reported on two studies that demonstrated improved posttest scores and decreased study time for experimental groups who used IVD as opposed to control groups who did not use IVD in an introductory biology class.

Many of the initial IVD programs were developed for medical education.

However, many nursing programs now exist, including programs about basic anatomy and physiology, basic and advanced life support, general nursing skills, hospital safety, infection control, monitoring and interpretation, and physical assessment and programs in specialty areas of nursing practice such as critical care, geriatrics, and emergency nursing.[5] An excellent resource for nursing software programs is the *Directory of Educational Software for Nursing* by Christine Bolwell. Now in its fourth edition, this directory describes available instructional software and is a great asset to educators who are responsible for making software purchases.

Other technologies that are similar to IVD include digital video interactive (DVI) and compact disk interactive (CD-I). DVI is designed to eliminate the videodisk and videodisk player.[10] All video and audio are stored in the computer on a CD-ROM. CD-I also stores the data on a CD-ROM. These three systems function similarly.

Compressed video is another version of interactive video communication that can be used in real-time meetings, training, and patient treatment. High-speed telephone lines or fiber-optic cables are used to connect one remote site to another. Dialing the phone initiates a two-way, interactive conference within seconds.

Special equipment is necessary to make this work. "At each site (host and end-user), the equipment is a self-encased, stand-alone unit that includes the following[19]:

- A robotized camera
- Two monitors: one to see the person at the end-user site and another for the person at the host site to preview any documents, graphics, or images that are to be shared
- A notebook-sized tablet that has a penbased stylus to maneuver the cameras, zoom in and out, and manipulate communication
- A codec (the "brain" of the system), which is a coder/decoder that compresses and decompresses the real-time audio and video images
- A table microphone
- A telephone

This technology can be used to connect patients to hospital or physician offices; conduct business meetings with audiences who are at numerous, distant sites; or hold educational programs that reach individuals or groups at multiple sites. This allows for reduced travel time and expenses, makes it possible to train staff on site, allows hospitals to network with other hospitals, extends services to rural communities, and provides services to community groups.

The primary drawbacks to using IVD continue to be the lack of standardization in the industry and the high cost. The compatibility problem is more acute in IVD because three different technologies (computer, videodisk player, and monitors) must work together. It is possible to make a substantial investment in equipment and then gain little from the equipment because little compatible software exists.

Whether IVD is purchased or produced, it is expensive. Developing a system in-house involves a team of professionals including the interactive producer,

FACTORS TO CONSIDER IN CAI SELECTION

Project and resource considerations

What is the nature of the lesson and the interaction (i.e., tutorial versus simulation versus drill and practice)?
What computer equipment will be used?
How much can be spent on development?
How much staff expertise is available?
How soon will the finished product be needed?
Is there a commercially available courseware on the market that would meet the needs of the staff development department?

Lesson considerations

What will be created?
Consider the nature and purpose of content. Consider whether it will be numeric-based, text-focused, or involve visual cues.
What educational approach will be taken (i.e., tutorial versus drill and practice versus simulation)?
How will the program be used both now and in the future?
For example, will it be a stand-alone lesson or will other modules be added to it?
What type of evaluation will be done?
For example, will the lesson provide feedback on each question or provide an overall measure of learning at the end of the program?
What equipment will be used?
Aside from the basic computer hardware, determine whether color, touch screens, high-capacity storage devices, synthetic speech, or videotape or videodisk players are needed.
Who will do the authoring?
For example, has the person had previous computer experience or authoring system experience? Could the author work as a team with a more experienced programmer?
What specific authoring system features are needed?
Having a detailed design plan helps in choosing the system that will provide the appropriate features.

Authoring system features

System requirements
Compatibility of the system's equipment with the peripherals; amount of RAM (random access memory) and video interfaces the authoring system supports
Nature of the developed courseware
Group or individual use; able to be used on a local area network (LAN)
Screen display features
Size and style of text, graphics capabilities, color, sound, animation, screen transition options, and ability to import graphics from other sources
Branching and input capabilities

Modified from Christensen MN, Murphy MA: *Comput Nurs* 8(2):73, 1990.

FACTORS TO CONSIDER IN CAI SELECTION—CONT'D

Linear, freeform, one per row, random pool, and list access; touch screen, videodisk, and voice input devices

Questioning strategies

Allows for multiple choice, matching, fill-in, true or false, yes or no, single-word questions; response options include text, numbers, click and touch area, keypress, moving objects, and menu options

Answer judging capabilities

Includes exact matches, string matching, numeric range, and free text

Feedback and response strategies

Time limits or answer limits to student response; feedback required or optional

User friendly

What levels are possible? Is extensive keyboarding necessary?

Recordkeeping and performance tracking

Can the system record and track student responses? Is all input or are only correct responses recorded? Can customized reports be easily created?

User support

Does the vendor provide adequate documentation (training manuals that are understandable)? What other types of support are available (e.g., telephone hot lines, support groups, or newsletters)?

instructional designer, content specialist, writers and editors, media producers, and packager.[8] If the training budget is slim, the manager must think carefully before investing in IVD.

Authoring Systems. If the decision is made to produce CAI programs in-house, the staff development department needs to select an authoring approach. The use of programming languages, such as C++, C, or Visual Basic, offers maximal flexibility but requires in-depth programming knowledge. Authoring languages, such as Basic Macromedia Director or Video Fusion, allow the user to enter text and create graphics through simple programming commands. Other capabilities include animation and other special effects; however, their features may be limited, and extensive learning time may be required to use them. "Authoring systems are predeveloped software packages (such as QUEST or COURSE OF ACTION), which guide the developer through the creating of a lesson in a logical relatively quick and easy fashion."[7] Depending on the user's knowledge and the features of the authoring system, a fairly sophisticated program can be developed in-house in much less time than with a programming or an authoring language.

Three major areas must be considered when deciding on an approach. These include general questions about the project and the staff development department's resources, the nature of the lesson to be produced, and specific authoring system features. The box provides an overview of the major issues that need to be addressed.

TEACHING COMPUTER SKILLS TO OTHERS

Training staff development personnel and other hospital staff in computer concepts and applications is also a part of the staff development educator's job. In approaching this task, it is important to consider the person doing the training and the way that the training experience should be designed. Training may be accomplished by the facility's information systems department, staff development educators, or area trainers such as preceptors. The information systems department may have computer expertise but lack the resources to devote time to orientation or continuing education computer programs. They may also lack the instructional skills to develop and deliver content in an understandable, non-threatening manner. Staff development educators may lack computer knowledge themselves. Adequate time should be devoted to training instructor staff to use the system. Flaugher[9] recommends the preceptor approach because it ensures on-site access to a resource person. Furthermore, the preceptor is familiar with the jargon, services, and work routines of the area and is in a better position to address application questions specific to this area. On-site preceptors are already recognized by the staff and may enjoy a greater degree of acceptance than an outside individual. Finally, these preceptors would be available for ongoing follow-up and reassurance. A combined centralized and decentralized approach might be the ideal way to provide the best training. Information systems' staff and/or staff development educators could provide the general knowledge of the system; area preceptors could provide unit-specific applications. Area preceptors would also need adequate time to become oriented with the system, including hands-on practice using a test system or dummy database.

Once trainers are identified, instructional design features can be addressed. Axford[3] emphasizes that computer training includes the cognitive, affective, and psychomotor domains of learning. On the cognitive level, learners require an overview of computer terminology, an overview of the particular system to be used, understanding of the system's relationship to the work, and access to a user or reference manual. On a cognitive level, educators may need to overcome resistance to change and computer phobia on the part of the staff. The learning environment must be nonthreatening, and positive advantages to using the system should be shared. In the psychomotor domain, basic keyboarding skills may be all that is required to operate the system. If technologies such as penlights and touch screens are used, this may not be an issue. However, trainees will need individual or paired practice at the computer terminal to fully master the psychomotor and cognitive aspects of the new system.[11] It is generally recommended that no more than two trainees work at a terminal and the trainer:trainee ratio should be 1:8.

Planning of a computer system should include determining who will do the training, the instructional approach to be used, the resource materials that are needed, who will prepare the reference materials, and the expected implementation schedule. Attention to these questions will make implementation easier for all concerned. Gonce-Winder, Kidd, and Lenz[11] wrote an overview article about the software and human consideration of computer system use. This article may serve as a useful reference for staff developers.

IMPLEMENTING COMPUTER FUNCTIONS

Thus far this chapter has focused on computer applications in staff development and ways to plan for computers. It is now time to discuss how to implement computers.

The first step is to decide which programs or features to implement first. The needs analysis serves as a guide. The next step is to gain administrative approval and devise a budget to support the project. Ideally, staff development personnel have done their homework, interviewed key people, and marketed the positive impact that the application will have on the organization. A formal proposal to the administrator also helps. This demonstrates commitment to the application and answers any questions or arguments that might be raised against it.

Next, the hardware and software packages that meet the needs and budget are selected. Staff members who will be responsible for using the technology are selected and trained. Even people who may not work directly with the hardware and software need to know something about the application. For example, if a computerized record-keeping system is implemented, the clerical staff will enter the data and the instructor staff, who will record attendance at programs, need to be familiar with the attendance forms.

This leads to the next step—the design of specific data entry forms and procedures to support the application. For a CAI application, this may involve developing a flowchart for use by the design team. For an administration function, such as computerized registration, a registration form and specific procedures for data collection, entry, reporting, and distribution are needed. Staff and hospital managers must be informed about the system and instructed in its use as related to their own operation. Also, application must be piloted before full implementation begins. This provides a chance to work out any "bugs" and make revisions before the old system has been scrapped.

Finally, it is necessary to provide for ongoing evaluation and revision of the system. This may be built into the department's quality-assurance plan to ensure that this important monitoring function is carried out regularly. The box summarizes the steps for implementing computer applications.

EVALUATING COMPUTER APPLICATION

Once the application is in place, it is important to determine whether the effort was worth the cost. Comparing outcomes with original goals helps evaluate the return on investment. The following lists some evaluation questions:

- Has productivity increased in terms of a greater or faster output of service?
- Have the quality and quantity of management information improved?
- Does it take less time to retrieve records?

IMPLEMENTING COMPUTER APPLICATION

Conduct an adequate needs analysis
Determine features to be implemented first
Obtain administrative approval and budget
Select hardware and software
Select and train responsible staff
Design data entry forms
Design internal policies and procedures
Inform and instruct staff and hospital managers regarding their role in the operation
Pilot the system
Make revisions and fully implement them
Provide ongoing evaluation and revision of the system

- Are records more accurate?
- Has storage space become less of a problem as records, files, handouts, and manuals are transferred to disks?
- Has transfer of knowledge been enhanced for program participants?
- Has it been easier for employees to access services because a computerized program is available at all times?
- Are educators freed from routine and repetitive tasks?
- Are users satisfied with the services delivered?

The answers to these questions determine whether the application is effective. They also provide information for future needs analysis. Evaluating current usage and satisfaction also assists in identifying issues to address in the future, such as the following:

- Does demand continue to outpace capacity?
- Are there applications that cannot be achieved with your current system?
- Does current use point out areas of future possibilities?
- What does the literature say about future technology?
- How may future technology be applied to the staff educator's situation?
- What is being learned from professional organizations and vendors?

The process is one of constant evaluation and change. Examining all of these avenues assists in identifying, assessing, and planning for future computer needs.

FUTURE COMPUTER TRENDS

One area of growing potential in the future of computers is expert systems. As a form of artificial intelligence, expert systems are hard to define precisely. They consist of computer software that assists human problem solving by using logic and heuristics (rules of thumb) to find solutions.

Expert systems are built by knowledge engineers who extract knowledge from experts and translate this knowledge to computers through one of the several expert system development tools available. The system usually consists of two parts, the knowledge base and inference engine. The knowledge base contains the facts, empirical knowledge, formulas, statistical probabilities, and rules that use this information as a basis for solving a problem. The inference engine is separate from the knowledge base. It combines knowledge in the knowledge base with information supplied by the user to arrive at a decision or a solution.[26]

Expert systems are significant because they manipulate knowledge rather than data.

Expert systems are currently being used in medicine (to assist in the diagnosis and treatment of diseases), science, and engineering. They have definite applications in nursing and nursing education. This can most clearly be demonstrated in the area of clinical judgment and decision making. In an expert system, "decision rules are combined into reference chains that indicate the path taken by the system to make a decision. This feature allows the user of an expert system to see into the workings of the system and has implications for educational uses of expert systems."[6] Learners can work forward on the learning chain to study which data are important to gather and cluster to arrive at a particular diagnosis. They can work backward in a chain to determine which data change first when a problem is developing. This allows for early intervention before a full-blown problem arises. The potential of the expert system as a powerful learning tool is obvious. Learners actually experience and work through an analytic process specific to their particular discipline. New nurses can draw on the expert system's theoretic knowledge base to *make* decisions. Experienced nurses can use the knowledge base to consider a range of possible alternatives. "By combining the nurses' clinical knowledge and judgment with the computer's capability to process data and theoretical knowledge, better clinical decisions may be made than either nurse or computer could make alone."[27] Expert systems also hold promise for rapid reference information for nursing professionals providing care outside of their specialty, perhaps in "pull" situations.[25]

The Creighton On-Line Multiple Medical Expert System (COMMES) demonstrates the many uses of an expert system in practice. COMMES has a component subsystem known as the *Nursing Diagnosis Consultant*. Ryan[24] describes the features of COMMES as follows:

To actually consult with the NDC, the nurse provides the NDC one or more patient signs or symptoms. Using an associative semantic network and heuristics, the NDC performs the following functions: (1) proposes one or more potential nursing diagnoses; (2) attempts to confirm the diagnosis by questioning the nurse concerning the presence or absence of additional defining characteristics within the given diagnostic category; (3) recommends confirmation or rejection of the suspected diagnosis on the basis of this additional information; (4) suggests additional potential nursing diagnoses for consideration, on the basis of the system's knowledge of the patient symptoms and its own associate semantic network; and (5) provides the nursing diagnosis definition and possible etiologies.

Application of expert system technology is not limited to staff nurses.

Managers can also improve their analytic abilities. As managers apply a set of ideas to on-the-job situations, they learn as if they had experienced the situation first hand.

Another exciting development is the use of artificial intelligence in CAI packages. This capability increases the interactivity of these applications and allows students to enter hypothetical situations and learn from the resulting solutions presented.

COMPUTER COMPETENCIES FOR STAFF DEVELOPMENT EDUCATORS

As technology continues to develop and enjoy wider use, staff educators will be challenged to not only keep pace but lead the way in integrating technology with practice. *Nursing informatics*, defined as the application of information science to nursing and patient care, has arrived as a specific discipline.[16] A nurse informatics specialist is recognized as a new career in nursing. The University of Maryland has graduate programs to prepare nurses for this new role.[23] Given the increasing computerization of nursing practice, a number of skills and competencies will be requisite for future staff development professional practice. Informatics competencies have been established at three levels of use for practicing nurses, nurse administrators, nurse educators, and nurse researchers by the International Medical Informatics Association (IMIA) Task Force on Education (Working Group and Nursing Informatics). The emphasis of these competency statements lies in the familiarity with a range of computer-based applications in practice, administration, and research and in incorporating computer technology into the education process.[20]

In a broader context, Armstrong[2] surveyed staff development educators about required computer competencies. Respondents identified the following as current requisites:
1. Ability to use the computer as an instructional tool
2. Knowledge about computer technology
3. Recognition of the nurse's role and issues with the computer in health care
4. Use of the nursing process in the development of computerized charting and care plans

Identified future requisites included the following:
1. Use of the computer as an instructional, documentation, and research tool
2. Evaluation of the effects of computerization in nursing
3. Involvement of computers with patient health education

SUMMARY

The challenge for staff development professionals is to become computer literate in the fullest sense of the word. They must research computer applications in hospitals, facilitate communication among various user departments, develop computer learning materials, conduct and evaluate computer training, and incorporate computer technology into their own practice. A world of exciting possibilities awaits.

REFERENCES

1. Adams N: CBT or not CBT? *Training* 30(3):74, 1993.
2. Armstrong ML: Computer competencies identified for nursing staff development educators, *J Nurs Staff Dev* 5(4):187, 1989.
3. Axford RL: Implementation of nursing computer systems: a new challenge for staff development departments, *J Nurs Staff Dev* 4(3):125, 1988.
4. Belfry MJ, Winne PH: A review of the effectiveness of computer assisted instruction in nursing education, *Comput Nurs* 6(2):77, 1988.
5. Bolwell C: *Directory of educational software for nursing*, New York, 1989, National League for Nursing.
6. Chase SK: Knowledge representation in expert systems: nursing diagnosis applications, *Comput Nurs* 6(2):58, 1988.
7. Christensen MN, Murphy MA: Authoring systems: finding the right tool for your courseware development project, *Comput Nurs* 8(2):73, 1990.
8. Dahmer B: When technologies connect, *Train Dev J* 47(1):52, 1993.
9. Flaugher PD: Training computer users, *J Nurs Staff Dev* 4(1):19, 1988.
10. Geber B: Whither interactive videodisc? *Training* 26(3):47, 1989.
11. Gonce-Winder C, Kidd RO, Lenz ER: Optimizing computer-based system use in health professions' education programs, *Comput Nurs* 11(4):199, 1993.
12. Holmes SA: Getting started: data management...beyond basics, *J Nurs Staff Dev* 9(4):202, 1993.
13. Holtzclaw BJ, Underman-Boggs K, Wilson ME: Mail by modem: the BITNET connection, *Comput Nurs* 11(5):242, 1993.
14. Howard EP: Use of a computer simulation for the continuing education of registered nurses, *Comput Nurs* 5(6):208, 1987.
15. Land L et al: Computer-assisted interactive video instruction in nursing (CAIVIN), *J Nurs Staff Dev* 5(6):273, 1989.
16. Lawless KA: Nursing informatics as a needed emphasis in graduate nursing administration education: the student perspective, *Comput Nurs* 11(6):263, 1993.
17. March J, Bernhards J: Software for training administration, *Train Dev J* 43(6):85, 1989.
18. McNeal GJ: Designing a test bank computer program, *Comput Nurs* 7(1):29, 1989.
19. Miller R: Compressed video, *Alliance* Mar 1994, pp 5-10.
20. Peterson HE, Gerdin-Jelger U, editors: *Preparing nurses for using information systems: recommended informatics competencies*, Pub No 14-2234, New York, 1988, National League for Nursing.
21. Reimer MS: Computerized cost analysis for the nursing skills laboratory, *Nurs Educator* 17(4):8, 1992.
22. Rizzolo MA: What's new in interactive video? *Am J Nurs* 89(3):407, 1989.
23. Romano CA et al: Levels of computer education for professional nursing: development of a prototype graduate course, *Comput Nurs* 7(1):21, 1989.
24. Ryan SA: An expert system for nursing practice: clinical decision support, *Comput Nurs* 3(3):77, 1985.
25. Saleem N, Moses B: Expert systems as computer assisted instruction systems for nursing education and training, *Comput Nurs* 12(1):35, 1994.
26. Schank MJ, Doney LD, Seizyk J: The potential of expert systems in nursing, *J Nurs Adm* 18(6):26, 1988.
27. Sinclair UG: Potential effects of decision support systems on the role of the nurse, *Comput Nurs* 8(2):60, 1990.
28. Sparks SM: Electronic networking for nurses, *IMAGE JL Nurs Scholarship* 25(3):245, 1993.
29. Sweeney MA, Gulino C: From variables to videodiscs: interactive video in the clinical setting, *Comput Nurs* 6(4):157, 1988.
30. Zemke R: 12 ways to "micro-manage" the training function, *Training* 20(7):46, 1983.

Computer Resources

ORGANIZATIONS

1. International Association of Information Systems Professionals (IAISP)
   104 Wilmot Road, Suite 201
   Deerfield, IL 60015-5195
   (312) 940-8800 FAX (312) 940-7218
2. American Nurses Association
   Council on Computer Applications in Nursing
   600 Maryland Avenue SW
   Washington, DC 20024
   (202) 554-4444
   FAX: (202) 651-7004
3. National League for Nursing
   National Forum for Computer Professionals in Health Care
   350 Hudson Street
   New York, NY 10014
   1-800-NOW-1-NLN
   FAX: (212) 989-3710

CONSULTATION ABOUT CBE

1. American Nurses Association
   Computer Nurse Directory
   An alphabetical listing by name, state, and functional area of nurses with computer expertise
2. Fuld Institute for Technology in Nursing Education (FITNE)
   28 Station Street
   Athens, OH 45701
   (614) 592-2511
   FAX: (619) 592-2650

Serves as a technical resource to member organizations by serving as a clearinghouse for current information and reviews of software and hardware and as a telephone support service; publishes a quarterly newsletter and offers an electronic bulletin board

3. Healthcare Interactive Video Consortium (HIVC) Project
   201 Silver Cedar Court
   Chapel Hill, NC 27514
   (919) 942-8731
   FAX: (919) 942-3689
   Offers computer expertise and technical support to its members in the area of interactive video and computer-based education

4. National League for Nursing
   Computer Consultation Bureau
   350 Hudson Street
   New York, NY 10014
   1-800-NOW-1-NLN
   FAX: (212) 989-3710

COMPUTER PUBLICATIONS

1. Computers in Nursing
   c/o JB Lippincott Company
   East Washington Square
   Philadelphia, PA 19105
   (215) 238-4200
   FAX: (212) 238-4266

2. Medical Disc Reporter
   c/o Stewart Publishing, Inc.
   6471 Merritt Court
   Alexandria, VA 22312
   (703) 354-8155

3. Nursing Education Microworld
   13740 Harleigh Court
   Saratoga, CA 95070
   (408) 741-0156

COMPUTER CONFERENCES

1. Interactive '96 Conference, organized through:
   Ziff Institute
   25 First Street
   Cambridge, MA 02141
   1-800-34-TRAIN
   FAX: (617) 393-3322

This annual 4-day conference is conducted for computing managers and trainers rather than strictly health care staff. It provides access to state-of-the-art computer technology and applications. A multitude of vendors are also available with their displays.

2. Interactive Healthcare Conference and Exposition, organized through:
   Stewart Publishing, Inc.
   6471 Merritt Court
   Alexandria, VA 22312
   (703) 354-8155
   FAX: (703) 354-2177
   This annual 4-day conference focuses exclusively on the use of interactive video in the health care industry.

3. Nursing Computer Symposium, organized through:
   National Institutes for Health
   Clinical Center, Nursing Department
   Division of Professional Development
   9000 Rockville Pike
   Bethesda, MD 20892
   This 1-day computer symposium consists of paper presentations but does not have vendor displays. It is held every 2 to 3 years.

4. Symposium on Computer Applications in Medical Care (SCAMC), organized through:
   George Washington University
   Office of Continuing Medical Education
   2300 "K" Street
   Washington, DC 20037
   (202) 994-4285
   FAX: (202) 994-1791
   This annual 3-day conference, offered in the fall of each year, includes plenary sessions, presentation of papers, and many vendor displays. The conference is interdisciplinary and includes a nursing track.

5. Fourteenth Annual International Nursing Informatics Conference, organized through:
   Rutgers, College of Nursing
   Continuing Education Program
   University Heights
   216 Conklin Hall
   Newark, NJ 07102
   (201) 648-5895
   FAX: (201) 648-1700
   This 3-day annual conference is geared to provide the latest information on the current use of computers in the health care delivery system. The program is specifically designed for a nursing audience.

ADMINISTRATIVE SOFTWARE PROGRAMS

1. EDU-EZ
   EDUCOS-II
   Educos Training Management and HRD Systems
   Automated Performance Technologies
   111 West 40th Street
   28th Floor
   New York, NY 10018
   FAX: 1-800-343-5797
2. The Education Manager
   CDR Applied Technology, Inc.
   Box 5076
   Madison, WI 53705
   (608) 255-8081
3. The Registrar
   The Scheduler
   Silton-Bookman Systems, Inc.
   20410 Town Center Lane
   Suite 280
   Cupertino, CA 95014
   (408) 446-1170
   FAX: (408) 446-0731
4. Ed-U-Keep
   JMT Enterprises
   15502 Highway 3, Suite M2
   Webster, TX 77598
   (713) 488-6674
   FAX: (713) 448-4584
5. TR Plus
   HRD Software
   22 Software
   Amherst, MA 10002
   1-800-822-2801
   FAX: (413) 253-3490

INTERACTIVE VIDEO COMPANIES

1. Actronics
   810 River Ave.
   Pittsburgh, PA 15212
   1-800-851-3780
   FAX: (412) 828-8987

2. Mirror Systems, Inc.
   2067 Massachusetts Avenue
   Cambridge, MA 02140
   (617) 661-0777

BAR CODE VENDORS

1. Avery Label
   777 E. Foothill Boulevard
   Azusa, CA 91702-1358
   1-800-441-2345 Ext. 545
2. Computype
   2285 W. County Road C
   St. Paul, MN 55113
   (612) 633-0633
   FAX: (612) 496-1650
3. Datacode Systems
   5122 St. Clair Avenue
   Cleveland, OH 44103
   1-800-345-5300
   FAX: (216) 498-3410
4. Watson Label Products
   3684 Forest Park Boulevard
   St. Louis, MO 63108
   (314) 652-6715
   FAX: (314) 652-5743

DATABASES FOR NURSE EDUCATOR USE

1. Educational Resources Information Center (ERIC)
   ERIC Processing and Reference Facility
   1301 Piccard Drive, Suite 300
   Rockville, MD 20850-4305
   1-800-799-3742
   FAX: (301) 948-3695
   Contains findings, projects, technical reports, speeches, unpublished man-
   uscripts, books, and journal articles in the field of education
2. Health Planning and Administration
   National Library of Medicine
   8600 Rockville Pike
   Bethesda, MD 20894
   1-800-638-8480
   FAX: (301) 496-6193
   Covers national and international journals and nonjournals in health care

planning, organization, financing, management, staffing, and related subjects

3. Medlars-on-line (MEDLINE)
   National Library of Medicine
   8600 Rockville Pike
   Bethesda, MD 20209
   (301) 496-6095
   FAX: (301) 496-0822
   Contains all aspects of biomedicine, including the allied health fields, as well as the biological and physical sciences, humanities, and information science as they relate to medicine and health care.

4. CINAHL ONLINE
   Nursing and Allied Health Databases
   CINAHL Corporation
   PO Box 871
   Glendale, CA 91209
   1-800-959-7167
   FAX: (818) 546-5679
   Covers current periodical literature relating to nursing, health care and administration, and other allied health disciplines; all major English-language nursing and selective allied health journals are indexed.

The Process
of Nursing Staff
Development

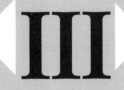

Learning Needs Assessment

11

The first step to designing an effective learning experience is to assess learning needs. Failure to assess these needs accurately can result in well-developed but potentially irrelevant offerings for learners and the organization; Mager[16] says, "If you're not sure where you're going, you're liable to end up someplace else."

Although most authors refer to the initial phase of the educational process as "needs assessment," these needs relate to learning. That is, staff development educators may uncover or verify other types of needs, but those needs are not the primary reason for assessment and do not relate to the learning design in the same way. Performance, personal, and human needs are the most common uncovered needs that are not learning needs. *Performance needs* refer to the lack of optimal performance at times related to causes other than a knowledge/skill deficit. For instance, an individual may know the way to perform but does not do so because of impediments in the worksetting such as lack of reward, supplies, or time. According to Mager,[16] the problem is a performance deficit, not a knowledge/skill deficit, and cannot be solved by a class.

A personal need is a desire to learn a topic that is not used on the job but is of interest to the individual. For example, an individual who works in a rehabilitation unit may want to attend a class about emergency triage. A *human need* refers to one of Maslow's hierarchy of needs—safety, security, belonging, or self-fulfillment. An important *safety* need may be learning an isolation technique or karate; an important *belonging* need may be the ability to speak Spanish. Personal needs and human needs are important[23] and deserve the attention of staff development educators. However, the ability to satisfy these needs through staff development activities may be limited. However, "disregard for the needs of the employees as individuals can serve as a deterrent in their motivation for continued learning."[22]

Need is typically defined as a deficiency or lack of something requisite, desirable, or useful. Mager and Pipe[17] have changed that definition for most staff development educators. *Discrepancy* is the preferred term for learning needs. A discrepancy is "a difference, a lack of balance between the actual and the desired."[17] It may indicate the difference between the present and the desired performance. For example, a professional nurse who is experienced in providing care to patients undergoing open heart surgery but has not functioned on a general surgical unit may have a discrepancy in acceptable performance on the latter unit. Discrepancy merely conveys a situation other than a perfect fit. Describing a nurse as having a deficiency conveys a negative judgment. Thus learning needs assessments reveal discrepancies between the present knowledge and skill performance and the organization's standards of desired knowledge and skill performance.

PERSPECTIVES OF LEARNING NEEDS ASSESSMENTS

Assessing learning needs is a crucial element for planning educational activities. Learning needs serve several purposes and strongly influence subsequent educational activities. Four perspectives of the value of learning needs assessments are timing, marketing, priorities, and data.

Timing

Cooper[5] addresses the issue of timing by saying, "Learning needs assessments are usually valid only for short periods of time, since needs change with modifications in practice." Timing suggests that needs assessments must be conducted to meet *current* learning needs. With the rapid changes of society in general and in health care in particular, needs assessment must capitalize on the fit between the need and current demands of practice. Thus timing assumes an even greater magnitude because learning needs "expire" or are reconfigured as time passes. For example, admissions of patients with burns may cause a need for classes regarding the area of burned patients and fluid and electrolyte balance. That need for information must be met immediately. However, 2 months later, there may not be any patients with burns and no immediate need for that knowledge. In essence, planning learning activities to correct discrepancies must occur in a fairly restricted time with attention to those changes in the environment that created the learning needs.

Marketing

Learning needs assessments also serve as a way to market specific courses and the value of the staff development department.[26] Conducting needs assessments provides information about topics that learners themselves may not have thought of as a need. The needs assessment makes learners aware of the topic's importance so that learners then desire to know about that topic and recognize the staff development department as a valuable resource to provide this needed knowledge.

According to Kidd,[14] "the main reason, of course, for the concentration on interests [needs] as a source for educational objectives is the close relationship that this seems to bear with gaining the attention of people and having them participate in educational endeavors." The needs assessment imparts awareness of a topic, which stimulates interest and leads to a desire to know more about that topic. This motivates learners to attend a learning experience. As a result, the needs assessment serves as a marketing device to get people to attend a course.

The manner in which needs assessments are conducted also relates to marketing strategies. If the questionnaire, for example, is carelessly designed and boring, learners may assume that the staff development class will be boring too. If the questionnaire is complex, long, and filled with five-syllable words, learners may assume the classes will be taught in the same manner. On the other hand, if the needs assessment form is interesting, attractively designed, and appropriately focused on the topics of interest to learners' clinical service, learners may assume the classes will be similar. Thus needs assessments are *always* a marketing opportunity.

Priorities

Staff development as a nursing service-based activity must be concerned with nursing service priorities. Some organizations have a policy that performance discrepancies identified by quality improvement audits have priority over discrepancies identified by other methods. Other organizations may try to enhance their capabilities for a specialty niche, such as cardiovascular care, so that all needs related to cardiovascular nursing have a higher priority than other topics. The development of a specialty unit for the rehabilitation of patients with neurologic disorders would set certain priorities for classes on that topic. Perhaps the need for cross-training of staff members so that they can safely practice on a variety of units dictates that certain topics have higher priorities. The flux in the nursing market influences the priorities of needs identified on assessments. Some organizations that had firm policies dictating that staff development classes must relate to job requirements may have policies allowing classes on personal and human needs during staff shortages and may eliminate these opportunities when no staff shortage exists. Harrison[10] suggests that "with a plethora of opportunities in the many new as well as more traditional sectors of the health-care industry, talented registered nurses will have their pick of places to contribute and grow." Inherent in these growth opportunities for nurses are opportunities to learn about topics in which they are personally interested and a mandate to remain knowledgeable and skilled to remain competitive. Some organizations have continued to place the highest priority on performance-based learning, such as in clinical assessment centers and unit-based self-learning modules, or to emphasize the needs of evening- and night-shift personnel.[4]

Staff development educators should be proactive in setting priorities, not just reactive in trying to meet priorities as set by nursing service. This is accomplished by persuasive reports and proposals for learning experiences that may not be on the high-priority list of others but which have been determined to be high priority by educators through the observation of learners or repeated problems on clinical units. Through cutting-edge programming, staff development educators can meet the learning needs of staff and the programmatic needs of the organization. However, "the staff development or continuing education department cannot respond directly to all of the learning needs that are identified."[19] As a result, staff development educators must determine which needs assessment finding must be developed first, has the greatest interest, is the most prevalent, and can be referred to another source or delayed.

Data

Finally and most obviously, learning needs assessments are crucial to providing useful data. The nature of the data may be broad (for example, physical assessments) or specific (for example, abdominal percussion sequence). Generally, the more targeted the data, the more useful the data are. It is important, however, to gather data about the health care environment, new and continuing services, learners' styles and learning preferences, actual current performance, and standards that influence practice. In organizations where staff are assigned to a shift, this source must also be considered.[7]

The most obvious source of standards influencing practice is the Joint Commission on Accreditation of Healthcare Organizations (JCAHO), but many others exist such as state nurse practice acts and other state regulatory agencies (for example, health departments and professional organizations). Professional standards of practice, current literature, and research reports are also important data sources that influence standards. Staff development educators are responsible for gathering data from many sources to validate the findings of needs assessments. Depending on only one source does not produce sufficient data to set priorities for learning activities.

Interrelationship

Timing, marketing, priorities, and data are interrelated in the structuring of needs assessments and the designing of subsequent learning experiences. For example, data from needs assessments may reveal a discrepancy that requires immediate action, that is, the immediate design of a learning experience. Learner participation in a high-priority class results in enhanced clinical performance and professional growth and satisfaction. The quick implementation of an excellent learning experience also markets the staff development department as an effective resource for meeting clinical nursing needs. This dynamic interaction of timing, marketing, priorities, and data is the challenge of needs assessment.

FRAMEWORK FOR IDENTIFYING LEARNING NEEDS

At first glance, assessing needs appears to be an internally focused standards- and performance-based activity. This may be true if time is a major constraint. On the other hand, that is not the comprehensive view of needs assessments.

Tobin, Wise, and Hull[22] identified a comprehensive model that results in a more accurate identification of needs than does the time-constrained approach. Fig. 11-1 shows comprehensive sources of needs and reflects the crucial influence that the needs assessments process has on subsequent activities of implementation and evaluation.

Health care agencies, specific communities, and individuals operate in a broad societal and universal context. Naisbitt and Aburdene[18] describe the ways global influences affect daily lives resulting in society shaping the community, thus influencing the health care organization. Health care and nursing personnel are also influenced by the community and society at large, and they influence needs within the organization. These needs influence the selection of assessment strategies that may affect learning activities. Specific agency, community, and health care personnel are sources of needs that contribute to an identification of organizational, health care, and individual needs. Organizational and individual needs require further elaboration in the context of health care needs; they both result in defined learning needs. These two data sets must be meshed to determine a consensus of needs and mutual goal setting for deciding priorities. After the implementation of learning opportunities to meet the identified needs, evaluation takes place. Evaluation of outcomes can be in terms of cost effectiveness, cost benefits, optimum health care for patients, and competency in practice for individuals. The feedback results in the consideration of needs generated by the agency, community, and health care personnel.

Bowman et al[1] refer to a synthesis of learner and organizational needs in a comprehensive needs assessment model. The topics identified in the needs assessment can be labeled as focus A, B, C, D, and E. They are then arranged in a grid depicting high and low priorities for the organization and learners. Fig. 11-2 shows the way these data are evaluated to determine which topics will be addressed in programs and implemented to correct discrepancies. In Fig. 11-2, focus B clearly has a consensus and high priority for both the organization and learners, whereas focus E shows no priority for either the organization or learners. Focus A shows needs for only the organization, and focus C shows needs for only the individuals. Focus D is a need with high individual priority and low organizational priority.

As a result of this analysis, focus B will be addressed in a learning experience, E will be ignored, and D and C should be implemented if the belief of the organization is to meet the needs of learners and the organization. On the other hand, if the organization's philosophy only stresses concern for the organization, focus A and focus B will be developed into a program, whereas focus D will not be a priority and focus C will be ignored.

Reaching conclusions or priorities about learning needs should also include another screening activity, as proposed by Mager and Pipe.[17] The process begins by asking whether a discrepancy exists and whether it is important (box). If a need is unimportant, it has a low priority when planning classes. It should also be asked whether this is a skill that the person once had. Another critical question is whether the skill is used often. Again, if a need is unimportant and sel-

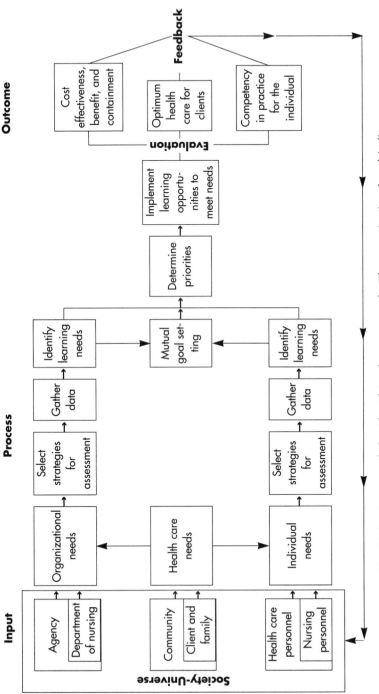

Fig. 11-1   Framework for identifying learning needs. The organizational and individual needs form the basis for mutual goal setting and priority determination. (From Tobin HM, Wise PSY, Hull PK: *The process of staff development: components for change,* ed 2, St Louis, 1979, Mosby.)

Focus	A	B	C	D	E
Organization need	X_H	X_H	—	X_L	X—
Individual need	—	X_H	X_H	X_H	X—
Consensus of needs	X_O	$X_{O,I}$	X_I	$X_{I,O}$	X—

Key: X = defined need
    H = high priority
    L = low priority
    — = no priority
    O = organization
    I = individual

Fig. 11-2   Establishing consensus and priority of individuals' and organizations' needs for learning.

DISCREPANCY ANALYSIS

1. Is there a discrepancy identified?
2. What is the value of the discrepancy? If it is frequently used and critical, it has a high priority. If it is critical but not frequently used, it may also have a high priority. If it is neither frequently used nor critical, it has low priority.
3. What is the cause of the discrepancy? Is it a knowledge discrepancy or a performance discrepancy?
4. If it is a knowledge discrepancy, did the person once know how to do the task? Does the person need a class or just a quick on-the-job review and a written procedure?
5. If it is a performance discrepancy, what is the cause? Is performance punishing or unimportant? Does nonperformance matter? Maybe what is needed is incentives to perform, job redesign, or positive feedback for performing. A class should not be designed for this.

Modified from Mager RF, Pipe P: *Analyzing performance problems: or "you really oughta wanna,"* Beaumont, Calif, 1970, Fearon.

dom used, planning efforts should not be focused on that need. Conversely, if a need is both important and frequently used, that need has a higher priority in planning efforts. Some skills are important but seldom used, such as cardiopulmonary (CPR) code protocols on a nonacute maternity unit. Although codes are not expected, if a CPR code is necessary, competent performance is critical. Translating such a need to programming is obviously a high priority. Two additional questions have major implications for staff development educators and both relate to peer and administrative support. These questions are as follows: What if a desired performance is punished? What if nonperformance is rewarded? This "need" is not resolved through teaching performers or nonperformers; rather, the need is for different feedback behavior by peers and administrators.

The process of identifying learning needs is time consuming, multidimensional, and complex. However, this task shapes all other educational activities in the staff development department.

LEARNING NEEDS ASSESSMENT STRATEGIES

Before various strategies are addressed, it is important to reiterate that using multiple sources to identify needs yields more accurate information about needs and priorities than only one source. A single source for assessing needs limits the usefulness of the findings by making it more difficult to set priorities. For example, if three different sources indicate a need for a class on pain management, that is a more definitive indicator of the need than if only a questionnaire indicated a need.

Additionally, it is important to consider the response rate (i.e., how many people filled out the questionnaire) for any needs assessment strategy. Response rates are influenced by the specific strategy and the way the strategy is implemented. Although many authors are wary about the ultimate response rate desired, it is safe to say the smaller the sample, the greater the consensus needed to be significant, and that the greater the number of responses (completed assessments), the more reflective the findings. However, this chapter is not intended to address the multiple research factors necessary to design or evaluate needs studies.

Finally, it is probably more cost effective to target one area or topic and develop that topic in depth than it is to conduct general assessments for a broader group. If identifying the specific needs of individuals is important, a target specific assessment is better than a broader assessment. In using these strategies, staff development educators should remember that "the literature describes various methods of conducting needs assessments for different populations and purposes. Many of the tools used and methods selected require further refinement and testing to establish the validity and reliability of instruments."[15]

The following strategies are presented as an overview of approaches for defining needs. For ease in referencing later, these needs assessment strategies are presented in alphabetical order.

Advisory Groups

Advisory groups are composed of people who represent the total population or target audience for staff development programs. This group should not exceed nine people and should meet regularly to be effective. A carefully planned agenda should be circulated before the meeting so that everyone arrives at the meeting with ideas for programs resulting from needs identified in their areas of practice.

Advisory groups can include internal and/or external members of the organization. For large staff development departments, it may be necessary to have several advisory committees for various types of programming. For example, there could be an advisory group for patient education activities that is composed of representative patients and home health care nurses and managers from within the organization. For designing learning experiences for surgical nursing, there could be another committee made up of representatives from the surgical units, surgical suite, and emergency department.

Advisory committees are especially useful as sounding boards for creative programming. If the committee includes experts in an area, that committee can identify programming needs, resources, speakers, and content.

The authority of advisory groups should be clear because an advisory group has different input than a decision-making group. Advisory groups must understand that all their ideas may not be implemented because of competing priorities, budget restraints, or time commitments. Whether used to create a list of cutting-edge topics or expand content in a defined area, advisory groups should be acknowledged for their quality of input.

Anecdotal Notes

Anecdotal notes reflect the observations of specific individuals, units, or clinical concerns. All entries should contain succinct, objective recording of data that reflect a comprehensive view of the individual or situation. A common administrative approach to recall meetings or troubling incidents is a "memo to the file," which is an anecdotal note. A series of these notes about an individual, a unit, or a clinical concern can reveal emerging themes that identify performance discrepancies. For example, a registered nurse may be technically competent but unable to communicate clearly in stressful situations. This need may only be evident when the manager is analyzing anecdotal notes over a period of months.

Brainstorming

Brainstorming as a strategy for needs assessment is conducted by convening a representative group of people who are willing to be free and open about discrepancies in their clinical areas. For example, the first group consideration could be "What classes would people in your clinical areas like to have?" One person records the responses on a blackboard or flip chart. The only rule is that ideas are generated without criticism or praise. An object can be passed among participants; as it is passed from person to person, each person quickly responds with the first idea that comes to mind. There can be several rounds, but the time frame should be tight so that the quality and quantity of output do not diminish. The second question could be "What method of teaching and learning would you suggest for the learning needs?"

Brainstorming is defined in Webster's dictionary as "a series of sudden, violent cerebral disturbances." This is an apt description of the way an individual feels in the process. This definition conveys inspiration, not necessarily logical relationships and synthesis. Brainstorming is a "freewheeling" approach in which outlandish ideas are encouraged. Even when problems (as opposed to general ideas) are being considered, the energy experienced in brainstorming can leave participants feeling energized. Because the approach is so "sudden" and "violent," it is especially valuable to summarize ideas at the meeting's end so that participants see their contributions as a group. Participants also enjoy choosing options from the wide variety of ideas generated. These ideas become the needs assessment and lead to the design of learning experiences.

Checklists and Reiterated Checklists

Checklists are sources of readily available data that indicate learning needs. They may be preexisting or need to be developed. For example, a preexisting checklist for orientation can be used to identify skills, knowledge, values, or a combination of these that are lacking in most orientees. These identified needs can then be incorporated into the routine orientation classes instead of added later as needs are identified.

Checklists that need to be developed can help identify topics for learning. For example, all first-line managers could be asked to identify five topics for a series of management classes. The topics can be listed and returned to all participants for priority rankings. This "reiterated list" can be compared with the tally from the first list to determine the priority of topics. The number of nurses identifying a topic on the first list should be validated by the ranking of the topic on the reiterated list.

Checklists are especially helpful in narrowing the focus of a broad course. For example, if nurses identified the care of patients using respirators as one of their needs, this broad topic should be narrowed to meet the exact aspects of care that are problems. For instance, a checklist of topics pertaining to the care of patients using respirators could indicate the specific highest priority as the content and skill in suctioning techniques.

Critical Incident Technique

This classic technique is based on a critical incident, for example, performing adequately during a CPR code.[8] A specific description of the incident comprises this strategy. An accumulation of incident recordings, when written properly, can reveal specific performance discrepancies. If this technique is to be useful with specific behaviors, there must be a guide for data entry to ensure that all elements are addressed. The following are usually recorded: date, "classification" of the incident, who was observed, what was said and done, and where the incident occurred. In addition, a listing of problems in correct performance could be recorded.

One use of this incident technique for needs analysis is an analysis of a CPR critical incident recording from every unit that had a code within a 3-month period. If each recording is well described and ends with a listing of problems encountered, this can be a valuable source of data for revising the CPR course and practice sessions required of all nurses.

Delphi Technique

The Delphi technique, like the nominal group process, is a specific strategy to obtain consensus and priority. Questionnaires are mailed to the targeted group, responses are summarized, and a new version of the questionnaire is sent to the same responders for additional response. The goal is to obtain a consensus about needs.[6]

For example, in a series of classes for first-line managers, managers could be sent a list of 20 statements related to management responsibilities and asked to respond to each statement in terms of its relevance and importance to them. Their statements and rankings would be tabulated and returned to them for rerating. The information from the Delphi technique can serve as the basis for design of the management course in terms of the priority of topics. Carter and Axford[4] used this approach to obtain a listing of essential knowledge and skills related to computer learning needs, a content area with numerous potential needs.

Focus Groups

Focus groups are designed to provide in-depth information regarding a specific concern or topic.[25] Focus groups are limited to between five and nine people and last about 1 to 1 1/2 hours. There is a leader and an observer who have planned the questions, but the group is allowed latitude in discussing these questions and may stray to other questions that are out of sequence. Sometimes the group discussion is taped with the participants' permission; other times the observer may take notes on important answers or ideas generated. This strategy is designed to maintain a close understanding of consumers by asking their opinions or soliciting their appraisals. Consumers' opinions are *always* valued in excellent organizations.

The focus group can have an informal but targeted discussion about what learners define as their needs. This approach allows for elaboration of ideas and refinement of statements to create more targeted suggestions. This approach is especially useful for including "grass roots" input into future plans or correcting past inadequacies.

Interviews

Interviews provide an opportunity for individuals to share in-depth views, expand on areas of particular concern, and provide examples to clarify their points. Interviewees may be prospective learners or managers of learners.

Interviews can be structured or unstructured. Unstructured interviews typically begin with a general question, such as "What do you think are the biggest problems with working with the new computer?" The interviewee's response then directs further questions. In contrast, structured interviews are guided by a specific list and sequence of questions. Structured interviews have a preestablished format for analyzing responses; unstructured interviews do not have a preestablished format and require more time to analyze trends. The interview technique is especially helpful in needs assessment when it is important to have a thorough understanding of each person's perception of the topic before proceeding to design learning experiences.

Literature Analysis

Remaining current with the literature in various areas of nursing is important to analyze trends and project learning needs for future programs. It can be valuable to delegate literature reviews to the staff development educator responsible for various areas of practice or to the advisory committee member from each area of practice.

For example, literature analysis indicated that the primary care model for nursing delivery was being replaced (or augmented) by the managed care model and that nursing was incorporating unlicensed assistive personnel to provide cost-effective comprehensive service. Awareness of a coming trend allows staff development educators to become knowledgeable about the new delivery system and educators' roles in helping staff adapt to a new system. As a result, the needs for new classes are identified early, and literature packets and films can be evaluated and purchased as the new system evolves.

Nominal Group Process

The nominal group process is a specific strategy designed to create consensus through the individual ranking of items and a pooling of scores.[6] This process is similar to the Delphi technique because its goal is to obtain consensus; this process differs in that it requires a convened group.

An assembled group defines needs by responding individually to a question and then sharing the individual responses with the entire group in a round-robin. No discussion is allowed. After all responses are shared and written on a flip chart, participants identify similarities and rank the responses with a modified list. Again, each individual responds in turn with a ranking. A pooling of scores creates the targeted needs and priorities. This structured process ensures an orderly process but limits creativity in responses. This process can also be time consuming if there are several small groups sharing their rankings. With one group of 8 to 10 people, the process takes about 2 hours.

This process can be a valuable needs assessment technique for exploring an emerging need. For example, the extent of the need for learning experiences related to ethical topics can be determined by the nominal group process. First-line managers can be asked to list the top 10 ethical problems on their units. A recorder writes on a flip chart as each manager states one ethical problem in turn. This continues around the circle until there are no new items to list. No evaluation or comments are allowed at this time. The meaning of each ethical issue is discussed only if clarification is necessary. Each person ranks the top 10 ethical problems listed. The recorder writes the rank beside each previously listed ethical issue and then mathematically computes the top 10 ethical issues.

Observations

When focusing on an individual's needs, "direct observation of work performance is probably the best method of identifying learning needs."[22] Direct observation has a major marketing influence because prospective learners know educators have at least "seen the trenches," even if they have never been in them. Clinically based staff development educators have a special opportunity to observe performance directly.

For the collected data to be meaningful, the observations must be purposeful and planned. On the other hand, observations may also be made serendipitously and have just as much value as those that were planned. Educational rounds (or grand rounds) provide opportunities for such direct observation.

Observation allows for the opportunity to verify or refute value and performance statements. For example, individuals in orientation may state that appearance is important and that they themselves portray a professional appearance. Direct observation can verify or refute such statements.

Incidental observations may also be useful. Tobin, Wise, and Hull[22] identified some questions to ask when making direct observations in the clinical areas (box).

In using observations as a technique for needs assessment, it is advantageous to use standards to determine the adequacy of performance. It is also necessary to have some validation of interrater reliability so that the report of discrepancies in performance on one unit is the same as the report by another staff development educator on another unit.

Position Analysis

Because all positions have some form of description that conveys typical duties or examples of function, analyzing performance in relation to the actual position description is a crucial technique for needs assessment. One source for needs assessment is an anonymous review of performance ratings, in essence, a tally of which behaviors are met and which are not. Another source for a comparison of position descriptions to performance may be input from a nurse manager. The individual who defines discrepant performance is certainly a third source.

Promotional workshops rely heavily on the analysis of position descriptions for the content and level of desired performance. In addition, new employees typically express most learning needs in relation to a specific position because that description forms the basis for their performance appraisal. As a result, position descriptions are a valuable source for indicating learner needs.

INCIDENTAL QUESTIONS USED DURING DIRECT OBSERVATION OPPORTUNITIES

Where are the registered nurses on the unit most frequently found?
How do the patients appear (e.g., comfortable and safe)?
How are nursing practice skills carried out?
What evidence of planning and organizing nursing care is present?
Does documentation reflect what is happening to the patient?
Are all personnel occupied, or do some seem unusually busy and others often not occupied?
Are the verbal and nonverbal communications conducive to effective working relationships, both between nursing personnel and between nursing and other hospital personnel?

Tobin HM, Wise PSY, Hull PK: *The process of staff development: components for change,* ed 2, St. Louis, 1979, Mosby.

Process Recordings

Process recordings are especially helpful in identifying learning needs related to communication. For example, on a psychiatric unit the process of recording a conversation with a patient may reveal learning needs related to therapeutic communication. Only in retrospect can the nurse and the preceptor or manager identify patterns of communication and ways those patterns may be improved. These recordings may consist of a verbatim report of a conversation recorded by another, or they may be recorded by the nurse after the conversation. Obviously these recordings serve a major purpose for supervision in psychiatric services. They can also serve a major purpose if used on a general medical or surgical unit to record interactions with an angry patient. After the incident, the process recording by the nurse involved may reveal patterns of response that exacerbated the angry responses of the patient and escalated a simple misunderstanding into a major conflict. Process recordings can therefore be a valuable strategy to identify learning needs.

Professional Standards

Professional standards influencing nursing may arise from numerous sources. These sources include professional associations (e.g., American Nurses Association), speciality associations (e.g., Association of Operating Room Nurses), accreditation groups (particularly the JCAHO), and state boards of nursing.

Loss of license registration or accreditation is a potential consequence of not meeting the standards mandated by these agencies. The goal of techniques used to identify learning needs is to alter discrepancies between present performance and performance according to standards set by the professional groups.

As these groups change their standards, new learning needs are created unless the current staff development programming is up to date. Staff development educators must constantly be vigilant about monitoring changes or proposed changes in standards so that educators have ample time to implement the mandated changes and provide needed learning experiences for nursing service staff.

Questionnaires and Opinionnaires

Questionnaires and opinionnaires are surveys that focus only on the respondent's opinion as opposed to the respondent's actual knowledge or skill. Questionnaires may be used with groups at an ongoing meeting or during an interview. These questionnaires may be distributed through another person (e.g., a clinical nurse specialist) or by internal or external mail. Closed-ended, open-ended, or sentence-completion formats may be used. Questionnaires can be used to rank needs, differentiate between new and experienced staff, provide data for follow-up surveys, and show changes over time.[2]

Considerable time is required to develop questionnaires with closed-ended questions, but less time is required to analyze the responses. Open-ended question or sentence-completion formats require less initial effort, but they are fairly time consuming to analyze because decisions must be made about the meanings of responses. The latter approaches typically yield more targeted data because respondents can use their own words to provide as little or as much information as they choose. Table 11-1 lists examples of questions used in both types of questionnaires. If the staff development departments provide education to staff members located throughout the community or to affiliated agency staff, a survey can be an effective way to obtain input.[13]

Rating Scales

The most common approaches to rating scales are a type of Likert scale or semantic differential scale. A Likert scale usually has response ranges from 1 to 5, with 1 representing the most or least and 5 representing the other extreme. These scales can be used to describe conditions, behaviors, or attitudes.

Semantic differential rating scales pose dichotomies such as good to bad, soft to hard, and fair to unfair. These scales are excellent for assessing attitudes. Sometimes the scales are presented on a line with one word at one end and the other word at the other end. The instructions are to place a mark at the point on the line that is most representative of the respondent's feelings.

Many course evaluations use a rating scale format. As with other evaluation techniques, these scales provide another source of assessing needs.

Records and Reports

Careful analysis of data from records and reports must be made because many of these records and reports reflect the organization's needs and not necessarily individuals' needs. Table 11-2 shows 10 of the most common records and reports used as sources for assessing learning needs.

Table 11-1   Question types commonly used in questionnaires

Name	Description	Example
Closed-end questions		
Dichotomous	A question offering two choices	Consultations are easy to provide, yes ( ) no ( )
Multiple choice	A question offering four choices	Choose the response most typical of you. My consultation skills are: a. at the beginning level. b. at the competent level. c. at the proficient level. d. at the expert level.
Likert scale	A statement to show disagreement or agreement	Consultation is an important part of my responsibilities. Strongly agree ___ Disagree ___ Neither ___ Agree ___ Strongly agree ___
Semantic differential	A scale set between two opposite words on which respondents choose their opinions	Consultation can be: Easy . . . . . . .Hard Simple . . . . .Complicated Fun . . . . . . .Boring
Rating scale	Rates an attribute from poor to excellent	Place a 1 by the highest priorities for your new role ___ Interpersonal relationships ___ Budgeting ___ Organizational structure ___ Performance appraisals
Open-ended or sentence-completion questions		
Completely unstructured	Questions have an unlimited number of possible answers	What is your opinion of consulting?
Word association	Words presented one at a time to which respondents mention the first thing that comes to their minds	What is the first thing that comes to mind when you hear the following? Entrepreneur Intrapreneur Staff development educator
Sentence completion	Incomplete sentences presented for participants to complete	When I choose a consultant, the most important considerations in my decisions are _____.
Story completion	An incomplete story presented, which participants are asked to complete	A few months ago we were having trouble in the new intensive care unit with the new interns. When I asked staff development for consultation, they _____.
Picture completion	A picture of two people talking, with one making a statement; respondents complete the second response	Two nurses are talking; one says "Don't ever hesitate to ask for consultation from staff development." The other person replies _____.
Thematic apperception test (TAT)	A picture presented to which respondents are asked to make up a story about what is happening	Show a picture of an educational setting and say, "Tell me a story about what is happening here."

Table 11-2   Records and reports commonly used as sources for assessing learning needs

Record/report	Types of data
Statistical reports	Common medical diagnoses, length of stay, nursing care hours
Patient record	Typical procedures, medications, nursing interventions
Patient surveys	Consumers' perceptions of care, specific incidents (positive and negative)
Minutes of meetings	Special shift-related problems, such as "sundowners" syndrome[4]
Nursing audits and quality improvement reports	Actual practice findings, documentation concerns
Infection control reports	Common infections, typical discrepancies in performances
Incident reports	Individual performance discrepancies, typical reportable errors
Employee records, including turn-over and absentee reports	Clinical areas of greatest turnover and absenteeism, level of participation in continuing education activities
Annual reports	Trend data of past accomplishments and future needs
Marketing reports	Trend data

These records and reports provide a rich source of data whether alone or combined. In some cases, such as incident reports, it is possible to separate learning and administrative needs readily. In other cases, it is more difficult to distinguish between these two needs. Of all the records and reports available in the typical hospital setting, quality improvement reports are the most useful. Based on actual practice findings and suggested remedies for deficiencies in standards, these reports are more accurate and detailed than any other single report. Although infection control reports and incident reports tend to be specific, they are both valuable sources of deviation from acceptable practices.

Forecasting data are evident in other reports such as annual and marketing reports. Analyzing new developments in light of current performances can predict learning needs for the future.

An advantage of records and reports is that other people have ready access to many of these documents. Therefore these documents are more readily accepted as "proof" of needs. In most cases staff development educators merely access these documents; they do not create them. This saves time, as does the fact that these records and reports are a readily available source of data.

Role Changes

Whenever new workers are introduced or roles are restructured, it is logical to assume that learning needs will emerge. For example, if the role of RNs was originally described in reference to inpatient services and that role converts to across settings, the role has changed substantively and learning needs will differ. Staff development must be prepared to address needs if the way in which service is delivered changes or if the way in which governance is structured is altered.[24] When assessment is conducted in a comprehensive and integrated manner, short- and long-term needs can be identified.

Services and Organizational Changes

Changes in the existing services of an organization also provide many indicators for learning needs. One of the most common organizational changes that dramatically affects learning needs is computerization of health records. As health care organizations become computerized, the demand for computing skills will be critical. This indicates a major learning need requiring staff development attention.

Major changes in services have historically created learning needs for nurses. These changes include alterations in technology and focused services. For example, an alteration in service-based technology affected postoperative care when light amplification by stimulated emission of radiation (LASER) surgery was introduced. Geriatric psychiatry is an example of focused services in a highly specialized practice. These examples of organizational changes result in learning needs. For a smooth transition these changes should be foreseen and learning experiences implemented, a situation that only occurs if the staff development director is a part of the executive team in nursing.

Simulations

Simulations, whether implemented via a computer or not, can be valuable as an assessment strategy. Combined with knowledge tests and other strategies, simulations can be especially valuable in areas in which critical thinking is demanded.[12] When protocols or critical paths exist, the use of simulations can show when discrepancies exist.

Slip Technique

The slip technique is similar to several oral techniques except that it uses a written format on slips of paper. Each participant is given a stack of paper slips (file cards also work well). After listening to a particular problem or issue, group members are asked to respond to a question by writing as many short answers as possible in a specified amount of time.[22] Each answer can be written on a slip of paper or file card, and the cards are separated according to the category of the answer. An advantage of this technique, which requires some judgment about creating answer categories, is that respondents can see the strength of a given response. That is, when slips of paper pertaining to different answers are put into a stack, the tallest stack is the most evident or most popular answer.

This strategy saves writing time for the group facilitator because the answers can be separated into different piles by renaming the answer categories.

One warning to educators is to save all the slips of paper. Throwing these pieces of paper away in front of participants shows a disregard for the suggestions given, whereas saving them shows that participants' ideas are valued.

Testing

Pretests are used for the following two purposes: "(1) To determine whether or not individuals have knowledge and skills that are prerequisite to participating in a specific learning offering and (2) to determine what the participants already know based on the objectives of the offering."[22] Posttests are means to determine information learners did not learn or the teachers did not teach. Posttests can identify potential needs for subsequent learning.

Many courses include pretests, posttests, or both that convey a simplistic view of testing. In truth, testing is complex and should include considerations regarding criterion- and norm-referenced grading, validity and reliability, pilot testing of questions, cultural biases or reading difficulty of the test, and use of a test blueprint to structure questions. The classic reference *Measurement and Evaluation in Teaching*[9] discusses the details of testing and addresses these issues specifically.

Data from tests should be assessed carefully to ensure that they truly reflect learning needs as opposed to a discrepancy in test-taking ability. If learners are comfortable with computers, it is advantageous to test with computers to facilitate the ease with which data can be analyzed and to provide feedback for learners.

Telephone Surveys

Hash, Donlea, and Walljasper[11] and Cannon and Waters[3] used the telephone survey technique with positive outcomes. In addition to constructing the questionnaire, they trained interviewers. They defined several advantages such as rapid responses, current need documentation, low refusal rate, high result reliability, low cost, and potential for a wide geographic sample.

Although this is not a typical strategy in staff development, it has some potential when printed surveys produce low response rates and individuals prefer to respond without work distractions. Some research suggests that interviewees tend to respond more accurately to sensitive questions during telephone interviews than during face-to-face interviews.[21]

Telephone surveys can be used to brainstorm for needs analyses. For example, a staff development educator could call each unit manager and say, "I appreciate how busy you are. What three topics would you like staff development to present that would make nursing care on your unit more efficient?" The call takes little time from the unit manager and may elicit excellent answers because the question was unexpected.

Prospective Versus Retrospective Assessments

Although retrospective data sources are more reliable and complete, they are oriented to problem solving. The need to solve problems is critical; however, a prospective data source would theoretically prevent problems in the first place. The prospective approach relies heavily on forecasting changes in the organization or trends in health care delivery systems. The data sources for prospective needs assessments include the following: strategic plans of the organization and nursing department, nursing research reports, advertisements for new technology or recently developed dressings or medications, frequently discussed trends in the nursing literature, new surgical techniques described in medical literature, training strategies used in the Fortune 500 companies[20] and described in training for business magazines, and changes within the community as described in local newspapers. Clearly, a recent example experienced by all health care related entities has been the projections about health care reform changes occurring throughout the next decade.

SUMMARY

Assessing learning needs is a comprehensive, complex process. It is the initial and most crucial step in planning staff development activities. Inaccurate or incomplete needs assessments can result in inadequate programming. Creating learning activities that meet the needs of learners and the organization is the outcome of effective assessments.

REFERENCES

1. Bowman B et al: Needs assessment: an information processing model, *J Contin Educ Nurs* 16(6):200, 1985.
2. Byrne MM: Using a survey to assess perioperative staff learning needs, *AORN* 49(1):307, 1989.
3. Cannon CA, Waters LD: Preparing for mandatory continuing education—assessing interests, *J Cont Educ Nurs* 24(4):148, 1993.
4. Carter BE, Axford RL: Assessment of computer learning needs and priorities of registered nurses practicing in hospitals, *Comput Nurs* 11(3):122, 1993.
5. Cooper S: *The practice of continuing education in nursing*, Rockville, Md, 1983, Aspen.
6. Delbecq AL, Van de Ven AW, Gustafson DH: *Group techniques for program planning: a guide to nominal group and Delphi processes*, Glenview, Il, 1975, Scott, Foresman.
7. Diaz DP: Promote recruitment and retention by meeting the unique learning needs of the off shifts, *J Contin Educ Nurs* 20(6):249, 1989.
8. Flanagan JC: The critical incident technique, *Psychol Bull* 51:327, 1954.
9. Gronlund NE: Measurement and evaluation in teaching, New York, 1981, Macmillan.
10. Harrison JK: Tuning in to the growth needs of registered nurses, *Nurs Econ* 5(6):297, 1987.
11. Hash V, Donlea J, Walljasper D: The telephone survey: a procedure for assessing education needs of nurses, *Nurs Res* 34(2):126, 1985.

12. Henry SB, Waltmire D: Computerized clinical simulations: a strategy for staff development in critical care, *Am J Crit Care* 1(2):99, 1992.
13. Kelly KC: Brief: management and leadership learning needs in a community setting—education and practice implications, *J Cont Educ Nurs* 21(2):90, 1990.
14. Kidd JR: *How adults learn*, New York, 1973, Association Press.
15. Kristjanson LJ, Scanlon JM: Assessment of continuing nursing education needs: a literature review, *J Contin Educ Nurs* 20(3):118, 1989.
16. Mager RF: *Preparing instructional objectives*, Palo Alto, Calif, 1962, Fearon.
17. Mager RF, Pipe P: *Analyzing performance problems: or "you really oughta wanna,"* Beaumont, Calif, 1970, Fearon.
18. Naisbitt J, Aburdene P: *Megatrends 2000: ten new directions for the 1990s*, New York, 1990, William Morrow.
19. O'Connor AB: *Nursing staff development and continuing education*, Boston, 1986, Little, Brown.
20. Peters T, Waterman RH Jr: *In search of excellence: lessons from America's best-run companies*, New York, 1982, Harper & Row.
21. Sudman S, Bradburn NM: *Asking questions*, San Francisco, 1983, Jossey-Bass.
22. Tobin HM, Wise PSY, Hull PK: *The process of staff development: components for change*, ed 2, St Louis, 1979, Mosby.
23. Valadez AM, Lund CA: Mentorship—Maslow and me, *J Cont Educ Nurs* 24(6):259, 1993.
24. Vogel G, Ruppel DL, Kaufmann CS: Learning needs assessment as a vehicle for intergrating staff development into a professional practice model, *J Cont Educ Nurs* 22(5):192, 1991.
25. Wise PSY: Needs assessment as a marketing strategy, *J Contin Educ Nurs* 12(5):5, 1981.
26. Wise PSY: Administrative angles: the focus group or let's give them what they want, *J Contin Educ Nurs* 18(4):137, 1987.

DONNA S. LEROUX   ◆   BETTY CODY

Curriculum Planning and Development

12

The design of a staff development curriculum must be responsive to the realities of today's nurses. The past approaches, in which teachers were the gatekeepers for acquiring knowledge and skills, must give way to a new curriculum design. In this new design, teachers become problem posers instead of problem solvers, facilitators, and nurturers. A well-planned curriculum prepares nurses to independently address real experiences encountered as employees.

CURRICULUM IN STAFF DEVELOPMENT

Throughtout the past several years, nursing curriculum design has moved from the authoritarian role of teaching, in which teachers act as information providers, demonstrators, and evaluators, to "emancipatory teaching,"[5] which creates a "teacher-student partnership" with "flexibility and individual differences in how and what one learns."[6] The structured, planned, and integrated curriculum approach has long been a part of academic education. The Tyler curriculum model has dominated many aspects of curriculum development in academic settings.[22] Tyler's model identifies four elements of curricula—philosophy, conceptual framework, objectives, and curriculum threads. This easy-to-use model is sequential, logical, and organized. It develops a philosophy from which stems a conceptual framework. Behavioral objectives and content are selected from this conceptual framework. Bevis[2] says that the Tyler model "is an ends-means model in that the ends (objectives) are first established and the means (content and teaching strategies) are then picked that will attain the specific ends."

This focus for academic curricula, however, has not gone unchallenged. At the 1988 National Nurse Educator Conference a curriculum that was less behavioral and rigid and more sensitive to individual learning needs and the needs of society was favored.[4] A curriculum based on learners' needs should facilitate each individual's acquisition of the knowledge and experiences neces-

Table 12-1   Comparison of educative-caring and traditional styles

Parameter	Educative-caring style	Traditional style (training and indoctrination)
Teacher role	Meta-strategist Problem-poser consultants Nurturers of curiosity, criticism, inquiry, caring, meaning making	Information provider Demonstrator Monitor of return demonstration Discussion conductor Validator that the "truth" has been learned
Purpose of model	To focus on teacher-student interactions and learning experiences desired To develop the individual into an autonomous and reflective thinker—one who can formulate goals and possess the means with which to do so	Ends-means model—to first establish ends (objectives) and to pick means (content and teaching strategies) to attain the specific ends
Curriculum definition	Interactions and transitions between and among teachers and students with the intent that learning takes place	A systematic group of courses, sequences of subjects, and planned experiences designed to achieve specific education goals[9] Teacher-proof curriculum with exhaustive list of objectives

sary to deliver patient care in an ever changing society.[9] This approach should provide for new and creative development of curricula and lead to exciting teaching strategies.[4] Table 12-1 compares traditional and new styles of teaching strategies.

The National League for Nursing[17] states the following:

The most significant reform involves process—the changed relationship to information on the part of faculty, student, and health care consumer. Technology has democratized information and in the process shifted the points of access and control from the professional to the educated public. With this shift then, the focus of education turns from content to: a)critical thinking; b) skills in collaboration; c) shared decision-making; d) social epidemiological viewpoint; and e) analyses and interventions at the systems and aggregate levels.

Bevis and Watson[6] define *curriculum* as "the interactions and transactions that occur between and among students and teachers with the intent that learning occurs." Once curriculum is viewed as interactions, the way those interactions take place and what they lead to become the essence of the curriculum. This is in stark contrast to "curriculum as a systematic group of courses, sequence of subjects, and planned experiences"[11] or Bevis' earlier definition[3] that a "curricu-

Table 12-1 cont'd   Comparison of traditional and educative-caring styles

Parameter	Educative-caring style	Instruction style (training and indoctrination)
Learning	Learning process in which individual cultivates the disciplined scholarship and experience necessary for expertise, including acquiring insights; seeing patterns; finding meanings and significance; seeing balance and wholeness; making compassionate and wise judgment while acquiring foresight; generating creative, flexible strategies; developing informed, skilled intenitonality; identifying with the ethical and cultural traditions of the field; grasping the deeper structures of the knowledge base; enlarging the ability to think critically and creatively; finding pathways to new knowledge	Learning process in which individual cultivates the disciplined scholarship and experience necessary for expertise, including a change in human disposition or capability that can be retained and that is not simply ascribable to the process of growth; a change in performance
Curriculum design	Use of criteria for identifying activities with inherent worth Determination of different types of procedures to implement the aims of education Focusing of the aims of education, which calls for the creation of meaning for the individual Choice and flexibility Direct experiences Discussion Evaluation involving frequent communication related to behavior and performance	Behavioral objectives
Teaching-learning process	Student-teacher→content→learning	Student←→teacher/content→learning

lum is the totality of learning activities that are designed to achieve specific educational goals."

There are many different definitions for curriculum and approaches to its design from a narrow perspective of subjects taught to a broader focus of total learner experience. The challenge for staff educators is to design curricula consisting of the appropriate interactions and transactions of emancipatory education while completely meeting the standards of the American Nurses Association[1] and the American Nurses Credentialing Center (ANCC). These standards for education design are based on the Tyler curriculum model.[22] Because adherence to these standards is critical for ANCC approval as a provider of continuing nurses education and is now implied by the Joint

Commission on Accreditation of Healthcare Organizations (JCAHO) Standard,[14] this is the format used to outline curriculum design.

CURRICULUM COMPONENTS

The task of designing a curriculum often raises many questions. These questions include the following:

- What guidelines should be used?
- What should be included?
- What should be omitted?
- Who gives input into the design?
- What factors should influence the final design?

Many factors and principles may be used as guidelines. Using the Tyler model as the focus for the major components,[22] emphasis is on principles of adult learning and other factors critical in developing staff.

The American Nurses Association's *Standards for Nursing Professional Development: Continuing Education and Staff Development* states that program design must be based on adult learning principles.[1] These principles, which are familiar to all staff development educators, guide design choices that reflect relevancy, learner involvement, and role expectations. The following paraphrases examples of adult learning principles from Knowles[15] that can serve as a basis for design and help planners incorporate content and methods relevant to adult learners:

- As people mature, they become more self-directed.
- Adult learners have a broad base of life experiences that influence new concepts.
- Adults like to link learning to evolving roles.
- Adult learners tend to have a problem-centered approach to learning.

A curriculum design may also consider factors proposed by Howey and Vaughn,[13] who state that the curriculum should be the following:

- *Interactive*: Principles of adult learning, health care trends, and mission and goals of the oranizations should all be interrelated.
- *Comprehensive*: Orientation, in-service education, and continuing education offerings should reflect the organization's mission.
- *Continuous*: Development of staff should be ongoing and targeted to various levels of experience from beginning orientation for immediate needs to advanced development for high levels of knowledge and skills.
- *Potent*: Development of staff should deal with practical, day-to-day problems so that staff can meet their performance expectations.

Curricula designed to incorporate these guidelines acknowledge the individuality of each learner, respond to needs of the organization and society, provide coping mechanisms for knowledge explosion and rapid technological change, and incorporate progressive methodology. A well-designed curriculum based on adult learning principles and adult development factors consists of a philosophy, conceptual framework, objectives, and curriculum strands, which are Tyler's four components of curriculum.[22] These components give direction, description, concepts, and process to curriculum development.

Philosophy

Philosophy is the staff development department's belief statement (see Chapter 4). The philosophies of the nursing and staff development departments serve as the basis for the curriculum and reflect perspectives on nursing, health care, the nurse as caregiver, and the education process.[18] Each staff development department creates its own series of courses, methods of teaching, approaches to facilitation of learning, and attitudes toward learners from its philosophy.

Conceptual Framework

The conceptual framework "delineates the substance, shape, and scope" of a staff development curriculum.[18] This framework is founded on the department's philosophy, which reflects the purpose and mission of the organization.[18] The conceptual framework provides for a common language and consistent teaching about clinical nursing practice. The framework specifies the ways, concepts address the components of orientation, in-service education, and continuing education. The box provides two examples of conceptual framework statements.[12]

All courses and classes within the curriculum must reflect and be consistent with the conceptual framework. The framework guides the curriculum and ultimately provides the design and sequence of courses.

EXAMPLES OF CONCEPTUAL FRAMEWORK STATEMENTS

1. In order to provide quality care for the individual with cancer and his family, education must be provided to meet the initial and continuing learning needs of nurses in oncology. The components of Nursing Staff Development include orientation, in-service education, and continuing education. Orientation and in-service education address those developing needs necessary for nursing service employees to function at a safe level with oncology patients. Continuing education prepares the nurse to provide comprehensive nursing care to the individual with cancer and his family.*
2. The conceptual framework for education in the Division of Nursing is performance-based development...Performance-Based Development consists of four major activities: assessment, learning, practice, and evaluation of performance criteria in the three realms of competence (technical/clerical, critical thinking, and inter-personal skills). These activities form the basis for unit and service-specific plans for orientation, continuing education, and remediation of problems.†

---

*From the conceptual framework of the University of Texas, M.D. Anderson Cancer Center, Department of Staff Development, 1986.
†From the conceptual framework of Hermann Hospital, Division of Nursing Affairs,

Table 12-2   Example of curriculum objectives: orientation program objective—to be able to deliver nursing care to the oncology patient based on oncology knowledge and skill

Course objectives	Class objective examples
Phase I (orientation)	
At completion of phase I, the staff nurse will be able to administer safe care to the individual with cancer.	Recognize life-threatening situations and respond appropriately.
Phase II	
At completion of phase II, the staff nurse will be able to apply basic principles of oncology nursing to the care of the patient with cancer.	Anticipate and initiate care for acute problems related to malignant disease.
Phase III	
At the completion of phase III, the staff nurse will be able to apply the nursing process to the holistic needs of the patient with cancer with in-depth clinical knowledge.	Implement appropriate nursing interventions to prevent or minimize the development of specific oncology emergencies.

NOTE: Class and course objectives are leveled to lead to the accomplishment of the program objective.

Objectives

Specific objectives for outcome behavior make up the third component of a curriculum. Objectives provide the mechanism necessary for the analysis and development of individual courses. Clear objectives result in experience and activities that relate to the curriculum's overall purpose. Objectives stated in measurable, valid, and observable terms clearly state the content to be learned, the way it is to be learned, and the behavior necessary for staff nurses to demonstrate that the information has been learned.

Three types of objectives exist in the staff development curriculum—program, course, and class objectives (Table 12-2). Program objectives state outcomes at the completion of an entire series of classes.[18] Course objectives are the means by which program objectives are completed. Class objectives are specific instances of actions that comprise the course objective. All objectives reflect desired behavior as defined in the conceptual framework and are usually easy components to develop.

Curriculum Strands

Certain ideas or concepts derived from the philosophy and conceptual framework permeate all programs, courses, and classes. These ideas and concepts are called *curriculum strands* or *threads* and make up the fourth curriculum component. Examples of curriculum strands that may be derived from a philosophy

Table 12-3   Example of horizontal and vertical strands

Horizontal strands	Vertical strands: objectives
Orientation	Recognize life-threatening situations specific to assigned clinical areas and respond accordingly.
Continuing education Basic oncology I	Identify oncologic emergencies for which all patients with cancer care are at high risk and respond appropriately.
Continuing education Basic oncology II	Implement nursing interventions to prevent or minimize the development of specific oncologic emergencies.

and conceptual framework based on Knowles' adult learning principles[15] are respect for learners, incorporation of experiential learning, needs assessment by learners, evaluation of progress by learners, problem-centered approaches to learning, and self-directed learning.

Curriculum strands are usually labeled as vertical or horizontal. Vertical strands are concepts included in all courses, for example, information literacy, collaboration skills, management of self and others, and critical thinking. Horizontal strands reflect major components of a curriculum found along a continuum.[18]

For example, the horizontal strand can be levels of expertise in oncology nursing and the vertical strand can be emergency care of oncology patients. The horizontal strand of expertise begins in the orientation classes and proceeds through basic oncology classes I and II. The vertical strand of emergency care begins with the recognition of life-threatening situations, proceeds to the identification and response to all life-threatening situations, and culminates in the implementation of interventions to prevent or minimize the development of the emergency (Table 12-3).

DEVELOPING A CURRICULUM

The description of each of the four curriculum components leads to the actual steps in the task of curriculum development. The responsibility for curriculum development belongs to staff department educators who use input from nurse learners and user groups such as nurse managers. Their representation on a planning committee ensures that the developed curriculum will be realistic, oriented, and consonant with the organization's mission and goals.

According to Bevis,[3] the steps and activities necessary in designing the curriculum are the following:

1. Analyze the organization's mission and goals.
2. Develop a philosophy and conceptual framework for staff development.
3. Develop curriculum purpose, objectives, and strands.

4. Organize the department's programs, courses, and classes.
5. Develop specific contents for programs, courses, and classes that are consistent with the overall plan.

A systematic approach to accomplish these steps is to ask relevant questions that will provide direction. Questions can be guided by the Context, Input, Process, and Product (CIPP) evaluation technique developed by Stufflebeam.[21] The CIPP approach guides the curriculum planning group in an organized consideration of all programs, courses, and classes.

Applicable context questions from Stufflebeam's model[21] include the following:

- What is the overall goal?
- What must be achieved?
- Who are the interested parties?
- What are community and professional standards?
- What are the current means for accomplishing the goal?

These and other probing questions help clarify beliefs, content, framework, and specific goals that result in developing a philosophy, a conceptual framework, a purpose, objectives, and strands.

Step 1: Analyze the Organization's Mission and Goals

The organization's mission provides the ultimate basis for the curriculum. However, the curriculum is also influenced by current trends in the community and professional standards.[16] The planning committee should carefully analyze these areas and include aspects that affect the curriculum. An analysis of the organization's mission, professional standards, and community directly and indirectly indicates the committee's outcome expectations of the curriculum.[10] Examples of expected outcomes are to "provide quality care for patients with cancer and their families" and to "further the understanding of cancer."[8] The analysis addresses the significance of staff education to the target population. This step is the foundation for curriculum development and is the precursor of the following steps.

Step 2: Develop a Philosophy and Conceptual Framework

The mission and goal of the organization and community as well as professional standards influence the philosophy and conceptual framework. (The actual development steps of a philosophy are addressed in Chapter 4.) The choices made in the curriculum directly depend on statements found in the philosophy. For example, if the philosophy states that emphasis should be on application of knowledge to the actual work environment, then the design of the curriculum must provide experiences that facilitate application of knowledge in clinical practice. Likewise, if the philosophy states that the educational environment should be nonthreatening and should acknowledge the individuality of its learners, the curriculum design must provide for a variety of instructional methods addressing individual needs and learning styles. National standards and trends also serve as guidelines for developing the curriculum. Examples include JCAHO standards for infection control, cardiopulmonary resuscitation (CPR), and fire safety.

The conceptual framework provides the actual structure for the staff development curriculum.[18] The conceptual framework should be based on the organization's clinical practice expectations and address the educational components required to facilitate the expected level of practice.[7] Therefore the first step in developing a conceptual framework is to identify, define, and integrate aspects of clinical practice. According to the missions and philosophies of organizations and departments, the qualities that are really valued in the practice of nursing should be defined. Second, external and internal influences affecting nursing practice should be carefully examined when the framework is formulated. Societal and professional expectations should be determined, legal standards and national standards for practice should be considered, and the expectations of staff nurses for their own practice should be identified.

Once practice issues are determined, nurse employees should be examined as learners. The learning needs of each nurse and the way and times that these needs can be best addressed are important to determine. At this point in the formulation of the framework, the teaching/learning process should be specified. After the practice issues and learners have been identified, the setting should be addressed. The place in which learning best takes place and the types of support the setting provides should be defined.

The framework articulates the expectations of the staff development department and defines its relationship to nursing practice. A well-synthesized framework directs the curriculum and determines the type of clinician desired and the way to facilitate the development of that clinician.

Step 3: Develop Curriculum Purpose, Objectives, and Strands

The purpose of the curriculum is the expressed intent of the conceptual framework. In a purpose statement, the following questions should be answered:

- What do we want to achieve with this curriculum?
- Where do we want to go?
- Do we want to increase disease knowledge or practice using critical-thinking and problem-solving techniques?

The answers relate directly to the conceptual framework. If the purpose is to develop problem-solving, critical-thinking clinicians, the curriculum should provide staff nurses with learning activities and opportunities for problem solving in patient care situations. If the purpose is to acquire knowledge about disease processes and technical skills, the curriculum must be arranged to provide staff nurses with current disease information and relevant skills. The purpose statement should tell staff development what to do with the curriculum.

The formulation of objectives according to Stufflebeam's model[21] indicates the end result of context evaluation. The behavior expected at the completion of the curriculum should be defined. Based on the philosophy, conceptual framework, and purpose statement, the knowledge, skill, and attitudes desired at the completion of each staff development component should be listed. Knowledge and skill levels and expected attitudes can be identified through an analysis of performance expectations for each staff level. Behaviors expected for a staff nurse and clinician I should be identified. Expected behaviors should be stated in program objectives (see Table 12-2). In Table 12-2 the program objective reflects an overall outcome behavior expectation. At the end of the orientation program (phase I), the expected behavior falls within the safe and competent category of behavior. However, the objectives for continuing education programs phase II and phase III reflect increased knowledge and expertise in a specific area of patient care. Program objectives direct learners to accomplish the curriculum purpose.

Objectives must be written in a style that uses active behavior terms. Numerous resources are available for this task and are not addressed here. Objectives should identify learners, state the behavior and degree of behavior expected, and outline the content included. Specific class objectives lead to overall course objectives. The course objectives are the stepping stones to achievement of the course's program objectives (see Table 12-2).

An even more explicit description of curriculum content is found in curriculum strands. Curriculum strands identify levels of content and specific concepts to be integrated into the curriculum. The model presented in Table 12-3 illustrates the components of orientation and major continuing education courses that are horizontal strands. For example, emergency care (the vertical strand) is addressed in every component but is expressed differently depending on the level identified in the component (see Table 12-3). In orientation, emergency care consists of content that will lead to the recognition of and basic responses to an emergency and the knowledge of and request for appropriate resources. However, emergency care is presented at an in-depth level when found in continuing education courses. Other examples of vertical strands that are included in all courses are information literacy, collaboration skills, management of self and others, and critical thinking.

Steps 4 and 5: Organize Courses and Classes and Develop Content

The final steps in curriculum design may be accomplished by asking applicable "input" questions, such as the following[21]:
- What design approach is logical?
- Does it meet the objectives?
- What design for organization will be based on the theoretic principles?
- What do the experts recommend for design?
- What design would best use existing resources?
- Will the design meet the learners' needs?

The answers to these questions will yield an organizational scheme for classes and courses in the curriculum. The organization of schematic needs facilitates an optimal amount of learning and implements the conceptual framework. There is, of course, no one right way to arrange courses. Some suggestions for course design order include the following[3]:

- Known to unknown
- General to specific
- Simple to complex
- Facts to principles to application
- Safe (competent) to expert

Almost any pattern selected will accomplish the purpose. The key factor in organization, however, "is how the format is used."[3] The sequence illustrated in Fig. 12-1 was planned for a particular group of nurses who were advancing through a career ladder program. This illustratioin is based on the fact that undergraduate oncology education is somewhat limited; therefore the level of cancer knowledge and clinical skills vary with each nurse who comes to an oncology practice setting. If the decision about the way to sequence the curriculum is based on knowledge of who the learner is, the conceptual framework, and learners' attaining skill and knowledge at the appropriate time, the curriculum sequence may use a variable combination of modes (for example, general to specific, known to unknown, and simple to complex). These modes should result in a clinician who proceeds from safe to expert levels of practice.

Determination of the sequencing of courses and classes is the responsibility of all faculty members, not just the original planning group. According to Bevis,[3] the faculty is in a better position to "envision" the complete curriculum pattern that will fulfill the department's goals and conceptual framework.

Sequencing and organization of courses should not become rigid. Feedback from learners and faculty members indicates whether learning has taken place and has been meaningful. Faculty should be ready to change the organization of courses in response to feedback.

NEED FOR ONGOING CURRICULUM COMMITTEE

It is helpful to establish a diverse, ongoing curriculum committee to maintain a vital curriculum. The purpose of this committee is to oversee the total curriculum to ensure that the design and content remain relevant to the changing needs of the staff. The committee ensures that new proposed courses meet existing standards and fall within the intent of the total curriculum. The committee also obtains evaluations of individual courses and makes changes in the curriculum to meet learner needs and trends in health care delivery. Goals for this committee change from year to year in response to departmental goals and strategic plans.

Nursing staff development educators may experience some turmoil when a curriculum approach is initially adopted. This evolution and upheaval from the "old" to the "new" is routine and must be expected to elicit response in the faculty and user group. The "new" approach can be marketed by helping all involved to understand the rationale and design of the entire curriculum.

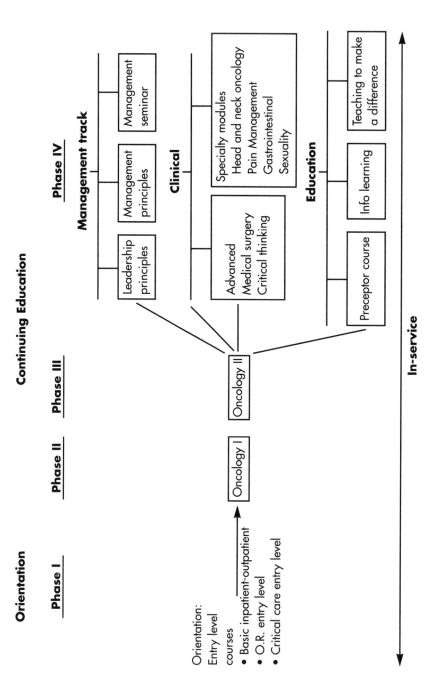

Fig. 12-1   Curriculum organization and sequence of courses is based on general to specific and competent to expert. Orientation centers on courses that give general information, which generally leads to a competent practitioner. Specific clinical, management, and education courses lead to specific knowledge and, it is hoped, an expert. In-service education addresses immediate learning needs of all learner levels and is shown as a continuum.

FUTURE CONSIDERATIONS

At the beginning of this chapter, emphasis was placed on reviewing emancipatory education described by Bevis and Watson[6] in contrast to the tylerian ends-means model of instruction.[22] This paradigm shift is indeed a revolution, but educators should carefully review and test this new approach. Education systems in the practice settings must model behaviors expected of nurses, that is, skilled, compassionate scholar-clinicians, capable of developing into autonomous and reflective thinkers who can formulate their own goals and possess the means to do so.[6] In addition, nurses must be skilled in collaboration, shared decision-making, and analysis of systems. It is also imperative that educators work with the American Nurses Association Council for Professional Nursing Education and Development to develop models incorporating the concepts of emancipatory education into curriculum and program design.

These are challenging and exciting times for staff development educators. Current authors who write about organization change and effectiveness emphasize the importance of people's commitment and capacity to learn at all levels of the organization.[19,20] The focus of curriculum will change from content to teaching people the ways to learn and to be contributing members of an integrated team.

SUMMARY

Curriculum planning and development are important aspects of a staff development department to focus programs, courses, and classes on the organziation's mission and goals. A curriculum that centers on the achievement of nurses' competency to provide high-quality patient care will contribute to the recruitment and retention of nurses. This is best accomplished when a curriculum committee continually updates the conceptual framework, objectives, curriculum strands, and programs in relation to the organization's philosophy and mission and the needs of the community it serves.

A well-planned and well-organized curriculum focuses on the product, that is, on well-developed staff nurses. The curriculum should be integrated, comprehensive, continuous, and potent so that it can become the blueprint that will encourage innovation, productivity, retention, and ultimately patient care at a high-quality level. With such curricula, staff development will no longer be only about the business of "survival."

REFERENCES

1. American Nurses Association: *Standards for nursing professional development: continuing education and staff development*, Washington, DC, 1994, American Nurses.
2. Bevis EO: *Curriculum building in nursing*, ed 3, New York, 1989, National League for Nursing.
3. Bevis EO: *Curriculum building in nursing: a process*, ed 3, St Louis, 1982, Mosby.
4. Bevis EO: *New direction for a new age: curriculum revolution—mandate for change*, New York, 1988, National League for Nursing.
5. Bevis EO, Murray JP: The essence of the curriculum revolution, *J Nurs Educ* 29(7): 326, 1990.
6. Bevis EO, Watson J: *Toward a caring curriculum: a new pedagogy for nursing*, New York, 1989, National League for Nursing.

7. del Bueno DJ: Nursing staff development: critical times, critical issues, *J Nurs Staff Dev* 2(3):94, 1986.
8. Department of Nursing Staff Development: *Staff development policy manual: conceptual framework*, Houston, 1986, University of Texas MD Anderson Cancer Center.
9. DeTornyay R: The curriculum revolution, *J Nurs Educ* 29(7):292, 1990.
10. Dolphin P, Holtzclaw B: *Continuing education in nursing*, Englewood Cliffs, NJ, 1983, Prentice-Hall.
11. Good CV, editor: *Dictionary of education*, ed 3, New York, 1973, McGraw-Hill.
12. Hospital Education Department, Division of Nursing Affairs, Hermann Hospital, Policy and Procedure, 1987, Hermann Hospital, Houston.
13. Howey KR, Vaughn JC: Current pattern of staff development. In Griffin G, editor: *Staff development*, Chicago, 1983, National Society for the Study of Education.
14. Joint Commission on Accreditation of Healthcare Organizations: *1994 Accreditation manual for hospitals*, Chicago, 1994, The Joint Commission.
15. Knowles M: *The adult learner: a neglected species*, ed 2, Houston, 1978, Gulf.
16. Moore TF, Simendinger EA: *Managing the nursing shortage*, Rockville, Md, 1989, Aspen.
17. National League for Nursing: *Vision for nursing education*, New York, 1993, The League.
18. O'Connor AB: *Nursing staff development and continuing education*, Boston, 1986, Little, Brown.
19. Peters T: *The Tom Peters seminar: crazy times call for crazy organizations*, New York, 1994, Vintage.
20. Senge PM: *The fifth discipline: the art and practice of the learning organization*, New York, 1990, Doubleday.
21. Stufflebeam DL: *Educational evaluation and decision making*, Itasca, Ill, 1971, FE Peacock.
22. Tyler R: *Basic principles of curriculum and instruction*, Chicago, 1949, University of Chicago Press.

Effective Teaching and Learning Strategies for Adults

13

Teaching and learning strategies enhance the outcomes of educational offerings and are the keys to learners' understanding and use of the presented content. Selection of a teaching strategy is based on the use of adult education guidelines and achievement of outcomes stated in the behavioral objectives for each class. Each teaching strategy is advantageous for certain outcomes and has considerations that influence its choice. Effective staff development educators use a variety of teaching strategies that are chosen for a particular group of learners or behavioral objectives.

FACILITATING LEARNING FOR ADULTS

Appropriate teaching and learning strategies are based on the concepts of adult learning, which imply that educators do not act as "imparters" of knowledge but rather as "facilitators" of learning (see Chapter 3). For convenience, Knowles' concepts are summarized as follows[11]:

- Adults have a need to know the reason they should learn something.
- Adults have a need to be self-directing.
- Adults have a greater volume and different quality of experience than young people.
- Adults become ready to learn when they experience a need to know or they need to be able to do something to perform more effectively and satisfyingly.
- Adults enter into a learning experience with a task-centered, problem-centered, or life-centered orientation to learning.
- Adults are motivated to learn by extrinsic and intrinsic motivators.

The concepts of adult learning need to be incorporated into all teaching and learning strategies for learning to occur and knowledge to be retained. These concepts of adult learning can be illustrated using the following example from a critical care course.

223

As an introduction to the critical care course, the staff development instructor discusses the topics and skills needed for successful performance in a critical care unit. Learners each identify one topic they need to learn, and the educator writes each item on a flip chart or chalkboard. Learners next identify skills they all need to learn; these are also written on the board. Learners can then identify attitudes or feelings necessary for nursing care (e.g., fearing death, being calm with distraught families, controlling panic in a crisis). This initial listing provides an indication of the preconceived notions of the learners about nursing in critical care units. This may also indicate the learners' priorities. The sequence of topics could be changed to meet the learners' needs and provide self-direction in the learning process. Identifying learning needs related to critical care nursing and obtaining some idea about their priorities helps the educator structure learning experiences that are problem centered for the learners.

After learners have listed their topics, the instructor may list other cognitive, affective, and psychomotor items and discuss their importance. This interaction of the educator and learners in listing topics sets the climate of adult learning by emphasizing that learners are expected to take an active part in the classes.

Involving the Senses in Learning

Staff development educators should plan a variety of teaching and learning strategies that involve the use of the senses, (i.e., seeing, hearing, feeling, touching). Generally, using only one teaching strategy or appealing to only one sense is inadequate because learners have a variety of learning styles. Educators who consistently rely on one strategy will only educate a portion of the learners. For example, a lecture without audiovisual enhancement and creative use of questioning will only stimulate the small number of adults who learn best by listening. Most learners require the stimulation of other senses for learning to occur. A usual estimation of the amount of learning that occurs through the use of various senses is listed as follows[22]:

- Reading: 10%
- Listening: 20%
- Seeing (observing): 30%
- Listening and observing: 50%
- Listening, observing, and discussing: 70%
- Listening, observing, discussing, and performing: 90%

The more senses used, the greater the retention of knowledge. Educators are encouraged to devise learning experiences that involve learners and use multiple teaching strategies. Sometimes learning experiences are built around a series of videotapes. Although videotapes incorporate auditory and visual stimulation, learners are not challenged to apply the information being presented and miss the valuable element of discussion found in other teaching and learning strategies. On more than one occasion, learners have complained that they are being "videotaped to death!"

Motivating Heterogeneous Learners

Most classes are composed of learners representing a variety of educational preparations and levels of practice. Benner[3] describes these levels as advanced beginner, competent, proficient, and expert. These heterogeneous learners should influence the way content is presented. A brief review of basic content at the beginning of a learning activity is appropriate. A long, detailed presentation of information that learners should already know is boring and adversely affects learners' motivation.[1] If learners' questions indicate that some members of the group require more detailed information on the basics, that information can be provided through reference material or self-study modules. Conversely, if learners' questions indicate that some learners are at an advanced level in content, they can be referred to research reports and advanced technical materials. The advanced level in content usually relates to physiology, physics, chemistry, computers, or monitors or other technical equipment. The design of the learning experience should include self-study materials at a more basic level and self-study materials at the extremely advanced level.

Experienced learners, or those at the advanced level in some aspects of the content or clinical practice, can be motivated by asking them to assist with the teaching. These learners should be encouraged to share their specialized knowledge and skills. Educators can help these learners develop teaching outlines and prepare audiovisual aids. This is a productive way to provide experienced learners with professional development and recognize their abilities. This also provides a role model for less experienced learners. Another way to help heterogeneous learners remain interested and retain more class information is to teach them proactive listening. Abruzzese[1] bases proactive listening on the rate with which thoughts are processed. The usual rate of speaking in casual conversation is approximately 250 words per minute, and the usual lecture rate is 125 words per minute. However, the usual capacity to process thoughts is 500 to 1200 words per minute.[10] The "lag time" between a teacher lecturing at 125 words per minute and the learner processing thoughts at 500 to 1200 words per minute leaves time for learners to reinforce the ideas being presented. For example, learners have time before the teacher proceeds to the next topic to repeat the dosage and side effects of a drug at least three times, think about patients who exhibited the same symptoms, or determine the reason that the fact just discussed differs from the information presented in basic nursing classes. Using the listening lag time this way enhances memory and understanding, motivates learners to remain interested, and prevents lapses of attention (for example, daydreaming, worrying about personal problems).

READING LEVELS AND LEARNING MATERIALS

Designing learning experiences for heterogeneous learners requires attention to the difficulty level of written materials; handouts used in class and self-directed learning modules should be assessed. If the reading level is too advanced,

Table 13-1   SMOG readablility formula conversion table

Total polysyllabic word count	Approximate grade level (+1.5 grades)
0-2	4
3-6	5
7-12	6
13-20	7
21-30	8
31-42	9
43-56	10
57-72	11
73-90	12
91-110	13
111-132	14
133-156	15
157-182	16
183-210	17
211-240	18

From U.S. Department of Health and Human Services: *Pretesting in health communications*, NIH Pub No 84-1493, Washington, DC, 1984, US Government Printing Office.[21]

learning will be impeded for less educated learners or learners whose primary language is not English. If the reading level is too low, many learners may become bored.

Several formulas have been developed to assess reading levels; two popular formulas are the SMOG Readability Formula and the Fry Graph Reading Level Index.[15] The SMOG Readability Formula is the easier of the two to use. The following explains the way this formula works:

1. Count off 10 consecutive sentences near the beginning, in the middle, and near the end of the text. If the text has fewer than 30 sentences, use as many as are provided.
2. Count the number of words containing three or more syllables (polysyllabic), including repetitions of the same words.
3. Look up the approximate grade level on the SMOG Conversion Table (Table 13-1).

After the reading difficulty level is determined, educators can determine the usefulness of the material for specific learner groups. For example, materials written at a twelfth grade level would be inappropriate for employees who have not completed high school or for whom English is not the primary language.

All teaching and learning materials should be clearly and precisely written and target the appropriate reading level. Writing well is difficult, but many books provide helpful guidelines. Two favorites are Zinsser's *On Writing Well*[27] and Sheridan and Dowdney's *How to Write and Publish Articles in Nursing*.[17] Although the latter pertains to writing for publication, the ideas are appropriate for writing self-learning modules or materials for classroom use. For example, Sheridan and Dowdney[17] suggest the following five simple rules:

1. Be concise; omit all unnecessary words, phrases, and ideas.
2. Be specific; avoid generalizations.
3. Use the active voice whenever possible.
4. Use strong verbs.
5. Use the simple, familiar word rather than the long or obscure word.

Many other suggestions are made in both books to improve writing for staff development teaching and learning strategies. The suggestions, strategies, and guidelines are especially helpful for writing self-study modules.

SELF-DIRECTED LEARNING MODULES

Self-directed instructional modules have become more popular throughout the past decade. These modules can be used to facilitate learning that requires knowledge acquisition and application. Modules can be purchased or developed by educators by using a specific format. Unless a module's content is specific to the health care facility, the availability of a commercially developed module should first be assessed. The purchase price is usually less than the cost of the time required by educators to develop the instructional module. The development of structured modules is described in detail by Miller[14] and O'Connor.[16]

A module is a self-contained learning activity that allows learners to progress at their own pace. Various strategies for learning can be incorporated into one module. For example, a module can consist of written content only or incorporate the written material, audiovisuals, and equipment that the learner is directed to use throughout the learning activity.

Module Format

A well-designed learning module usually consists of the following:
- Overall purpose of the learning activity
- Behavioral objectives
- Learning resources contained within the module (e.g., written content, audiovisual equipment)
- Directions for use of the module
- Pretest
- Exercises with feedback that provide for application of knowledge throughout the module
- Posttest with feedback

Successful use of instructional modules depends on a variety of variables. Some of these include the following:
- The modules should be stored in an area that is readily accessible to learners.
- Space should be available for use of the module.
- Time should be provided for the learning activity.
- Reinforcement of knowledge acquired through the module should take place in planned classroom or clinical activities.

- The module content should be assessed periodically and updated as needed. The module components (for example, written pages, equipment) may be damaged through continual use and require a dedicated staff of educators to keep in good repair.

Although some adults may be self-directed in their use of assigned learning activities, others may require more structure for the learning process. Scheduling a room and a time for the use of the instructional module may be necessary for learners who are not as motivated or lack experience with this type of learning.

Use of Self-Learning Modules

There are various ways to use self-directed modules—self-directed, formal contract, or group projects. A self-directed learning project is usually initiated solely or in part by the learner and is based on an identified need to acquire and apply specific knowledge. The strategies used in this type of learning can vary. The educator facilitates learning by helping the learner choose the appropriate strategy. The educator intervenes at specific intervals to offer feedback and encouragement and to help the learner evaluate the outcome of the learning project.

The formal learning contract requires the learner to state in writing the knowledge to be acquired, resources to be used, time needed to acquire the knowledge, evaluation criteria to be used in assessing knowledge acquisition, and method to demonstrate the outcome.[12] The learner and educator usually sign the contract and agree to meet periodically to discuss the learner's progress.

The group project facilitates learning for a small group of learners. The contract may be written according to the previously described format, indicating each learner's specific area of responsibility, or the contract can be an informal, verbal agreement with the educator. The group project can be designed so that all the completed individual parts combine to form one larger product or outcome.

Self-learning projects can be used to facilitate in-depth learning for individuals without discriminating against the learning needs of the larger group. Self-learning projects can be used for the following learners:

- Learners who lack basic information essential for gaining a higher level of knowledge.
- Advanced level clinicians who have assessed role-development needs related to knowledge deficits.
- Small groups of new staff members who lack the knowledge already possessed by experienced staff members.
- Small groups of staff members who want to participate in a project but who lack specific knowledge to enable them to complete the project. For example, a group may require knowledge in standard development and formatting before they are able to develop a specific standard of patient care.

Self-directed learning projects are an excellent strategy for motivated learners. However, learners who have not identified the need to learn or lack the motivation and time to follow through with the project will not meet learning outcomes with this strategy. Educators must also be committed to providing consistent and adequate time for self-directed learners. If educators do not follow through with this commitment, learners will be discouraged and lack the motivation to continue.

TEACHING STRATEGIES MATCHED TO BEHAVIORAL OBJECTIVES

Self-directed learning modules and other teaching and learning strategies for adults are enhanced by well-written behavioral objectives. These objectives contain a behavioral word in the cognitive, psychomotor, or affective domain, which helps educators select specific teaching and learning strategies that will facilitate the attainment of desired outcomes. The box contains examples of objectives and related strategies in each domain to show the ways teaching strategies flow from objectives.

EXAMPLES OF TEACHING STRATEGIES MATCHED TO BEHAVIORAL OBJECTIVES

Cognitive domain

Objective: Identify three causes of fluid dehydration

Strategy: A method that allows for knowledge acquisition, such as programmed instruction, lecture, or videotape

Objective: Discuss the rationale for protective room isolation

Strategy: A method that allows for application of knowledge, such as group discussion, games incorporating discussion, or role playing

Objective: Develop three nursing interventions for a patient with the nursing diagnosis of impaired skin integrity, related to immobility

Strategy: A method that allows for the application of knowledge, such as computer-based instruction, a game, or group problem solving based on a case study

Psychomotor domain

Objective: Demonstrate the correct procedure for drawing medication into a syringe

Strategy: A method that allows learners to actually carry out a skill, such as demonstration with return demonstration, or video demonstration that pauses to let learners practice the procedure and is followed by return demonstration

Affective domain

Objective: Examine feelings related to caring for an ill elderly person

Strategy: A method that allows learners to acquire greater knowledge of their own value systems, such as a values clarification exercise, video simulation of a patient care situation followed by group discussion, or role playing followed by discussion of feelings generated by the role

---

Objectives for complex program offerings proceed from simple to complex and incorporate the cognitive, psychomotor, and affective domains. Teaching strategies in turn should reflect methods for initial knowledge acquisition (for example, a lecture) and progress to strategies that encourage application and synthesis of knowledge (for example, group work, games, role play).

QUESTIONING TO MATCH BEHAVIORAL OBJECTIVES

Questioning is an effective teaching strategy that can be matched to behavioral objectives. Questioning can be effectively integrated into the lecture format, self-directed learning, discussion, and clinical practice. By asking questions, educators can ascertain the learners' basic knowledge, comprehension, and abilities to apply and synthesize knowledge and judge the appropriateness of actions in various situations.[4] The box shows some examples of questions matched to cognitive objectives.

Questioning is an excellent way to involve learners as active participants in the learning process. When questions are used at appropriate intervals throughout the educational offering, they become a very effective strategy.

SPECIFIC TEACHING AND LEARNING STRATEGIES

Matching teaching and learning strategies to objectives and judiciously asking questions that assist learners to attain higher-level objectives are always challenging to staff development educators. Sometimes environmental constraints are an equal challenge and can lead to creative ways to use various teaching strategies.

Creative Teaching Strategies

Some creative teaching strategies incorporate a self-learning format in a manner that is cost effective *and* enjoyable for the learners. The following lists some examples of these:

- *"What's New?" solitaire posters*: A small poster labeled "What's New?" is placed in a designated spot on the unit. Affixed to the poster are small, folded cards. A question is typed on the outside of the card with the answer typed on the inside. Learners read the question and flip the card for the correct answer. The poster should be left on the unit for approximately 2 weeks to facilitate learning by all staff members.[18]
- *Fact sheets*: When information that does not require an explanation or a discussion is given, a fact sheet detailing the information can be posted or distributed.[5]
- *Newsletter*: This format is very useful to disseminate essential, factual information to all staff members. The education department can develop its own newsletter or request space in the facility's nursing staff newsletter.[13,2]
- *Portable educational carts*: Mobile carts displaying fact sheets and equip-

---

QUESTIONS MATCHED TO COGNITIVE OBJECTIVES

Questions to ascertain knowledge
- When should you wash your hands when giving patient care?
- What is the next step in this procedure?
- Identify the chambers of the heart.

Additional questioning words that can be used to ascertain knowledge are *name, define, describe, who, what,* and *how.*

Questions to ascertain comprehension
- Compare two methods of protective room isolation.
- Explain the rationale for flushing a central venous device with heparin.
- Why would serum calcium levels increase in an immobilized patient?

Additional questioning words that can be used to ascertain comprehension are *contrast, predict, explain, illustrate, which,* and *why.*

Questions to ascertain application
- How would you intervene with Mrs. G, a depressed patient?
- Identify two nursing diagnoses for Mr. W, a patient with diabetes.
- Why should a patient be turned frequently after surgery?

Additional questioning words that can be used to ascertain application are *demonstrate, construct, and* solve.

Questions to ascertain synthesis
- Develop a patient care plan for Mrs. A, a patient who has undergone open heart surgery.
- Formulate a plan for responding to an angry family member.
- How would you as a preceptor provide support and direction to a new graduate who is repeatedly making the same mistakes?

Additional questioning words that can be used to ascertain synthesis are *suggest, create, synthesize,* and *derive.*

Questions to ascertain judgment
- Select the most appropriate way to teach a patient how to change an ostomy pouch.
- Defend your method for intervening with a child who will not eat.
- What is the most approprate way to develop a self-learning module?

Additional phrases or words that can be used to ascertain judgment are *select on the basis of, decide,* and *judge.*

---

ment are another useful way to educate. The carts stay on a unit for a specified time so that learners can use them whenever time permits. If validation of learning is required, the staff development educator can provide posttests about the content.[8,24]

Except for the newsletter, all these methods use an accompanying sign-in sheet to allow learners to document their use of the learning activity.

Literature Search on Teaching Strategies

Professional literature is rich in the area of teaching strategies. Learners and educators can brainstorm to identify different ways to accomplish selected projects. The information can be used to develop and maintain a departmental list or file of teaching-learning strategies for general use or specific topics. This list can be referred to often. Whenever possible, a variety of ways to meet the same instructional objectives should be offered, and learners should be allowed to choose activities. This is possible even in mandatory training. For example, accredited cardiopulmonary resuscitation (CPR) training generally requires standardized written and performance tests. Beyond these usually nonnegotiable aspects, the way learners prepare for the tests may be discretionary, especially for recertification. Different approaches that may be made available for learner selection include manuals, programmed instruction, and other written materials for self-study out of class; computer-assisted instruction or simulation; lecture/discussion; movies or videotapes; demonstration of skills; and supervised practice with feedback. Participants may feel comfortable enough with the content to simply take (challenge) the tests without special preparation.

Programmed Instruction

This strategy, also known as *programmed-based instruction* and *programmed unit of instruction*, can be used as a single strategy or with other learning strategies. The content can be presented in a written format or by computer-based instruction.

Programmed instruction provides information in instructional units called *frames*. Each frame contains a discrete area of content followed by a question requiring immediate recall. If the answer is correct, learners are directed to continue with the learning activity. If the answer is incorrect, learners are directed to review the content again before proceeding.

Programmed instruction can also be branched. This format enhances learner interest and provides individualized learning. Branching refers learners to expanded repetition of content if they answer a question incorrectly or refers learners to more advanced content if they answer a question correctly.[6] With computer-based instruction, branching can occur automatically.

Programmed instruction is a realistic way to learn. One study demonstrated that learners who used programmed instruction scored higher on a posttest than those who attended a lecture about the same topic.[9] However, the design of the programmed instruction unit is extremely important. Educators who lack experience in instructional design should consider purchasing programmed instructional units that encompass branching and are tested for reliability.

Demonstration

Demonstration is a live enactment of a skill or an action that provides visual, auditory, and tactile learning. This method provides learners with the opportunity to see and practice a skill while providing a rationale for the action.

Demonstration is used primarily to teach psychomotor skills such as patient procedures. This method can also be used to teach interactive skills such as interviewing, patient teaching, and classroom or clinical teaching.

If possible, demonstrations of skills should take place in a skills laboratory or the clinical area of practice. This allows learners to closely associate the procedure with the environment in which it will be practiced. If this is not possible, the classroom can be used. Equipment required to demonstrate the skill and a practice mannequin or learner volunteer should be available. Learners should never be required to imagine the application of a procedure to a patient situation because of lack of equipment. Staff development budgets should include adequate funds for equipment purchases and replacements.

Adequate time should be allowed during demonstrations for learners to practice the demonstration using a skills checklist. The learners should be paired if a group of learners is involved. In these situations, one learner observes the other learner while using the skills checklist to verify accurate performance; the learners then switch roles. This method reinforces learning and allows the educator to interact with the entire group.

When demonstration is used to teach interactive skills, the procedure is quite similar. After a discussion of the rationale for the skill and its methodology, the skill is demonstrated. A skills checklist that delineates important aspects of the interaction can be used quite effectively. Mimicked demonstration in this case can be carried out using groups of three learners. Two learners take the part of the nurse and patient; one learner is the observer and uses the checklist. Roles are exchanged until each learner has had an opportunity to practice the skill.

Classroom and clinical teaching strategies can be taught in the same manner. A skills checklist is used for each teaching strategy demonstrated.

Effective use of demonstration as a teaching strategy always includes learner feedback. Learners must understand their strengths in performing the skill and the aspects that require further development.

Lecture

Lectures are useful for providing new information such as a new policy, treatment protocol, or concept related to professional practice. Lectures allow for the transmission of information in a short time to a large group of people. The sequencing of content is controlled by the educator to promote understanding by the learning group. The material presented is usually not available from a single resource but requires the educator to synthesize content in a logical format from several resources.

However, without the inclusion of other strategies, the lecture format is not effective because learners become passive observers. Lectures can be quite effective when combined with discussion, questioning techniques, and visual aids.

When combining these additional techniques, educators should assess the specific subcontent areas in the material. Questions related to the application of subcontent areas should be posed to learners before proceeding with other content. When learners do not respond as expected, further discussion and questioning techniques are necessary.

Visual aids are an effective adjunct to lectures when the content on the visual aid reinforces the point being made. The visual aid is *not* a substitute for the content, nor should it distract from the content.

Games and Simulations

Games and problem-solving exercises can also be used to reinforce the lecture content. These strategies allow for active learner participation and enjoyment while enhancing learning, especially when dull content is presented.

Games and simulations provide an opportunity to apply knowledge that has been previously learned or to gain insight and value clarification.[7] These strategies are particularly useful with a heterogeneous group of learners. The variety of learning obtained with these strategies can range from simple to complex and can encompass psychomotor, cognitive, and affective learning objectives.

A game can involve one learner, two individuals, or a team. The purpose of the game is for learners to make a choice when presented with alternatives that provide varying rewards. Wolf and Duffy[25] identify three essential elements inherent in a game. That is, games must be competitive, provide learner participation, and have a specific structure. Games must also provide the following specific elements: specific roles for each player, a description of the interactions to occur between players, the rules governing play, and the criteria for winning.[6]

Games can be used at the outset of a class as an icebreaker or to motivate learners. Games can be used during a learning experience to stimulate discussion, especially when the game relates to player interactions. At the end of a learning experience, games can be used to provide an opportunity to apply knowledge. Several types of games are listed in the following:

1. *Single player*: These games are usually modeled after a crossword puzzle, tic-tac-toe, or solitaire. They are played with pencil and paper or on the computer. In computer tic-tac-toe the computer acts as the second player.

2. *Team*

a. *Board games*: Popular board games can be converted into nursing games with ease. The most popular are adaptations of *Trivial Pursuit*. This game format can be used to teach leadership skills or fluid and electrolyte balance. Geyer and Korte[8] have used this game to teach nursing diagnoses. When *Trivial Pursuit* is used as a format, the game board is drawn on a transparency and projected onto a screen, playing pieces are made of cardboard, and dice can be purchased or borrowed from another game. The preparation time for this game is approximately 3 hours, which is as long as the time spent to prepare a 1-hour class. The game is played by the actual rules for *Trivial Pursuit*. Questions may be answered by individuals or teams of people depending on the group size. The playing time is approximately 30 minutes.

b. *Competitive games*: The least expensive type of competitive game involves two teams. The educator asks a question and whichever team answers correctly gets a point. This can be used with virtually any area of content.

c. *Card games*: Sisson and Becher[18] described a card game for the identification of basic dysrhythmias. A team chooses a card that is face down. The team asks the educator various questions pertaining to the card to which the educator can answer "yes, no," or "sometimes." When the team has enough information, the instructor asks the team to identify the dysrhythmia.

Many games based on a nursing format are available for purchase. Educators must decide whether it is more cost effective to purchase or develop a game. The cost of either approach should be seriously considered. Generally, the competitive game can be developed with little cost. Games such as *Trivial Pursuit* can be time consuming to develop, but considering the number of times it can be used and the knowledge application inherent in the game, it may be cost effective. Games are an excellent way to stimulate learner motivation and provide active participation.

A simulation is an actual enactment of a real-life situation. Each player assumes a role that must have an expected outcome. The simulation can occur on videotape, in which case learners respond to specific questions related to the content, or the simulation can be live, in which case the learner has specific roles with objective outcomes. Simulations can be an effective method with which to teach cardiac arrest code management, nursing processes, and ethical issues. When the learners experience a situation through simulation, they have a clearer understanding of the variables inherent to the situation and can relate them to clinical practice. Simulations can also be used to teach psychomotor skills such as dressing changes and bed baths. A simulation allows for realistic learner involvement. Learners actually experience a real-life situation or its consequences. Zeanah[26] describes the enactment of a mock trial based on actual trial situations. Although simulation development and enactment are expensive, the potential cost savings to the organization are significant if documentation improves and litigation decreases.

Computer-Assisted Instruction

Computer-assisted instruction (CAI) is actually a type of self-directed learning. Learners may use a form of programmed instruction with branching or an interactive program containing simulations. Interactive video, which uses audiovisual simulations and requires learner responses, allows for the greatest amount of learning and application.

The uses of this format are diverse. CAI can be used to teach basic content, stimulate critical thinking, permit learner application of knowledge, stimulate learner inquiry, or provide a test of knowledge.[16] This teaching strategy is particularly useful for teaching content to per diem or agency nurses, part-time employees, and individuals who work evenings and nights. The testing component provides validation of learning, which is extremely important for situations in which the availability of instructors is limited.

Several variables should be considered before using CAI. These include the cost of hardware and software, space availability, lack of software standardization, hardware maintenance, and lack of software developed for professional use.[19] These problems seem to be resolving. Although cost remains a concern, the savings in instructor time is great. Various companies that produce CAI are creating products compatible with a greater number of computer systems. The interactive videodisk programs currently available are frequently designed for a professional audience.

Panels, Symposiums, Seminars, and Debates

A panel is a discussion of a specific content area by a group of experts. Each member of the panel presents specific information followed by a discussion among the members. The discussion is more effective when learners also discuss the content with panel members. The discussion can be guided or moderated by a nurse educator who uses questions written on cards by the participants.

This strategy is more useful for higher levels of learning because basic knowledge may not be thoroughly covered by the panel members. A few questions should be prepared ahead of time to start the discussion. The moderator should be skilled in guiding the question-and-answer portion so that no one panel member or participant dominates the discussion.

The symposium can be used for a small group of learners, usually 10 to 20 members. The symposium can meet only once or repeatedly at specified intervals. A central theme is chosen, and experts present content related to specific parts of that theme. The presentations are usually followed by a question-and-answer period, or the entire presentation can consist of questions and answers.[16]

Speakers' repetition of content is always a concern. Educators can decrease repetition by carefully explaining the assigned content area to each speaker. Learners may have limited experience in posing questions to experts; therefore staff development educators should have several questions ready or assign specific questions to certain learners to start the discussion.

A seminar is a small discussion group that provides an opportunity for knowledge integration at a high level. Learners are given reading assignments to complete before attending the seminar. They are also provided with questions that will form the basis of the seminar's discussion. The seminar leader directs the group in discussing the questions and adds additional questions to stimulate a higher learning level. The seminar format is useful in teaching professional development, administrative abilities, and ethical and legal issues. The seminar leader must be committed to guiding the group through a discussion of all assigned questions so that the seminar learning objectives are met. Groups can become involved in discussing one particular question and forget that there are other questions to explore.

Debate is composed of a series of planned speeches relating to a specific subject. There are two teams, each taking opposing views related to the theme. Presentations are timed, and rebuttals are presented by each team. This strategy is particularly useful when presenting controversial issues. Debate stimulates learners to carefully consider both sides of an issue in an intellectual, objective manner. Staff development educators must be very specific when identifying the content areas to be debated. Educators should develop a specific statement or solution to a problem and then ask the debaters to defend or oppose it.

Grand Rounds and Case Studies

Usually grand rounds involves the presentation of a specific content area centering around a particular patient case study or patient care issue. The presentation is generally 1 hour, with 10- to 15-minute presentations given by each presenting staff member. This is an excellent strategy to provide staff nurses with an opportunity to share their specialized knowledge with peers and develop their public-speaking abilities. Educators should encourage presenters to develop an article for publication if the content presented in grand rounds is exceptional.

The case study is a thorough discussion of a patient and related health problems. Questions related to the case are posed to stimulate learners to apply knowledge and consider specific issues. Case studies are particularly useful at the end of a learning activity because they stimulate learners to apply the knowledge they have just learned. The case study should be as real as possible to allow easy learner identification with the patient situation. Learners should be reminded of confidentiality and patients' rights to privacy.

CLINICAL TEACHING

Effective teaching in the clinical area can be accomplished by using several of the strategies previously discussed, but it usually includes demonstration and questioning using a problem-solving format. The educator, clinical nurse specialist, or preceptor also serves as a role model for less experienced nurses while demonstrating complex patient care skills.

Demonstration

New procedures and equipment can be demonstrated at the bedside and in the classroom. Teaching these techniques in the clinical area allows learners to more easily perceive the variables that must be considered when performing a procedure or using equipment. The return demonstration by learners is frequently accompanied by some monitoring of criteria. These criteria are similar to a skills checklist and meet requirements for monitoring activities mandated by the Joint Commission on Accreditation of Healthcare Organizations (JCAHO). Monitoring is accomplished by having another nurse (perhaps a peer) observe as learners carry out the procedure. Learning is reinforced as each learner becomes acutely aware of the performance criteria.

Frequently, new employees and occasionally experienced employees require demonstration of a procedure or equipment pertaining specifically to their patient care assignment. In these situations, teaching and learning can be effectively accomplished by guiding learners through the procedure. Rather than the educator actually demonstrating the technique, learners are verbally directed through the procedure with minimal manual assistance from the educator. The nurse's hands-on involvement in the learning process reinforces learning. This technique is most effective and necessary because many procedures cannot be performed twice on an actual patient. In addition, the opportunity to carry out the procedure, especially if it is an unusual one, may not be available in the near future.

Using Questions

The use of judicious questions to assist learners in problem solving is effective in the clinical area. This strategy can be used effectively with any new employee (for example, nurse, nursing assistant, health care technician) and with experienced staff who seek information or guidance from the educator.

Questioning should be used at the outset of the clinical day to help new employees organize their assignments and prioritize the needs of each patient. The following sequence of questions can be used in this situation:

- What are the clinical problems of the patients you are assigned to care for today?
- What are the primary nursing diagnoses of each of your patients (for nurses only)?
- How do you plan to organize your patient care for the day? Why?
- Which of these patients will you provide care for first? Why?

As employees respond to each question, they are challenged to apply learned knowledge to a specific clinical situation. Educators can facilitate learning by effectively reinforcing correct knowledge applications and clarifying knowledge deficits, asking additional questions, and referring learners to appropriate resources.

Experienced clinical employees also frequently ask for advice about patient care. In an emergency situation, educators should respond with the information immediately. Not all situations are emergencies, however, and usually educators can use questioning techniques to assist experienced employees to discover appropriate answers for themselves.

Frequently the answers can be found in reference manuals already available on the clinical unit. Employees should be encouraged to use these resources. Questions can be asked to ascertain an employees' knowledge after using the resource. Educators may be tempted to always provide an immediate answer to employees' questions. If this is done, learning will be minimal and the same questions will be asked repeatedly.

Role Modeling

Role modeling can be used as a teaching and learning strategy when helping a nurse provide care in a complex patient care situation. Accompanied by a clinical expert, the nurse is assigned to care for a patient. First, the learner observes the manner in which the expert provides care. The expert explains the rationale for each action and asks questions to ascertain the learner's understanding of the actions. The learner is then given increased responsibility in the care situation while the expert gradually withdraws. Finally, the learner should be given total responsibility for the patient's care, using the expert as a resource.

This strategy allows the learner to actually see the correct manner in which care should be provided. At the same time the clinical expert can assess the learner's understanding of the clinical situation.

OTHER TEACHING STRATEGIES

This discussion of teaching strategies would be incomplete without mentioning two strategies that do not easily fit into any of the other categories.

Humor

Humor has the potential to stimulate thought processes, thereby acting as a motivating factor that can stimulate learners to explore new ideas and evaluate the relationship among concepts.[23] Humor cannot be used with ease by every educator or for every learner. A humorous strategy that works with one group of learners may fail with another. Therefore educators who are comfortable using humor should carefully assess each group before using this strategy.

Humor can be interspersed in self-directed learning and CAI in the form of cartoons and humorous quotations or sayings. Humor should always reinforce learning and *never* distract from it.

Humor can be used in games and simulations and as an icebreaker at the beginning of a lecture. Some educators use props, such as funny hats or clothing, which are related in a humorous way to the content being discussed. This approach works for people who are comfortable "dressing up" in front of an audience and chose the props to make a specific point.

Closed-Circuit Television

Some creative educators use their facility's patient education closed-circuit television system to provide staff development programs. This type of television system uses a computer format and can be programmed 24 hours in advance, thereby providing programs continuously. By using an existing system, the education department may realize a cost savings. However, there will probably be a need to purchase additional television sets that should be placed in areas accessible only to staff members. The savings in instructor time and increased access by the evening and night shifts to expert teachers will more than pay for the cost of closed circuit televisions.

Tribulski and Frank[20] have described their successful use of this system. The only difficulty described was that initially, the televisions could be tuned to other channels, thereby allowing popular television shows to be viewed instead of the staff development programs. This can be rectified by having a special peg inserted to deter channel changing. Because the peg can be removed, the authors recommend the purchase of sets with only one channel.

Educational television is useful for teaching mandated material, policy and procedure changes, leadership development, preceptor development, and clinical decision making. Validation of knowledge is accomplished through testing.

SUMMARY

Creative educators can effectively use the many teaching and learning strategies alone or in combination to accomplish stated behavioral outcomes. Recognizing that basic strategies have provided the impetus for developing newer and more effective strategies, educators should freely experiment with variations. Enjoyable and innovative strategies can overcome existing learner and environmental barriers to learning, thus ensuring the acquisition of essential knowledge.

REFERENCES

1. Abruzzese RS: How to have an effective in-service education in a small hospital, *Trainex Nursing Rounds* 1(1):19, 1976.
2. Anderson L, Rainey SM: Using a newsletter to deliver the message of cost containment, *J Contin Educ Nurs* 24(6):271,1993.
3. Benner P: *From novice to expert: excellence and power in clinical practice*, Menlo Park, Calif, 1984, Addison-Wesley.
4. Craig JL, Paige G: The questioning skills of nursing instructors, *J Nurs Educ* 20(5):20, 1981.
5. Crawford S et al: Comparing fact sheets and lectures to provide investigational drug information, *J Nurs Staff Dev* 6(1):35, 1990.
6. Dyche J: *Educational program development for employees in health care agencies*, ed 2, Murfreesboro, Tenn, 1988, Tri-Oak.
7. Evans ML: Simulations: their selection and use in developing competencies, *J Nurs Staff Dev* 5(2):65, 1989.
8. Geyer KA, Korte PD: Creativity in nursing staff development, *J Nurs Staff Dev* 6(3):112, 1990.
9. Goldrick BA: Programmed instruction revisited: a solution to infection control inservice education, *J Contin Educ Nurs* 20(5):222, 1989.
10. Hersey WD: *Blueprints for memory*, New York, 1989, American Management Association.
11. Knowles MS: Adult learning. In Craig RL, editor: *Training and development handbook: a guide to human resource development*, New York, 1987, McGraw-Hill.
12. Knowles MS: *The modern practice of adult education*, Chicago, 1980, Follett.
13. Mierzwa IP et al: A newsletter: an innovative teaching strategy, *J Nurs Staff Dev* 5(5):238, 1989.
14. Miller PJ: Developing self-learning packages, *J Nurs Staff Dev* 5(2):73, 1989.
15. National Cancer Institute: *Pretesting in health communications*, NIH Pub No 84-1493, Washington, DC, 1984, The Institute.
16. O'Connor A: *Nursing staff development and continuing education*, Boston, 1986, Little, Brown.
17. Sheridan DR, Dowdney DL: *How to write and publish articles in nursing*, New York, 1986, Springer.
18. Sisson PM, Becker LM: Using games in nursing education, *J Nurs Staff Dev* 4(4):146, 1988.
19. Sparks SM: *Computer-based education in nursing*, US Department of Health and Human Services, Lester Hill Monographs, No. LHNCBC 90-1, 1990.

20. Tribulski JA, Frank C: Closed circuit TV: an alternative teaching strategy, *J Nurs Staff Dev* 3(3):110, 1987.
21. US Department of Health and Human Services: *Pretesting in health communications*, NIH Pub No 84-1493, Washington, DC, 1988, US Government Printing Office.
22. Weinland JD: *How to improve your memory*, New York, 1957, Harper & Row.
23. White LA, Lewis DJ: Humor: a teaching strategy to promote learning, *J Nurs Staff Dev* 6(2):60, 1990.
24. Williams J: The mobile educational crash cart: self-directed learning supplement that meets staff needs, *J Contin Educ Nurs* 17(2):59, 1986.
25. Wolf MS, Duffy ME: *Simulation/games: a teaching strategy for nursing education*, New York, 1979, National League for Nursing.
26. Zeanah PD: An introduction to legal aspects of nursing: the mock trial experience, *J Nurs Staff Dev* 1(2):26, 1985.
27. Zinsser W: *On writing well*, New York, 1980, Harper & Row.

◆　■　◆　■　◆　■　◆　■　◆　■

Evaluation in Nursing Staff Development

14

One attention-getting, effective way to demonstrate the value of a staff development department is through evaluation strategies that document an increase in the quality of patient care and a decrease in the cost of services. These data can be gleaned from impact evaluation strategies and are in sharp contrast to the reports of activities used to justify the existence of the staff development department (that is, by the number of classes taught or the number of learners attending classes). Robinson and Robinson[28] distinguish between these methods, calling the former "training for impact" and the latter "training for activity." They maintain that training for impact implies an attention to a partnership between education and service. Education is related to the need for learners to perform more efficiently. Training for impact is a service environment that supports changes taught in learning experiences; the results are measured in terms meaningful to service managers. On the other hand, training for activity describes those staff development departments that are "minicolleges." Such departments count their worth by the number of students and courses offered. They are "crises colleges" that respond to all requests for learning experiences irrespective of the cause of the learning deficit. These departments rarely measure outcomes in the service area.

Evaluation of learning experiences in terms of their affect on the organization presupposes that the staff development department has identified its clients as the managers of the patient care units who send nursing personnel to the learning experiences. The success of the learning experience (in terms of changes in behavior on the clinical units) depends as much on these manager clients as it does on the design and implementation of the learning experience.[33] Successful staff development programs are those in which positive relationships are formed with clients so that learning experiences are designed to solve problems and assist in the provision of high-quality patient care. Relationship building is a high priority for successful staff development programs if success is defined as a high degree of positive change in behavior on clinical units. Staff development educators are often masters in the art of "influence without authority."[5] Such educators are able to design learning experiences that are supported by clinical managers and result in positive evaluations of changes in clinical practice.

Phillips[24] calls this a results-oriented approach for human resource development and says it is characterized by the following:

- Programs are usually not undertaken unless tangible results can be obtained.
- At least one method to measure the results of a program is included in the program design.
- All educators should be committed to measuring the results of their efforts.
- Management is involved at all phases.
- An active effort is made to increase management commitment and support of learning activities.

Thus evaluation is not regarded as an activity occurring at the end of a learning experience but rather as an activity that is a part of the design of all phases of a learning experience.[35]

For example, if learning experiences are designed to meet a need within the nursing service department, the need is evaluated to determine the gap between current performance and required performance. The gap is further evaluated by a cause analysis. If the cause of the performance deficit indicates that an educational experience can alleviate the need, an immediate evaluation step is to collect baseline performance data so that performance after the learning experience can be measured against the baseline data. After collecting baseline data, the next step is to select an evaluation instrument. The 10 categories in which evaluation instruments fall are as follows[20]:

1. Interviews
2. Questionnaires
3. Focus groups (that is, group discussions)
4. Critical incident reports
5. Work diaries
6. Performance records
7. Simulation role plays
8. Observations
9. Written tests
10. Performance tests

Before choosing any tool, staff development members should consider the following five questions:

1. Will the instrument answer your questions?
2. Does the instrument suit the evaluation design?
3. Is the instrument valid?
4. Is the instrument reliable?
5. Is the instrument practical?

Placing the evaluation instrument within a framework before its initial use is helpful.

OVERVIEW OF TERMINOLOGY AND EVALUATION SYSTEMS

The quantity and quality of evaluation methods are often hampered by the terminology used in evaluation. For example, some authors refer to the evaluation of changes that take place in the work setting as *impact evaluation*, whereas others refer to such an evaluation as an *outcome evaluation*. Still others refer to it as *long-term evaluation*, as opposed to *short-term evaluation*, which takes place immediately after the learning experience. Others might refer to it as *summative evaluation*, as contrasted to *formative evaluation*.[10] Therefore the terms used in the literature on evaluation should be reviewed and placed in the proper perspective.[13]

In contrast to Tyler's overemphasis[34] on objectives as the shaper of evaluation, Scriven[30] used the terms *formative* and *summative* evaluation. Formative evaluation occurs during the learning experience process and is used to change some of the content or methods in which the content is presented. Summative evaluation, on the other hand, occurs on completion of that learning experience and is used to make judgments about the value of that learning experience in changing the learner's behavior. Scriven is also associated with "goal-free" evaluation, which emphasizes that some learning experience outcomes are outside the realm of goals and objectives. Sometimes these are unexpected benefits or deficits that occur from the learning experience. Scriven says that in evaluation more attention should be paid to these outcomes instead of always focusing on objectives and goals.[30]

Norm referenced and *criterion referenced* are two additional terms often referred to in evaluation. Norm-referenced evaluations relate the achievement of a learner as compared with other learners. An example is a test given to screen applicants for a position, such as unit secretary, in which the highest scorer gets the position. This is seldom used in staff development education. Criterion-referenced evaluations are those in which the criteria for success are preset and all learners must achieve a certain score or competency in a new skill. Most evaluations in staff development education are criterion referenced, and in many organizations this is evident in competency-based learning centers. del Bueno has been a powerful influence in the establishment of clinical assessment centers, which are part of performance-based development systems. These systems are designed to provide a review of old skills or practice of new skills, and they include learning experiences intended to increase interpersonal skills or clinical decision making.[8] Assessment centers focus on criterion-referenced tools that contain critical elements to evaluate learners on frequently used and important activities.

Other terminology often used in evaluation originates from Stufflebeam's context, input, process, and product (CIPP) model for evaluation.[11,12] In context evaluation the assessment of needs, problems, and opportunities within the decision maker's domain is continuous and provides a rationale for choosing objectives. Context evaluation also identifies unmet needs and unused opportunities and diagnoses problems that keep needs from being met or opportunities from being used. In input evaluation, alternative means for achieving specified objectives and potential costs and benefits of competing strategies are assessed while staff and facilities needed for implementation are considered. In process evaluation the learning experience is continuously assessed so that improvements can be made. Process evaluation provides information necessary for monitoring the learning activity so that its strengths can be preserved and its weaknesses can be modified if not eliminated. In product evaluation the actual outcomes of the learning experience are examined in comparison with the intended goals or objectives.[11]

Guba and Lincoln[12] have described a "fourth-generation" evaluation system that considers the claims, concerns, and issues of the stakeholders (that is, people who will be affected by the evaluation) and uses a constructivist methodology to derive the tools or questions to be used in evaluation. Constructivist methodology aims "to develop judgmental consensus among stakeholders who earlier held different, perhaps conflicting constructions.... The effort to devise joint, collaborative, or shared constructions solicits and honors the inputs from the many stakeholders and affords them a measure of control over the nature of the evaluation activity."[12] Swenson[32] says fourth-generation evaluation "can provide focus through the use of anecdotal information, contextual reference, and personalized responses. The reader... experiences the phenomenon vicariously. A good evaluation makes the situation so clear that the reader feels like a part of the inquiry."[32] The fourth-generation model illustrates how complex evaluation models can become.

On the other hand, Pulley[25] advocates a type of evaluation called *responsive evaluation*. The emphasis here is on responding to the organizational needs and environment. The evaluator would be interested in shaping evaluation strategies for "both/and" instead of the old "either/or" approach. Responsive evaluation can be qualitative and quantitative, summative and formative, and process and outcome focused. The major focus is on responding to the needs of the organization and skillfully using the appropriate evaluation strategy required by the exigencies of the occasion. Responsive evaluation recognizes the political aspects of evaluation. Pulley[25] suggests that responsible evalutation is made up of the following five steps:

1. Identify decision makers.
2. Identify the information needs of the decision makers.
3. Systematically collect quantitative and qualitative data.
4. Translate the data into meaningful information.
5. Involve and inform decision makers continuously.

ROBERTA STRAESSLE ABRUZZESE EVALUATION MODEL

A simple evaluation model is exemplified by the Roberta Straessle Abruzzese (RSA) model, which was developed by Abruzzese[1] for use in conceptualizing evaluations. Figure 14-1 displays the RSA model as a hierarchical triangle with simple to complex levels of evaluation, frequencies of implementation, and cost factors. The first level is process evaluation, commonly called the *happiness*

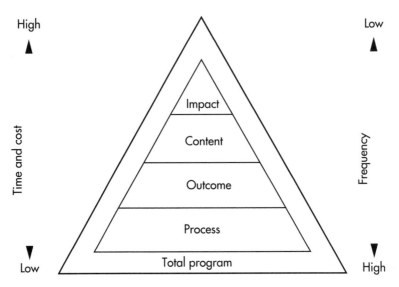

Fig. 14-1 RSA evaluation model. (Courtesy Roberta S. Abruzzese, Garden City, NY, 1978.)

index, which is a required part of all educational programs. The second level is content evaluation, which is a measurement occurring immediately after the affective, cognitive, or psychomotor skills-learning experience. The third level is outcome evaluation, which is a measurement of changes in performance on clinical units. The fourth level is impact evaluation, which is the operational result on the organization, such as a reduction in cost or an increase in the quality of patient care. (Items to be evaluated at each level are listed in the box). The space between the inside triangle and the outside triangle represents total program evaluation strategies that encompass and summarize all other types of evaluation (as in an annual report).

Not every learning experience or specific program needs all four levels of evaluation. This would be neither cost effective nor time efficient. A 1-day workshop about time management could not be expected to have an impact on the organization as a whole or on the quality of patient care in the entire organization. Therefore attempting to perform an impact evaluation of that workshop would not be wise. An integrated course for all nurses hired to work in critical care areas, such as coronary care, intensive surgical care, emergency departments, postanesthesia rooms, and dialysis units, would be expected to decrease staff turnover in those units and could thus be evaluated for an overall cost savings to the organization (that is, an impact evaluation).

The four levels of evaluation of the RSA model are similar to the four levels proposed by Kirkpatrick[18] for trainers in business and industry. Kirkpatrick[18] uses the terms *reaction, learning, behavior or skill application,* and *impact or results.* In his terminology, *reaction* evaluation refers to the learners' opinions

RSA EVALUATION MODEL

Process evaluation

General happiness with the learning experience; sample items to evaluate are:
- Faculty
- Objectives
- Content
- Teaching and learning methodologies
- Physical facilities
- Administration

Content evaluation

Change in knowledge, affect, or skill on completion of a learning experience; some tools for evaluation are:
- Self-rating scales
- Pretests and posttests
- Group work exercises
- Return demonstrations
- Multiple-choice examinations

Outcome evaluation

Changes in practice on clinical units following a learning experience; some changes might be:
- Integration of a new value
- Habitual use of a new skill
- Creation of a new product
- Institution of a new process

Impact evaluation

Organizational results attributable in part to learning experiences; some examples might be:
- Quality of patient care
- Cost-benefit or cost-effectiveness results
- Decreased turnover of nursing personnel
- Fewer risk-management incidents

Total program evaluation

Congruence of goals and accomplishments; these can be demonstrated by:
- Critique of advisory committee
- Annual reports to administration
- Reappraisal of goals for next year

Courtesy Roberta S. Abruzzese, Garden City, NY, 1978.

about the learning process; this is the same as measuring customer satisfaction. *Learning* evaluation is the measurement of the amount of learning achieved on completion of the learning experience. *Behavior* evaluation examines what learners can do as a result of the learning experience. *Impact or results* evaluation measures the effect of the learning experience on a unit or department; in Kirkpatrick's opinion,[17] this has the highest value.

The frequencies of use of each of the four levels of evaluation were summarized for 150 training directors from business and industry in 1987. Most (77%) used process evaluation for most of their programs (81% to 100%). However, few trainers were using impact evaluation; about 6% indicated they used impact evaluation on most of their programs. More than 59% did not use impact evaluation at all.[28] A survey in 1990 of six large corporations found that instead of performing impact evaluations, they surveyed trainees.[31] Even in the 1990s, impact evaluation remains little used, as Kirkpatrick meant it to be. However, if staff development departments are going to demonstrate their worth, there must be a greater use of all four levels of evaluation.[9, 27]

Process Evaluation

The first level of evaluation is process evaluation, which measures learners' satisfaction with the learning experience. The requirements of the American Nurses Association Credentialing Center (ANCC) specify the items to be included in process evaluation as follows[2]:

- Learner's achievement of each objective
- Effectiveness of each educator or learning facilitator
- Relevance of the content to the stated objectives
- Effectiveness of teaching and learning methods
- Appropriateness of physical facilities
- Learner's achievement of personal objectives

If the adult learner is not satisfied in these aspects, learning of the content will be hampered. Adults prefer a comfortable learning environment and want to be asked their opinions about the overall learning experience. Although creating one process evaluation form that can be used for all learning experiences is tempting, adapting the form individually for each learning experience is more effective. Learners can rate objectives more easily if each objective is written out instead of only having the objective number for evaluation.

Positive and negative questions should also be equally represented on process evaluation forms. Asking questions such as "What can be done to improve this learning experience?" elicits many suggestions for improvement. Sometimes staff development educators become very upset on seeing all the suggestions for changes after working diligently to prepare excellent courses. Therefore process evaluation questions should provide learners with an opportunity to express positive and negative responses.

In addition, process evaluation questions should not be biased. For example, asking "What part of the workshop, if any, was most interesting to you?" is less biased than "What part of the workshop was most interesting?" Also, questions should elicit personal responses and not opinions about the learners' reactions. For example, asking "To what extent did the workshop leader encourage you to ask questions?" elicits more personal responses than "Did the workshop leader encourage participants to ask questions?" The answers to the questions should not be dichotomous but should allow for a range of answers as in a Likert scale (see Chapter 11).

Another method of arranging answers on a scale is to use an even number of options such as *excellent, good, fair*, and *poor*. With this scale, learners are forced to choose negative or positive answers and can not choose a middle option, which is neither positive nor negative, as they may in a five-item (or uneven) number of options. Whenever learners mark all options to one side or the other or straight down the middle, the ratings are usually merely a "halo effect." Such responses are not valid indicators of the ratings of each of the items being evaluated.

Patton[22] suggests that for some learning experiences, more creative questions can be used in process evaluations, such as the following:

- Compared with other workshops you have taken, how would you rate this workshop?
- Compared with your expectations, how would you rate this workshop?
- Compared with other learning facilitators, how would you rate the educator for this workshop?
- Compared with your usual sources of information, how would you rate this workshop as a source of information?
- Compared with your personal ideals for what you should get out of a workshop, how would you rate this workshop?
- Compared with other learning experiences offered by the staff development department, how would you rate this workshop?

Process evaluations should not be used at the end of every 1- to 2-hour skill training class but should always be used at the end of a 1-day or longer workshop or whenever staff development educators want to particularly ascertain learners' opinions about the learning process. Process evaluations should always be used at the end of a series of classes (for example, at the end of orientation classes or a critical care course). Some questions, however, may not be used on every process evaluation. For example, if the only classroom available for most staff development learning experiences is crowded and not well ventilated, asking learners to rate the physical facilities on a process evaluation is not necessary. That would merely highlight for learners that the classroom is less than optimal. Such a question serves no real purpose unless the staff development educator is trying to collect data to build a case for obtaining a more comfortable classroom.

Learners need not sign a process evaluation. In fact, answers are more likely to reflect learners' true feelings if process evaluations are not signed. Usually a statement that signatures are optional is one way to invite anonymity and still allow those who wish to do so to sign their names.

Staff development educators or others who serve as learning facilitators should also be given an opportunity to complete a process evaluation. Usually the educators have pertinent remarks about the workshop that will help improve future classes.

A common error in evaluation is not to allow enough time at the end of a workshop to fill out the evaluation forms adequately. The process evaluation forms and content evaluation forms should always be completed within the workshop time. Furthermore, a discussion at the beginning of the workshop about the types of evaluation forms to complete at the end of the learning experience helps focus learners on completion of the forms. Another commonly used method to ensure completion of evaluation forms is to exchange the workshop contact-hour certificate for the evaluation form as learners leave the workshop.

Content Evaluation

Content evaluation measures the degree to which learners have learned the information imparted during the learning experience. This evaluation of knowledge, skill, affect, or a combination of these takes place immediately after the learning experience. The purpose of content evaluation is to determine whether learners have achieved the objectives of the learning experience. Therefore the tools used in content evaluation relate to the objectives and are usually criterion-referenced rather than norm-referenced evaluations. In staff development the desire is to know the level at which learners have achieved objectives (scores are referenced to preset criteria) rather than the way one learner compares with another as in norm-referenced evaluations.

The tools or forms used for content evaluation reflect the purpose of the evaluation. Common tools are self-rating scales, pretests and posttests, group work exercises, return demonstrations or competency-based assessments, and tests or scales for measuring affective changes.[21] The most effective tools for evaluation are simulations or case studies that require learners to apply knowledge to specific cases. The most commonly used evaluation tools, however, are multiple-choice examinations. Some state nurses' associations even deny contact-hour approval for courses not evaluated by multiple-choice examinations. Most teacher-made multiple-choice examinations are neither reliable nor valid.

Multiple-choice questions usually test only the immediate recall of knowledge. Multiple-choice examinations should be constructed from a test blueprint with a certain percentage of questions related to each of the topics presented and with careful attention to the level of the questions to be effective.[3] Robinson and Robinson[28] recommend developing content examination questions that determine whether learners have developed the necessary skills and knowledge to be competent in their clinical practice. They recommend using pilot-testing questions and the establishment of standards to ensure that those who score high are indeed able to perform at a satisfactory level.

Asking learners about the information they obtained from a workshop and what they plan to do with that knowledge in their clinical practice is a far better way to achieve content evaluation than giving a multiple-choice question examination. According to research by Wake,[36] the intention to use content in clinical practice is the best predictor of the ability to use the new information in practice. Therefore content evaluation is most effective when it relates to specific problem solving such as simulated problems found in clinical practice.[15]

Knowledge tests and competency demonstrations must constantly be checked against clinical practice so that the tests remain valid, that is, that the tests relate to patient care practices. One problem with repeated courses, such as a 150-hour content and practice course in critical care nursing, is that the longer the course is taught, the more difficult the knowledge and demonstration evaluations become. Educators become so familiar with the content and skills required in critical care that they keep adding more and more content and skills for beginning nurses to learn. When questioned, the educators insist that all the information and skills are absolutely essential. However, they make no distinction between the knowledge and skills required of nurses who are new to the critical care areas and the knowledge and skills expected of experienced nurses in critical care areas. This example shows the way evaluation tools lose their validity and become so difficult that few new nurses can be successful on the evaluations. In addition, the course and evaluation may no longer be cost effective because an excessive number of hours are demanded for completion.

Outcome Evaluation

The third level of the evaluation hierarchy is outcome evaluation; this is defined as a measurement of changes that persists after the learning experience. Most outcome evaluations should occur about 3 to 6 months after an extensive learning experience and should be used as a follow-up of learners on their clinical units. Some tools used to measure outcomes are questionnaires for learners and their managers, observations of practice, audits of changes in behavior, and learner self-reports.

Figure 14-2 shows an example of a self-report for learning experience outcomes. This form was used after a series of 1-day workshops about management for first-line managers. One problem with the use of self-reports for evaluation is that learners often give themselves lower ratings after the learning experience than before. For example, at the beginning of a workshop, learners are asked to rate their competence in therapeutic communication with patients and families; they may rate themselves at level 6 on a scale of 1 to 10 (with 1 being at the beginning skill level and 10 being at the expert skill level). After learners spend 10 hours in the workshop, they discover techniques for therapeutic communication and other facets of communication such as listening, writing procedures, providing patient education, and imparting empathy. If learners are asked about their ability in communication at the end of the workshop, their new knowledge about the topic may lead them to rate themselves lower on the 1 to 10 scale. For that reason, some self-evaluations should be "then and now" or "preclass and postclass" evaluations.[14] The self-rating is done at the end of the learning experience. Questions should be stated as follows:

- How would you rate your knowledge and skills in therapeutic communication at the beginning of the workshop?

Beginning skill				Intermediate skill				Expert skill	
1	2	3	4	5	6	7	8	9	10

- How would you rate your knowledge and skill in therapeutic communication now?

What I learned in the workshops was useful to me because it:

a. Increased the quality of my leadership by:

b. Increased my productivity as a manager by:

c. Increased cost-effectiveness on my unit by:

d. Increased the quality of patient care on my unit by:

e. Increased safety or risk management on my unit by:

f. Made me feel better about (raised my morale about):
   • Myself by:

   • My work envirnonment by:

   • Nursing in general by:

g. Was interesting to me at the time, but I don't remember any specifics.

h. I prefer not to comment.

Fig. 14-2   Self-evaluation of learning outcomes of management workshops.

Beginning skill				Intermediate skill				Expert skill	
1	2	3	4	5	6	7	8	9	10

Using the then and now format tends to produce a more accurate evaluation of the increase in knowledge and skill than does a preclass and postclass self-report.

Outcome evaluations should not ignore affective learning, although these evaluation strategies may be more difficult than those for cognitive and psychomotor evaluations. King[16] gives an excellent description of learning experiences that explore affective concepts such as "dignity, cooperation, trust, acceptance, respect for individual differences, compromise, and truth" and evaluation strategies that consider four orientations to affective evaluation. The four orientations to affective evaluation as described by King[16] are psychometric, behavioral, counseling, and traditional.

The psychometric orientation involves the use of Likert scales, semantic differential scales, or Thurstone scales. Likert scales are usually devised on a five-point scale—strongly agree, agree, undecided, disagree, and strongly disagree. The semantic differential scales use two words that are opposites (for example, weak and strong, kind and cruel) and ask learners to rate their feelings on a seven-point scale. The Thurstone scales depend on expert judges to provide a weight for each item that indicates an opinion about a series of statements on one topic.

The behavioral orientation toward affective evaluation for outcomes involves the observation of learners on their clinical units or the completion of rating scales, checklists, or anecdotal records. The counseling orientation involves the use of interview skills to determine feelings and attitudes. The traditional orientation involves the use of multiple-choice questions that elicit affective responses or the use of essay examinations.

Robinson and Robinson[28] also describe evaluation strategies for nonobservable results such as identifying changes in values, beliefs, and cognitive decision making. Affective evaluations are easier to construct if they are developed around the teaching strategies of simulation, role playing, games, and case studies. The problem is always to present a nonthreatening environment, anonymity, or both so that learners do not give socially acceptable false answers instead of their true feelings or beliefs.

Outcomes or changes in behavior that persist do not solely depend on the quality and quantity of the earlier learning experience. Using new knowledge, values, or skills requires a clinical practice environment that is conducive to their use and supports and encourages the use of the new knowledge, value, or skills.[4] Robinson and Robinson[28] emphasize that educational experiences will not have positive outcomes unless the work environment is conducive to changes in practice. Therefore outcome evaluations should consider what learners learned and the setting in which they practice. The new knowledge, skills, and values are most vulnerable immediately after the learning experience. Rackham[26] indicates that 87% of learning experiences are lost if not reinforced and encouraged in the work setting. Structured on-the-job training and reinforcement on the clinical unit may be most useful if the staff development educators are involved in the training and evaluation of unlicensed assistive personnel.[15]

Outcome evaluations must be compared with performance before the learning experience and must be reported meaningfully to be useful. Baseline data should be compared with clinical practice 6 months later to determine whether a change has taken place (that is, whether competency has improved). Before the learning experience the staff development educator and manager of the clinical unit should decide the criteria to be used to determine whether the learning experience was successful. Questions should be designed or observation checklists devised so that the educator, learner, and manager all know what will be evaluated and which criteria will be accepted as an indication of successful outcomes. Questions or checklists should contain the essential elements of actions to be improved or changed and should be stated in behavioral terms. A question such as "Has the learner improved the ability to communicate effectively with patients' families?" is too broad to be measurable. In this question the meanings of the words "improved" and "communicate effectively" are unclear. A better evaluation will be made if the desired behaviors necessary for effective communicating are listed and the manager and learner rate the learner on these elements.

Goal-attainment scaling is one method of establishing an outcome-oriented tool that presents behavior changes specifically related to a learning experience. Baseline data can be obtained; then a rating immediately after the learning experience and at set intervals can be made. The scale contains behaviors desired (ranging from the least to most favorable performance) and allows for both self-rating and rating by the manager if desired.[6]

Observation by the staff development educator is another way to use a performance checklist, but this is very time consuming and may not be the most cost-effective use of a staff development educator's time. If learners are assigned to preceptors, the preceptors can collect data for outcome evaluations, thus enabling more outcome evaluations to be completed. Outcome evaluations should not be used for all classes. Each year a few programs that are extensive and teach many new skills and values and much knowledge could be chosen for outcome evaluation. Evaluating a few learning experiences well is better than evaluating many inadequately.

Impact Evaluation

The fourth level of evaluation is impact evaluation, which measures the organization's results such as decreases in patient falls or in pressure ulcers that become large and require excessive care, a decrease in cost-benefit ratios, or an increase in cost effectiveness. Learning experiences alone cannot result in organizational impact. Many other factors, such as the work environment, encouragement to continuously improve quality, and readiness to change, influence the success of educational programs on the organization or patient care.[4]

Impact evaluations, which are similar to outcome evaluations, should only be implemented for a few extensive programs that have the possibility to influence changes on a unit, department, or the organization as a whole. These evaluations require complex designs that have more in common with formal research than with standard evaluations. Rossi and Freeman[29] refer to these as "evaluation research" because they have as much rigor as a research design, cost about as much, and require the same type of meticulous data collection. This partially explains the reason so little impact evaluation is implemented.

Total Program Evaluation

Total program evaluation measures the congruence of goals and accomplishments for the staff development department. Often this is accomplished by periodic reports to the administration about cost, participants, curriculum, and activities. Other ways to accomplish program evaluation are by critiques of advisory committees, formal reports such as those required for management by objectives, or cost-benefit and cost-effectiveness reports.

THE CERVERO MODEL

The RSA model forms a theoretic basis and rationale that helps staff development educators choose types of evaluations appropriate for diffferent programs. Another model that seeks to determine outcomes and the contributing factors influencing those outcomes is the Cevero Model.[4]

This model tries to determine whether continuing education classes make a difference. Most people in staff development believe that their courses do make a difference, but that a relationship is difficult to demonstrate.

Some of the difficulty in demonstrating a relationship between a class and an outcome is that there are so many intervening variables. Perhaps Malcolm Knowles[19] described it best when he identified at least four reasons it is difficult to evaluate course outcomes:

- The number of variables affecting human beings are too numerous.
- The measuring instruments are not subtle enough to detect the important outcomes.
- The intensive scientific methods require a considerable investment of time and money.
- The most important worth of the program is the satisfaction of the consumer.

Cervero's model attempts to work with these difficulties.

Cervero states that single measures of a program are certainly not going to demonstrate the program's worth in terms of patient outcomes. The assumption has to be that changes take place within the social environment. That means learners can like the learning experience (process evaluation), learn new content or skills (product evaluation), and still not change behavior in the clinical area (outcome evaluation). Multiple measures of other variables that influence the outcome need to be examined. The factors (independent variables) other than the program itself are characteristics of the proposed change, individual professional, and social systems. The dependent variable is change in practice; the hoped-for result is consumer outcome (see box on p. 247).

This model leads to the realization that characteristics of each of these variables can influence the patient care outcome. A dynamic program instructor, motivated learner, and type of change expected may all influence the outcome. For example, if the learner is not motivated, there will not be a change no matter how strong the program's instructor or content. Even if the characteristics of these three variables are conducive to change, nothing will happen unless the service unit itself is conducive to change.

These variables were examined in doctoral dissertations and other writings such as those by Wake,[36] Warmuth,[37] Daley,[7] and Peden, Rose, and Smith.[23] Their findings indicate that the influential characteristics of each variable identified by Cervero are subject to manipulation that will influence patient care outcome.

SUMMARY

Implementing evaluation strategies becomes increasingly difficult as programs are evaluated from the bottom to the top level of the RSA evaluation model. Process evaluation is the simplest to perform, requires a minimum amount of time and money, and is expected of nearly all education programs. Content evaluation requires more skill in tool development and more time to develop and administer evaluation procedures. Content evaluation also costs a moderate amount to implement. Outcome evaluation requires greater skill in devising strategies, much time to perform well, and knowledge of baseline data establishment and the collection of valid samples of behaviors before and after learning experiences. In addition, outcome evaluation requires a considerable amount of money in terms of time (that is, salaries). Impact evaluation is the most difficult, time consuming, and costly of all evaluations. It is more similar to research than to learning evaluations. Effective impact evaluation requires considerable skill in data collection and evaluation, and it often requires the help of a statistician or research designer. The RSA model for evaluation provides a simple way to understand the terms used in evaluating. As different terms or types of evaluations are created, they can be compared with the terms in the RSA model. This provides a framework for understanding evaluation terms even if the same terms are given different meanings.

Evaluation is an important part of the staff development department activities and documents their worth to the nursing service department and the organization as a whole. The Cervero model shows great promise in adding to the documentation of the worth of staff development activities. Outcomes can become more powerful through examination of the four variables of program, participant, change, and social system, in addition to the behavior change that leads to patient outcomes. This model should become more common and be used to negotiate with members of the administration so that the affect on patient care outcome can be enhanced.

REFERENCES

1. Abruzzese RS: *Critical reviews: evaluation in continuing nursing education*, Atlanta, 1982, Southern Regional Education Board.
2. American Nurses Association Board on Accreditation: *Manual for accreditation as a provider of continuing education in nursing*, Kansas City, Mo, 1986, The Association.
3. Bloom BS et al: *Taxonomy of educational objectives: handbook I—cognitive domain*, New York, 1956, David McKay.
4. Cervero RM: *Effective continuing education for professionals*, San Francisco, 1988, Jossey-Bass.
5. Cohen AR, Bradford DL: *Influence without authority*, New York, 1990, John Wiley & Sons.
6. Daley BJ: Goal-attainment scaling: a method of evaluation part one. *J Contin Educ Nurs* 18(6):200, 1987.
7. Daley BJ: *The interrelationship of knowledge, context and clinical nursing practice*, doctoral dissertation, New York, 1993, Cornell University.
8. del Bueno DJ, Weeks L, Brown-Stewart P: Clinical assessment centers: a cost-effective alternative for competency development, *Nurs Econ* 5(1):21, 1987.
9. Geber B: Does your training make a difference? Prove it, *Training* 32(3):27, 1995.
10. Grant P: Formative evaluation of a nursing orientation program: self-paced vs. lecture-discussion, *J Contin Educ Nurs* 24(6):245, 1993.
11. Guba EG, Lincoln YS: *Effective evaluation*, San Francisco, 1981, Jossey-Bass.
12. Guba EG, Lincoln YS: *Fourth generation evaluation*, Newbury Park, Calif, 1989, Sage.
13. Holzemer WL: Evaluation methods in continuing education, *J Contin Educ Nurs* 23(4):174, 1992.
14. Howard GS: Response-shift bias: a problem in evaluating interventions with pre/post self-reports, *Evaluat Rev* 4(1):91, 1980.
15. Jacobs RL, Jones MJ: *Structured on-the-job training: unleashing employee expertise in the workplace*, San Francisco, 1995, Barrett-Koehler.
16. King EC: *Effective education in nursing: a guide to teaching and assessment*, Rockville, Md, 1984, Aspen.
17. Kirkpatrick DL: *Evaluating training programs: the four levels*, San Francisco, 1994, Barrett-Koehler.
18. Kirkpatrick DL: *A practical guide for supervisory training and development*, ed 2, Reading, Mass, 1983, Addison-Wesley.
19. Knowles MS: *The modern practice of adult education*, Chicago, 1980, Follett.
20. Marrelli AF: Ten evaluation instruments for technical training, *Tech Skills Training* July 1993, pp 7-14.
21. Nilson C: *Training program workbook and kit*, Englewood Cliffs, NJ, 1989, Prentice Hall.
22. Patton MQ: *Practical evaluation*, Beverly Hills, Calif, 1982, Sage.
23. Peden AR, Rose H, Smith M: Transfer of continuing education to practice: testing an evaluation model, *J Contin Educ Nurs* 23(4):152, 1992.
24. Phillips JJ: *Handbook of training evaluation and measurement methods*, Houston, 1987, Gulf.
25. Pulley ML: Navigating the evaluation rapids, *Train Dev J* 48(9):19, 1994.
26. Rackham N: The coaching controversy, *Train Dev J* 33(11):14, 1979.
27. Robinson DG, Robinson JC: *Performance consulting: moving beyond training*, San Francisco, 1995, Barrett-Koehler.
28. Robinson DG, Robinson JC: *Training for impact: how to link training to business needs and measure the results*, San Francisco, 1989, Jossey-Bass.
29. Rossi PH, Freeman HE: *Evaluation: a systematic approach*, Beverly Hills, Calif, 1985, Sage.
30. Scriven M: *The methodology of evaluation*, AERA Monograph series in curriculum evaluation, No. 1, Chicago, 1967, Rand McNally.
31. Shelton S, Alliger G: Who's afraid of level 4 evaluation? A practical approach, *Train Dev* 47(6):43, 1993.
32. Swenson MM: Using fourth-generation evaluation in nursing, *Evaluat Health Prof* 14(1):79, 1991.

33. Svenson RA, Rinderer MJ: *The training and development strategic plan workbook*, Englewood Cliffs, NJ, 1992, Prentice Hall.
34. Tyler RW: *Basic principles of curriculum and instruction*, Chicago, 1950, University of Chicago Press.
35. Waddell DL: The effects of continuing education on nursing practice: a meta-analysis, *J Contin Educ Nurs* 23(4):164, 1992.
36. Wake MM: *A study of instruction and nurses' intentions to change practice*, doctoral dissertation, Milwaukee, 1986, Marquette University.
37. Warmuth JF: In search of the impact of continuing education, *J Contin Educ Nurs* 18(1):4, 1987.

ROBERTA S. ABRUZZESE ◆ BETH QUINN-O'NEIL

Orientation for General and Specialty Areas

15

Orientation is probably one of the most critical activities implemented by a staff development department. At the same time, this can be the activity that is alternately applauded and dreaded by newly hired nurses, staff who transfer, and staff development educators. Orientation must be a positive experience. First impressions set the tone for most learning experiences and can influence the attitudes of new employees. Orientation is especially important because it influences subsequent attitudes toward the entire organization. An orientation experience that makes new staff members feel welcome, safe, valued, and excited about learning opportunities sets a positive attitude and contributes to employees' productive adjustment in their new workplace.

Orientation is defined by the American Nurses Association (ANA) Council on Continuing Education and Staff Development in their 1994 *Standards for Nursing Professional Development: Continuing Education and Staff Development* as "the means by which new staff members are introduced to the philosophy, goals, policies, procedures, role expectations, physical facilities, and special services in a specific work setting."[2] The goal of high-quality orientation programs is to provide a transition to practice in a new organization by enhancing the competencies of new employees in an efficient and cost-effective manner.

QUALITY AND EFFICIENCY IN ORIENTATION

For the orientation experience to be positive, staff development educators should devote a sufficient amount of time to updating the program. They must improve the content, integrate a variety of teaching methods, prepare new self-learning modules, and enhance clinical experiences that provide a transition to successful nursing practice in a new organization.

Some staff development educators think of orientation classes as drudgery because they see orientation as a series of simple explanations about the same

259

basic information.[18] Other educators view orientation as one of the most challenging programs to manage because the content is always changing as procedures and policies change, learning needs and learning styles of the learners are
always different, and the integration of lectures, self-study modules, and clinical
experience differs for each learner. The orientation program is never stagnant.
As soon as one combination of classes and clinical experiences is in place, the
combination should be adapted. A new combination should usually be in place
within the year. Orientation classes that meet the needs of heterogeneous learners challenge the ingenuity of staff development educators. Because the emphasis is on assisting new employees to contribute to high-quality patient care, the
value of orientation is measured by outcomes demonstrated on the clinical units.

Centralized and Decentralized Content of Orientation

The emphasis on outcomes in clinical practice necessitates a combination of
centralized and decentralized orientation experiences. Consequently, educators
need to determine which learning experiences should take place in the staff
development department's classrooms and which on the clinical units.

The cognitive, psychomotor, and affective content needed by every nursing
service employee, regardless of the assigned unit, belongs in the centralized orientation program. Although this differs for each organization, some common
topics include the following:

- Philosophy and mission of the organization
- Philosophy and mission of the nursing service department
- Job description and performance expectations
- Patient populations served
- Patients' rights
- Services provided for patients
- Continuous quality-improvement plans
- Personnel policies (for example, health policies and parental leave)
- Employment policies (for example, sick leave and vacation time)
- Hygiene factors (for example, pay periods, parking, and work schedules)
- Mandatory educational topics (for example, fire, safety, and cardiopul-
  monary resuscitation [CPR] reviews)
- Infection control program
- Physical plant of the organization
- Specialty resources (for example, ethics committees and pastoral care ser-
  vices)

During centralized orientation, learners should be assessed for their competencies with common activities such as medication administration for nurses.
Only clinical activities common to most units should be taught in the centralized
portion of orientation.

Activities and content pertaining to specific clinical units are best taught on
the unit. The use of clinical educators or preceptors is most efficient and effective for unit-based orientation. The clinical educators or preceptors are responsible for determining which critical elements of practice on their unit are fre-

quent, high risk, or both. For each element a criterion checklist must be used to evaluate new nurses. Self-learning packages that provide the cognitive and affective content for the psychomotor skills may also be needed. Clinical educators are also responsible for the content and skills needed for nurses to work in other units within their specialty.

Cross-Training Staff

Cross-training staff may be necessary or desirable to support changes in patient care delivery or for budgetary purposes. An example of the need for cross-training that results from changing health care delivery systems is the cross-training of staff members who work in obstetrics. The use of one room for *l*abor, *d*elivery, *r*ecovery, and *p*ostpartum (the LDRP concept) has created a necessity for staff members within the labor and delivery, nursery, and postpartum units to be trained in all aspects of caring for mothers and newborns.

Other units may be clustered by division or clinical specialty for the purpose of reassigning staff to meet patient activity needs. In the era of managed care, decreased length of stay, and decreased patient volume, cross-training to home care or community service can also be an option. Some examples of clusters include the following:

- Intensive care unit, emergency room, and telemetry unit
- Labor and delivery, postpartum, and nursery
- Medical and surgical specialties
- Specialty intensive care units
- Postanesthesia and same-day surgery units
- Coronary care units and "step-down" units
- All outpatient clinics

When cross-training is needed during orientation, clinical experiences should be provided in each area that an individual may be regularly assigned. The extent of the cross-training experience depends on the frequency of the assignment. For example, if the LDRP concept is practiced, nursing staff members must become proficient in each aspect of LDRP practice. If reassignment is rare, the experience can be brief. Commonalities of practice in each area should be identified and incorporated into orientation classes. Activities that are frequent, high risk, or both should be taught first; other activities that are less frequent or not high risk should follow.

Communication for Effective Orientation

Communication is crucial to the success of orientation on individual units and in the staff development department. A system of communication should exist between the department that processes new employees and the staff development department. Everyone involved with new employees should know the date of orientation, time and location of the first day of orientation, and standard requirements throughout orientation.

Staff development department members should be provided with standard

Table 15-1 Suggested time frames for orientation

Category of new employee	Time frame
Nurse with experience in same clinical area	2 to 3 weeks
Experienced nurse entering new clinical area	3 to 6 weeks
Recently graduated nurse	6 weeks or more
Inexperienced new employees in specialty areas	8 weeks or more
Managers	2 to 4 weeks
Secretaries	2 weeks or more
Ancillary personnel (depending on experience)	2 to 4 weeks

information about each newly hired employee, including basic education, work experience, and any concerns or special needs that can be addressed at orientation. One way to ensure orientation proceeds smoothly is to set up periodic meetings to discuss common concerns and update different departments about procedural changes that may have occurred or orientation content and methodologies that may have been altered.

Educators should be aware of the curriculum and clinical experiences provided by local schools of nursing and departments within the organization when planning an orientation. Participation at joint professional meetings between educational and service organizations can facilitate this awareness. Educators should strive to maintain open communication with affiliating nursing faculty from these schools.

Suggested Time Frames for High-Quality Orientation

The time allotted for orientation depends on the organization's philosophy, financial conditions, and the new employee's ability to achieve orientation goals. The cost of orientation is high in terms of time, money, and lowered productivity. Curran[7] calculated the cost of orientation to be as high as $20,000. This figure includes the cost of advertising for, hiring, and processing a new employee, in addition to the salaries of the new employee, educator, and preceptor during orientation.

Orientation should be based on individual needs; however, the reality of cost containment dictates that the nursing department create time limitations. Therefore educators must be creative and plan efficient orientations, while including all critical skills and experiences necessary within that specified time. One example of time frames permitted for various types of new employees is provided in Table 15-1.

There should be written policies permitting these time frames to be altered according to individual need. Changes can include shortening or lengthening orientation.

Learning Activities Based on Learning Styles

The organizers of many orientation programs use self-study modules, performance-based assessment centers for skill demonstrations, videotapes, films, and audiotapes to remain efficient and within the specified time frame. Although these methods may save time for staff development educators and relieve the boredom of repetitious lectures, there must be a judicious mix of these methods with lectures and clinical experience. Not all learners are self-directed, nor do all learners have the reading comprehension skills needed to enable them to efficiently use self-study modules. This is especially true for learners from other cultures or for whom English is not their primary language.

In a study by Flewellyn and Gosnell,[15] 110 registered nurse orientees in six general hospitals were asked to rank their preferred methods of learning. The top five methods chosen were clinical experiences, preceptors, teacher demonstrations, skill laboratories, and lectures. Three methods were almost equally preferred for sixth place—reference readings, self-learning packages, and videotapes. Skill checklists, seminar groups, and audiotapes were the least preferred learning methods. The most preferred methods involved other people working with orientees. Self-learning packages and laboratory experiences were rated low by some orientees because they had not had experience with those methods; those same methods were rated low by recent graduates because the graduates had had too much experience with them. Although further research is necessary, staff development educators acknowledge many learners prefer methods of teaching that include interpersonal interactions. Orientation classes are always a challenge because new groups can differ from previous groups. Methods of learning preferred by one group may not be effective with another group.

ORIENTATION MODELS

Throughout the past 25 years, six basic models have been used for the orientation of nursing service personnel. Aspects of each model often overlap with those of other models. These six models are listed as follows:

- Traditional lectures and buddy system
- Contracts and self-directed study
- Internships and rotations
- Preceptors and mentors
- Competency-based orientation
- Performance-based development system

Some aspects of each of these models may be used in an orientation program. For example, preceptors are commonly used with self-directed study or performance-based learning. Often preceptors are used with the traditional lecture model. Lectures are a part of most models.

Traditional Lecture and Buddy System

The traditional orientation model consists of routine lectures given in the classroom by a parade of speakers from various services. Basic procedures regarding the procurement of medications and supplies are reviewed, in addition to lectures related to documentation. The nursing staff on the units are responsible for orienting new employees to the work setting.[29] The staff members chosen to orient new nurses on the unit are usually people who have been employed the longest, have demonstrated knowledge of the system, and make new employees feel welcome. Their responsibility is to show new employees the ways to complete tasks in a given clinical setting.

Staff members who function as buddies for new employees do not receive formal preparation for their roles and may not always be attuned to needs of new employees. If several staff members on a unit function as buddies, the newly hired employee may be assigned to a different person each day. This results in inconsistent style, clinical expertise, and performance expectations.

The orientee or unit manager must assume responsibility for keeping track of the orientee's progress in completing critical procedures and skills if there is not a consistent individual overseeing the new employee's daily assignments. This orientation model may work for experienced individuals who are assertive and can verbalize their needs. Neophyte nurses do not always fare as well in this model because their learning needs are usually complex, and they need to learn more than the way to function on a specific unit.

Contracts and Self-Directed Learning

Contracts and self-directed learning are orientation strategies used in conjunction with traditional lectures and clinical experience on an orientation unit or the assigned clinical unit. Learners are encouraged to make contracts with staff development educators or unit instructors. These contracts include the activities that learners will perform within a specified time frame to accomplish orientation objectives.[33] Orientees may choose a variety of self-directed learning activities to fulfill the contract. Some orientees may choose a self-learning module; others may decide to demonstrate that they have already mastered the required competence.[13]

The most extreme form of contract orientation was a program initiated by Hilliard[21] for new graduates. New graduates were told that they had received excellent preparation for nursing so that they were capable of taking their places on the nursing units as beginning clinicians. Orientees were given a 1-week orientation to the organization and handed a manual outlining the competencies expected of graduate nurses. Orientees were expected to complete all objectives listed in the manual within 6 weeks and pass an examination with a score of 80% or higher. Most units to which the orientees were assigned diligently helped orientees complete all the objectives. This project became a team effort of pride to ensure that the new nurse became proficient. No follow-up of this contract method is reported in the literature. The assumption is that the follow-up has also been integrated into other models of orientation.

Internships and Rotations

Internships in the 1970s were primarily designed for newly graduated nurses and provided a time of transition to the work setting.[16] Internships lasted from 3

to 6 months and sometimes involved rotations to clinical units in medical, surgical, obstetric, psychiatric, and pediatric units. Weiss and Ramsey[36] described an
interagency internship program consisting of the following rotations:

- 2 weeks of hospital orientation
- 1 week of support services
- 8 weeks on the medical-surgical unit
- 2 weeks of a chosen elective
- Shift rotation to evenings and nights
- 1 week of critical care

Sometimes these internships were linked to programs of biculturalism in an
effort to combat reality shock, as described by Kramer and Schmalenberg.[23]
These extensive programs for new graduates were modified in the 1980s with the
introduction of competency-based orientation programs.

In the 1980s, internships and rotations were extended orientation programs
designed to gradually introduce new employees (usually graduate nurses) into a
specific area of clinical practice. A common area for internships is critical care.
The internship program combines general orientation and a critical care nursing
course. Newly graduated nurses participate in formal classes and a supervised
clinical practicum. Nurse interns may rotate among several critical care units as
part of their clinical experience. Because this is more of an educational than an
orientation experience, clinical assignments can be correlated with class content.

During internships, nurse interns also work on the evening or night shift.
Each intern's clinical experiences are closely monitored by an instructor and a
preceptor. A gradual increase in autonomy and independent practice should be
built into the program because nurse interns will be expected to function as staff
nurses on their assigned unit after completing the program.

Internships are costly.[30] Although internships appear to improve retention,
they must be carefully evaluated in an environment of cost containment.[24]

Preceptors and Mentors

In the late 1970s the preceptor concept for orientation became popular and
formalized through specific classes to teach selected experienced nurses about
being clinical preceptors. Preceptor programs are considered a satisfying and
effective orientation method, especially for the orientation of new or relatively
inexperienced nurses.[27]

A preceptor is a member of the nursing staff who is specifically designated to
participate in the orientation of newly hired employees. Preceptors receive formal training in programs lasting between 1 and 3 days. The content of these
courses is fairly consistent and includes principles of adult learning, teaching
techniques, evaluation methods, and a variety of topics dealing with interpersonal skills.

An orientee is assigned to one preceptor and, if possible, works the same
schedule as that preceptor. Preceptors facilitate the orientation and assimilation
of newly hired employees into the work setting. Preceptors serve as teachers and

provide orientees with the clinical experiences needed to acquire the skills to function as members of the nursing staff. Consistency in style and expectations exists because this method provides a one-on-one relationship between preceptors and orientees. This one-on-one relationship prevents orientees from becoming confused or completing orientation without achieving the necessary objectives.

Preceptors play a key role in the evaluation process. Performance problems can be identified early and corrected. Preceptors can establish goals with orientees and meet with their orientees at given intervals to discuss progress toward meeting the goals. Unit managers are told about progress by the preceptor.

Another vital role that preceptors play is to help new employees "gain entry" into the unit. Preceptors guide and advise orientees about unit norms, culture, unwritten policies, and expectations. This important function should not be overlooked because acceptance by staff members is often based on an individual's ability to "fit in" with the group and rather than clinical expertise.

Preceptors require support from unit managers and staff development educators. In addition to initial classes, preceptors may need assistance if difficult learning situations or personality conflicts arise. Because the relationship between the preceptor and orientee is short term and eventually becomes a peer relationship, it may be difficult for preceptors to evaluate orientees or handle situations that create conflict. On those occasions the manager, staff development educator, or both must provide guidance or actively intervene to resolve the problem. Preceptors should have the opportunity to improve their skills by attending workshops and consulting with staff development educators.

Preceptors occasionally become frustrated in their roles because of staffing, patient assignments, or other responsibilities such as being the charge nurse. Some of these problems can be eliminated by providing an alternate or associate preceptor for each new employee, especially during the months when most staff take vacation. Preceptors should set realistic expectations. Educators must work closely with preceptors to provide support if patient and unit demands seem overwhelming. This preceptor approach to orientation is considered an effective method of orientation, and studies have shown that it decreases nursing staff turnover, especially in the first year of employment.[17]

Precepting is a formal (that is, assigned) and relatively short-term relationship; mentoring has traditionally been an informal (that is, by choice) and relatively long-term relationship that develops between an experienced clinician and an inexperienced newcomer or protege. In situations in which role modeling is critical, such as in management or advanced practice settings, this mentoring method works well for orientation.

Competency-Based Orientation

Competency-based orientation is a method that focuses on the end results of orientation, that is, the ability of a newly hired employee to perform expected job responsibilities. This method is practice oriented and emphasizes the performance of tasks and not necessarily the acquisition of knowledge. Acquisition of knowledge is demonstrated as applied to performance in the clinical area. This method of orientation provides structure for orientees, preceptors, and educators because tasks and learning activities are clearly identified. Several essential components to competency-based orientation exist.

Assessment of Skill and Knowledge Level of Newly Hired Employees. The skill and knowledge level of an individual should be evaluated before beginning the clinical component of orientation. This evaluation determines preexisting competencies and facilitates the planning of the clinical orientation. Evaluations can be accomplished by skills laboratories, clinical simulations, and testing.

Competency Statements. These statements are similar to behavioral objectives but differ in that they concentrate more on the individual's abilities rather than on their knowledge. The number and type of objectives and competencies are based on the individual's job description and clinical assignment. There should be general departmentwide competencies (for example, documentation and infection control) and unit-specific competencies.

Critical Behaviors. These criterion-referenced behaviors demonstrate successful achievement of skills. They include checklist behaviors, completion of forms, and ability to follow procedures.

Learning Resources. These include various activities provided to orientees to help achieve the intended objectives and skills. These activities include classes, readings, and clinical experiences. Learners can be provided with options and choose from a number of resources.

Time Frames and Target Dates. Time frames and target dates are not an essential component of competency-based orientation but are helpful in providing a guide for orientees and preceptors. Time frames also prevent timid orientees from delaying the achievement of competencies. Certain competencies must be successfully demonstrated before a certain date so that orientees are encouraged to complete the required competencies (Fig. 15-1). The many advantages to competency-based orientation are listed as follows:

- Clear guidelines are presented for everyone involved in orientation
- The amount of time spent in orientation for experienced or skilled nurses decreases because once all competencies are achieved, orientation ends[8,9,34]
- New employees who cannot achieve the competencies can be identified early and remediation and further clinical experiences can be planned for them[1]
- Orientation is cost effective if implemented correctly because unnecessary material is eliminated from orientation
- Accrediting agencies require competency to be established and validated during orientation and on an ongoing basis

Skill	Objective	Resources	Evaluation	Target date
1. Documentation	Documents patient assessments on "Nursing Admission Assessment Record"	1. Attendance at orientation class on documentation or 2. Completion of self-learning module on "chart" forms	1. Completes patient admission, filling in all sections of "Nursing Admission Assessment Record"	End of week 1
2. Medication administration	Administers medications safely to a "district" of patients, observing hospital policy and procedure	1. Pharmacy component of IV certification course 2. Self-learning module medication administration policy 3. Clinical experience with preceptor or instructor	1. Achieves a grade of 80% or better on the NLN pharmacology examination 2. Demonstrates an awareness of the significance of medication administration by looking up unfamiliar drugs 3. Administers medications to a group of assigned patients, observing hospital policies and procedures 4. Documents medication administration and controlled substance usage, observing hospital policy and procedure	End of week 2

Fig. 15-1 An example of a competency-based orientation tool.

- Orientation blueprints and competency logs provide excellent documentation of new employee orientation that can be included in personnel records

Performance-Based Development System

A refinement of competency-based orientation is the performance-based development system. This model uses the concept of assessment centers for competency-based learning. These centers provide opportunities for new employees to demonstrate their competencies in various skills, and they also provide an opportunity for cross-training. Competencies in various areas of practice can be validated in the assessment center before employees are expected to float to another unit. This increases the level of safety for employees, promotes confident practice on different patient care units, and is cost effective to staff units as patient census fluctuates.[10] The assessment center also provides experienced staff members with opportunities to review and update their skills. The centers contain self-learning packages, audiotapes and videotapes, small group exercises, and games. These resource centers have been used for team building and preceptor training.

The performance-based development system focuses on both managerial and clinical competencies. Criteria-based performance standards are developed by using del Bueno's model[10] of three interlocking circles in a square (Fig. 15-2). The three circles denote technical skills, interpersonal skills, and critical thinking skills; the square represents the situation or context within which the skills are

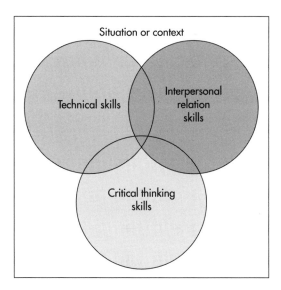

Fig. 15-2 Dimensions of competent performance. (From del Bueno DJ, Weeks L, Brown-Stewart P: Clinical assessment centers: a cost-effective alternative for competency development, *Nurs Econ* 5[1]:21, 1987.)

performed such as the clinical unit, shift, and organization. Evaluated technical skills can consist of many skills used in competency-based models. Interpersonal skills can be assessed through scripted role-play simulations based on common interactions on the clinical units. Critical thinking skills can be assessed in relation to clinical decision making, priority setting and revising, problem solving, and care planning. This is accomplished by viewing videotaped scenarios of common problems in clinical practice and by priority-setting exercises.

Although the performance-based development system is expensive to initiate, the system has many cost-effective benefits. This system is especially beneficial for large medical centers (that is, more than 400 beds), which have many new orientees each year. However, the system can be beneficial if shared by several smaller organizations. The system has been used to reduce learning time for critical care units and can produce revenue by charging other organizations a fee for their employees to use the system.

The Joint Commission on Accreditation of Healthcare Organizations (JCAHO) requires all staff members to competently perform their jobs. The task of competency validation begins in the preemployment phases and includes validation of education, licensure, and other credentials. Organizations must have policies and procedures in place to clearly outline skills that must be completed during orientation and skills that can be deferred to a later time during employment. In addition, validating skills after an individual transfers to a different clinical area or is promoted is also necessary.

The JCAHO does not mandate the competencies that must be validated, nor do they specify time intervals for ongoing validations. Also each organization is not required to establish its own standards and comply with these standards.[22] A well-defined competency-based orientation program that includes generic and unit-specific competencies is an excellent first step in this process.

The six orientation models are characterized by the predominant factors used in each. Traditional lecture and buddy system, contracts and self-directed study, internships and mentors, and competency- and performance-based systems provide aspects of the orientation that can be integrated in any organization's orientation program.

INDIVIDUALIZED ORIENTATION PROGRAMS

Some groups of learners deserve special adaptations of orientation models to meet their learning needs. These groups include new graduates, refresher-course graduates, foreign-educated nurses, and expert nurses.

New Graduates

A great deal has been written about the orientation needs of new graduates. A review of the literature from 1971 to 1985 by Schempp and Rompre[31] indicated that transition programs for new graduates have long been a concern of staff development educators. Descriptions of internships have been in the literature since 1972 and appear to be the earliest efforts to plan transition programs for new graduates. The use of preceptors, competency-based orientation models, and flexible time allotments are strategies that have also been used successfully. Some additional content and learning experiences may need to be added to the orientation for special group needs. Examples are assertiveness techniques, bicultural training, clinical simulations, and preparation for license examination.[6]

Assertiveness Techniques. This content is necessary for dealing with not only other professionals but also other nursing personnel who may eventually be supervised by the graduate. A relatively young registered nurse may have difficulty directing older, experienced employees and may be intimidated by them. Ample resources to design learning experiences that teach nurses to be assertive rather than passive or aggressive in their interpersonal relationships have existed since the 1970s. Two favorite books found in most libraries are Clark's *Assertiveness Skills for Nurses*[5] and Herman's *Becoming Assertive: A Guide for Nurses.*[20]

Components of Bicultural Training. This aspect can be initiated near the close of the scheduled orientation period and should continue for several months to provide graduate nurses with assistance and strategies to handle "reality shock."[23] The bicultural training program usually consists of six 1½-hour sessions that encourage new graduates to share their feelings related to being a new nurse.[31] Sometimes this is accomplished by sharing diary entries.[4] Two 1-day workshops about conflict resolution often include the first-line manager for each new graduate nurse so that positive interpersonal interactions may increase. Schmalenberg and Kramer[32] reported that bicultural training helped newly graduated nurses maintain their professional role orientation, choose bicultural role behaviors, institute effective changes, perform better on the clinical units, and remain members of the organization.

Staff development educators should recognize the need for bicultural training programs and integrate aspects within their current orientation model. Programs must be planned to integrate aspects of reality shock and include input from the learners themselves in the design of various aspects to effectively meet the needs of new graduates. Another type of bicultural orientation needs to be considered for nurses who were educated in another country.[26] Frequently, these nurses report to orientation only a few days after arriving in the United States. For these nurses, orientation content should be expanded to include issues regarding nursing practice in the United States, preparation for taking registered nurse licensure examinations,[6] and tips for living and working in the organization's geographical area.

Clinical Simulations. These simulations can be presented in the form of case studies, simulations such as a "mock code," computer instruction, or interactive video. These simulations provide graduate nurses with opportunities to test judgment skills in a nonthreatening environment. Other programs recommended for new graduates include internships and externships. Both provide guided work-study programs that extend beyond the normal orientation period.

Externships are also offered by many acute care facilities for nursing students during the summer before students enter their last year of a nursing program. The externship program provides students with an opportunity to work closely with a registered nurse preceptor, usually for 8 to 10 weeks. Externs are assigned to one clinical unit and follow their preceptor's schedule. The programs use established objectives, and an educational component in the form of weekly seminars and extern presentations usually exists. Some state boards of nursing allow externs to document on the patient record with the proviso that the notes be cosigned by the preceptor.[28]

These programs are excellent opportunities for students to improve clinical competence and confidence and allow students to see the reality of nursing practice from a somewhat sheltered perspective. Participation in one of these programs should be of benefit to the nurses after they graduate and enter the practice setting.

STAFF MEMBERS WHO TRANSFER

Staff members transfer to different units within the same organization for a variety of reasons. Some transfer for promotions; others transfer for a new challenge. In the era of cost containment and decreasing numbers of acute care beds, staff members also transfer to remain employed. Although staff members who transfer do not require orientation to the organization, they do require an orientation to the new clinical setting. This orientation should include a review of unit philosophies, policies, and activities such as the quality improvement program. Unit-specific competencies must be reviewed with the transferring nurse and time frames established for the completion of these skills. If additional theoretical experiences are necessary to prepare the nurse to work with the new patient population, the transferring nurse and unit manager must be aware of this. Dates for classes and time frames for attendance need to be coordinated with the completion of the unit-specific competencies.

Transferring employees should be assigned preceptors for the orientation period. If possible, this should be a senior preceptor on the unit. The staff development educators can play key roles in facilitating transfers by helping the preceptors and nurses to select clinical experiences that provide exposure to critical unit-based skills in the shortest amount of time.

Refresher Course Graduates

Graduates of nurse refresher courses also have special needs for orientation. The nurses are similar to new graduate nurses in that they feel insecure in their performance of psychomotor skills and priority setting. They differ from new graduates in that they may have years of experience providing a basis for understanding the content and clinical practice provided during the nurse refresher course. Many of them have been away from the clinical practice of nursing for

5 to 25 years. Most of these nurses state their reasons for inactivity as family and child-rearing responsibilities, although it may be assumed that some of them were dissatisfied with nursing practice.[35]

In planning to supplement the learner experiences of nurse refresher graduates in orientation, staff development educators need to consider the following factors:

- Length of the refresher course
- Ratio of classroom time to clinical practice time
- Content of the course
- Emphasis of the course on basic skills or systems review
- Purpose of the course for a general overview of current nursing or an evaluation of competency-based performance

Nurse refresher courses range from 30 to 250 hours and a median of 130 hours. The ratio of clinical experience to content lectures also varies. Some courses have as much clinical practice as classroom content lectures[35]; however, a common ratio is 1 hour of clinical experience to every 3 hours of classroom lecture.

Some nurse refresher courses are similar to adult health undergraduate courses, which provide a review of the treatments, medications, and nursing care of the various organ systems (for example, cardiovascular, respiratory, and renal). Other nurse refresher courses are merely a survey of current nursing practice and are similar to a senior nursing issues course that reviews topics such as legal issues and trends in nursing practice delivery systems. Some nurse refresher courses require many self-directed learning experiences,[19,25] whereas others do not require homework or evaluations. Obviously, the needs of nurse refresher course graduates from each type of course differ.

The purpose and emphasis of the nurse refresher course also provides an indication of learning deficits that need to be remedied during orientation. If the course intended to provide an overview of current nursing practice, the needs of these nurse refresher graduates differ greatly from the needs of those who graduated from a course built on the principles and practices of the competency-based evaluation of knowledge and nursing skills.

Similar to newly graduated nurses from undergraduate programs, nurse refresher graduates tend to be extremely anxious about their clinical skills and experience reality shock. Nursing may have changed drastically since they last practiced in a hospital setting. Many of these nurses are amazed at the preponderance of critically ill older people, same-day surgical procedures, and technological changes. Nurse refresher graduates may need some of the educational components suggested for nurses who have just graduated from undergraduate programs (that is, assertiveness techniques, components of bicultural training, and clinical simulations).

Expert Nurses

New employees who are practicing at the proficient or expert level, as defined by Benner,[3] and who have graduate degrees still require orientation to familiarize them with the philosophy, policies, and procedures of the health care organization. These individuals benefit from a competency-based model of orientation, since the length of orientation can be tailored to the time needed to complete the critical competencies.

Those involved in planning orientations should develop an orientation schedule for these nurses that includes required or mandatory topics and a quick introduction to clinical practice on their assigned unit or areas of practice. This short orientation decreases frustration on the part of new employees, preceptors, and educators. DiMauro and Mack[12] concurred with this need for the special orientation of expert nurses in saying that (with respect to clinical nurse specialists) "newly hired CNSs...have unclear ideas about how to establish themselves in their new role. They will go through a period of role transition before successfully undertaking all the roles and functions as defined by the employing agency." Furthermore, DiMauro and Mack[12] state that "a job description defining specific preparation and skills for CNSs and a comprehensive orientation program are significant factors that promote role integration." The comprehensive orientation referred to contains criterion-referenced competencies for each role of the CNS—education, clinical practice, consultation, and research.

Expert nurses also have other special needs that should be included in their orientation content. Topics to be considered for orientation of expert nurses include introduction to the librarian and information about performing computer searches, available reference books, details about the organization's review board and ongoing research studies, introduction to the grants management office, and support provided for research studies. Expert nurses should also be encouraged to share their expertise by planning to function as preceptors or instructors as the need arises. They need to be introduced to faculty from schools of nursing who use the organization for clinical experiences. Expert nurses, similar to extremely smart children, are often neglected because people assume they can provide learning experiences for themselves. Although this may be true, orientation educators can help these nurses by providing opportunities for future involvement.

SPECIALIZED ORIENTATIONS

Specialty units (for example, critical care, emergency, perioperative, and obstetric divisions) have special orientation needs. The integration of knowledge and practice in these areas is crucial. Unless new employees are experienced nurses in that specialty area, sufficient time must be allotted for new theoretical and clinical teaching. The preparation for a specialty unit should be separate from the general orientation provided for all new employees.

The content for specialty units is based on specialty nursing organization standards such as the core curriculum for the critical care units or emergency departments.[34] Topics should be tailored to the patient population served by the organization. Essential or high-priority content is identified by the nurses practicing in those areas and clinical instructors. This essential content should be incorporated into the specialized classes for nurses who practice in the specialty areas.

Topics that are common to several specialty units, such as cardiac monitoring, should be taught in combined centralized classes, with clinical practice reinforced in the specialty unit. Many large organizations have lengthy integrated courses for preparation to practice in specialty units. The specialty content should be separated from content belonging to only one specialty unit. The orientation to each specialty unit should include specific topics and usually can be taught on the unit itself.

Preceptors and unit managers should be aware of the class content so that weekly content goals can be established for the orientees. For example, if orientees attend a class about the management of the ventilator-dependent patient, each orientee should be assigned to provide care to a patient on a ventilator. In the operating room, orientees should be given specific assignments based on their progress through the curriculum.[14] As the technical preparation for each surgical specialty is presented, orientees should be assigned to cases in that specialty room. The integration of content with clinical practice provides a more effective learning experience than if all content classes are presented first and orientees are later assigned to the clinical units.

The orientee or preceptor must keep track of clinical experiences. The unit manager should provide every opportunity for orientees to obtain needed experiences. For example, if an orientee in the labor and delivery unit needs experience with patients who have undergone cesarean sections, that orientee should be reassigned to obtain the experience. Integrating the content taught in the centralized classes, content taught in the decentralized classes, and opportunities for supervised clinical practice is challenging to all educators and requires ongoing communication.

Orientation to Evening and Night Shifts

If nurses are required to rotate to evening and night shifts, information about clinical practice during those shifts should be included in the content of the general orientation of all nurses. Diaz[11] points out that staff who usually work on evening or night shifts fall into three categories—those who love working those shifts, those who must work those shifts, and those who are required to work those shifts. The learning needs and readiness to learn of these groups differs.

Nurses who are permanently assigned to the evening or night shift should receive extra orientation classes during their assigned shift. Experienced staff from the shift should be appointed as preceptors and should attend the formal preceptor training program. There should be a designated period during which the new employee will be considered an orientee on the shift and not be counted as a staff member. If several orientees rotate to the evening or night shift at the same time, a member of the staff development department should be an available resource. Providing learning experience to people working these shifts has always been a challenge for staff development. It is usually necessary to bring educational services to each unit. These unit-to-unit learning activities often involve the use of audiovisuals and self-learning packages. Educators can plan time for clinical teaching in group sessions, but they must always be flexible and sensitive to unit needs.

Orientation for Agency Personnel

Organizations that use people from supplemental personnel agencies must provide orientation to these individuals. This can be accomplished by orienting an agency representative to the organization's procedures. This individual will be responsible for orienting agency personnel and providing documentation to the organization when personnel complete the programs. Independent-learning modules can also be used for this purpose.

Orientation requirements should be the same for agency personnel and employees. The agencies should provide the organization with documentation of the following:

- Completion of the organization's orientation
- Completion of mandatory topics (for example, infection control, fire safety, and CPR)
- Copies of all certifications and test results (for example, pharmacology, cardiac monitoring, and IV therapy)
- Other contractual requirements (for example, malpractice insurance)

It is the responsibility of the agency and the nurses provided by the agency to maintain annual requirements for mandatory classes such as basic cardiac life support (BCLS).

ORIENTING ANCILLARY NURSING PERSONNEL

All ancillary nursing personnel need orientation. Ancillary personnel who are promoted or transferred also require orientation to their new roles. In addition to personnel and employment policies and classes about mandatory topics, these new employees need orientation content and clinical experiences based on their job descriptions.

For example, unit secretaries should attend formal classes about the following:

- Structure of the organization
- Interactions with other patient care departments
- Telephone courtesy
- Transcribing of orders
- Ordering of supplies
- Scheduling of procedures
- Special needs of patients and families
- Use of special equipment (for example, computer and fax machine)

Unit secretaries also need to be provided with a supervised clinical experience to practice these skills. They should be assigned to work with another secretary on a unit similar to the one for which they have been hired.

Nursing assistants also require formal classes based on the skills and expectations outlined in their job description. The extent and length of these classes depend on the previous education of new employees. Nursing assistants who have completed training programs at trade schools or other institutions need to be oriented to the organization's policies and procedures. They also need validation of their skills. Clinical orientation should be scheduled with another experienced nursing assistant; the overall process should be supervised by the unit manager or unit educator.

MEETING REGULATORY AGENCIES' REQUIREMENTS

The orientation period should be used to provide all mandatory topics, including personnel orientation. The importance of annual compliance with regulatory agency requirements should be stressed at the time of orientation. Nursing orientees can be scheduled to attend these classes with all other newly hired personnel. Application to patient care areas can be made at other times by preceptors or instructors.

Many organizations have opted for monthly classes to satisfy mandatory requirements. These education days are an efficient way to provide mandatory content, but this can also become very costly if staff members are provided with an entire off-duty day and extra clinical coverage is required. Other methods of providing programming for these topics include independent-learning modules, unit-based audiovisuals, and self-assessment tests. A key component to the success of compliance with mandatory education is to enlist the assistance of unit managers in raising staff awareness and to offer a variety of options to meet these requirements. However, the importance of meeting mandatory requirements of regulatory agencies is first presented in orientation.

Documentation of orientation and an individual's completion of orientation is required by the JCAHO. (An example of a form for documentation is shown in Figure 15-3.) Documentation regarding the successful completion of the orientation process is also important from a risk-management perspective.

Skills checklists or competency blueprints and logs can be added to personnel files. If the organization requires that nursing staff members have "certifications" such as BCLS, intravenous therapy, or chemotherapy review certifications, these should also be included as part of the record. When these certifications are obtained at other organizations, evidence of course completion should be in the file. If competency blueprints are bulky and cumbersome, an orientation summary sheet can be developed that includes a list of the competencies, dates of required completion, and signature. This is considered adequate documentation.

Although all organizations have probationary periods for new employees, adequate documentation of the progress or problems of employees who are terminated during orientation is still wise. These individuals do not have recourse through the organization's grievance procedure but can protest such decisions through outside agencies such as the Equal Employment Opportunity Commission (EEOC).

	Performed correctly				
	Yes	No	Instructor's initials	Date	Comments
Section V nursing form					
Admission _____					
Discharge _____					
Transfer _____					
Charting					
Patient care notes _____					
Patient daily care flow sheet _____					
I & O sheets _____					
Care plans _____					
Transcribing orders:					
Order entry _____					
Medication administration record _____					
Kardex _____					

Fig. 15-3   An orientation checklist summary.

SUMMARY

The qualities of a successful orientation are listed as follows:
- Integrates adult learning principles in all aspects
- Considers learners' needs
- Considers staff's learning styles
- Assists employees to enhance their strengths
- Assists employees to remedy discrepancies in performance
- Prepares new employees to function safely
- Covers essential content efficiently and cost effectively
- Minimizes the anxiety of new employees
- Promotes assimilation into a group
- Promotes pride in nursing and in the organization
- Provides a sense of accomplishment for educators, preceptors, managers, and newly hired staff

Orientation is one of the most important activities of the staff development department. It influences the attitudes of new employees on all subsequent experiences. Successful orientation programs require extensive communication with other departments and continuous updating of content and design. The model chosen by the staff development department for orientation influences the structure and content of individualized orientations for various groups of nursing service personnel. Requirements of regulatory agencies and the ANA's standards[1] provide guidelines for ensuring high-quality orientations. The goal of the orientation program is to enhance the competencies of nursing service personnel so that employees may continuously improve the quality of care provided to patients within the organization.

REFERENCES

1. Alspach J: Designing a competency-based orientation for critical care nurses, *Heart Lung* 13(6):655, 1984.
2. American Nurses Association: *Standards for nursing professional development: continuing education and staff development*, Washington, DC, 1994, The Association.
3. Benner P: *From novice to expert: excellence and power in clinical practice*, Menlo Park, Calif, 1984, Addison-Wesley.
4. Borovies DL, Newman NA: Graduate nurse transition program, *Am J Nurs* 81(10):1832, 1981.
5. Clark CC: *Assertiveness skills for nurses*, Wakefield, Mass, 1978, Contemporary Publishing.
6. Colombraro GC: NCLEX-RN preparation: enabling candidates to pass, *J Contin Educ Nurs* 20(6):261, 1989.
7. Curran C: *The nursing shortage and the healthcare industry's response: the results and findings of the Commonwealth Report*, paper presented at Resource Application Staff Development Workshop, New Orleans, Feb 4, 1990.
8. del Bueno D, Altano R: Competency-based orientation: no magic feather, *Nurs Manag* 15(4):48, 1984.
9. del Bueno D, Barker F, Christmyer C: Implementation of a competency-based orientation program, *Nurse Educ* 5(3):16, 1980.
10. del Bueno DJ, Weeks L, Brown-Stewart P: Clinical assessment centers: a cost-effective alternative for competency development, *Nurs Econ* 5(1):21, 1987.
11. Diaz DP: Promote recruitment and retention by meeting the unique learning needs of the off shifts, *J Contin Educ Nurs* 20(6):249, 1989.
12. DiMauro K, Mack LB: A competency-based orientation program for the clinical nurse specialist, *J Contin Educ Nurs* 20(2):74, 1989.
13. Donahue MA: New employees negotiate contract for orientation, *Cross-Reference* 6:6, 1976.
14. Edgar T et al: *Blueprint for orientation: a manual for perioperative educators*, Denver, 1988, AORN.
15. Flewellyn BJ, Gosnell DJ: Comparison of two approaches to hospital orientation for practice efficacy and preferred learning methods of registered nurses, *J Contin Educ Nurs* 16(5):147, 1985.
16. Gibbons LK, Lewison D: Nursing internships: a tri-state survey and model for evaluation, *J Nurs Adm* 10(1):31, 1980.
17. Giles PR, Morna V: Preceptor program evaluation demonstrates improved orientation, *J Nurs Staff Dev* 5(1):17, 1989.
18. Haggard A: *Hospital orientation handbook for nurses and allied health professionals*, Rockville, Md, 1984, Aspen.
19. Harris BS, Nesheim WW: Self-study reentry program for inactive nurses, *J Contin Educ Nurs* 20(6):268, 1989.
20. Herman S: *Becoming assertive: a guide for nurses*, New York, 1978, D Van Nostrand.
21. Hilliard M: *Orientation and evaluation of the professional nurse*, St Louis, 1974, Mosby.

22. Joint Commission on Accreditation of Healthcare Organizations: *1994 Accreditation manual for hospitals: scoring guidelines: section 4: orientation, training, and education of staff,* 2, Chicago, 1993, The Organization.

23. Kramer M, Schmalenberg C: *Path to biculturalism,* Wakefield, Mass, 1977, Nursing Resources.

24. Kotecki CN: Nursing internships: taking a second look, *J Contin Educ Nurs* 23(5):205, 1992.

25. Macdonald K, Freise W: Home study refresher courses for RNs and LPNs, *J Contin Educ Nurs* 20(6):272, 1989.

26. Maroun M, Serota C: Demanding quality when foreign nurses are in demand, *Nurs Health Care* 9(7):361, 1988.

27. Morrow KL: *Preceptorships in nursing staff development,* Rockville, Md, 1984, Aspen.

28. New Jersey Board of Nursing: *Guidelines for externship (work-learn) program for nursing students,* Trenton, NJ, 1986, The Board.

29. O'Connor AB: *Nursing staff development and continuing education,* Boston, 1986, Little, Brown.

30. O'Friel J, Bealieu A.: The nurse internship experience: a dynamic learning environment for the novice, *J Nurs Staff Dev* 9(1):26, 1993.

31. Schempp CM, Rompre RM: Transition programs for new graduates: how effective are they? *J Nurs Staff Dev* 2(4):150, 1986.

32. Schmalenberg C, Kramer M: Bicultural training: a cost-effective program, *J Nurs Adm* 9(12):10, 1979.

33. Schmidt MC, Quaife MC: Orientation by contract, *Superv Nurse* 5(10):38, 1974.

34. Stewart SL, Vitello-Ciciu J: Designing a competency-based orientation program for the care of the cardiac surgical patient, *J Cardiovasc Nurs* 3:34, 1989.

35. Warmuth JF: Reentry programs for nonpracticing nurses. In Cooper SS, editor: *The practice of continuing education in nursing,* Rockville, Md, 1983, Aspen.

36. Weiss SJ, Ramsey E: An interagency internship: a key to transitional adaptation, *J Nurs Adm* 7:36, 1977.

Professional Issues in Nursing Staff Development

IV

JANE KREPLICK BRODY ◆ ROBERTA S. ABRUZZESE

◆ ■ ◆ ■ ◆ ■ ◆ ■ ◆ ■

Ethical and Legal Issues in Nursing Staff Development

16

Ethical and legal issues in nursing staff development occur on two different but interconnected levels. One level involves the cultivation of legal and ethical knowledge and abilities of the nursing staff. The other relates to the ethical and legal concerns pertinent to the instructional activities of staff development educators (Fig. 16-1).

On the first level, educators must assess and enhance the competencies of the nursing staff to practice within ethical and legal parameters. Newly employed nurses come to the organization with widely divergent backgrounds; therefore formal instruction in ethics and law, in addition to opportunities to develop moral decision-making skills, are needed to achieve desired competencies. While staff development educators integrate new staff into the work environment, educators need to convey the ethical and professional values of the employing organization. New nurses need to be oriented to the organization's resources available to assist nurses who have ethical and legal concerns (for example, ethics committees, ethical rounds, nursing ethics groups, and risk management departments).[27] Staff development educators can work with management to foster an organizational climate in which ethical and legal aspects of care are well incorporated into nursing practice. If policies and procedures are being updated, staff development educators should be members of the committee so that ethical and legal concerns can be integrated into all learning experiences. For example, if the committee is reviewing the process of change of shift report, committee members should consider whether certain items are important; physical care, such as IV rates and laboratory tests should only be reported; and psychosocial information about the patient and family should be discussed. The addition of psychosocial information can help prevent ethical and legal dilemmas from arising.

On the second level, staff development educators must serve as role models by practicing ethically and legally. Educators are expected to integrate legal and ethical concepts in all classroom and clinical teaching, in addition to conducting themselves in a manner supportive of professional ethical values.[7,36] If staff mem-

283

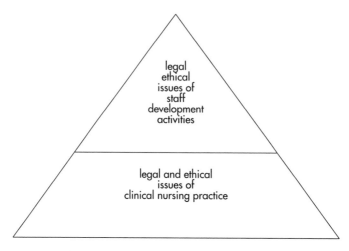

Fig. 16-1 Levels of Legal and Ethical Issues

bers are not treated with respect and fairness by educators in their own organization, staff members may be less likely to treat their patients respectfully and fairly.

This chapter explores ethical and legal issues on both levels of staff development. Ethical and legal concepts and concerns are discussed separately for clarification purposes, although considerable overlap between the levels occurs.

ETHICAL ISSUES
Theories of Ethics

Ethics is a form of philosophical inquiry that provides guidance in choosing a course of action in matters affecting basic social values and human welfare. Normative ethics structures and uses the standards of conduct developed by a community (for example, the nursing profession) to aid in selecting, justifying, and judging behavior. Ethical theories provide the framework for normative ethics and are usually divided between theories focusing on the outcome (consequentialist/teleological) and theories emphasizing action (deontological/principled) as the critical element in choosing and evaluating a behavior (Table 16-1).[35]

Consequentialist/Utilitarianism/Teleological. Consequentialist ethical theories base the rightness or wrongness of an action on the consequences or *Telos* (end). Actions that bring about the best results are the most ethical. Utilitarianism is a specific type of consequentialism and can be summarized as "the greatest good for the greatest number."[37] Utilitarian theory is based on the writings of Jeremy Bentham (1748-1832)[10] and John Stuart Mill (1806-1873).[22] Utilitarianism proclaims that the right action is the action that produces the greatest human happiness and well-being in comparison to alternative actions. The concepts of moral rights and duties, which permeate the ethical thinking of most nurses, do not enter into utilitarian justification as much unless these concepts support the

Table 16-1 Comparison of ethical theories

Consequentialist/Teleological	Deontological/Principled
Outcome oriented	Act oriented
Utilitarianism:	Multiprincipled:
Principle of utility	Nonmaleficence (do no harm)
(greatest good for the greatest	Beneficence (do good)
number	Autonomy
	Justice

greatest utility.[11] For example, if a decision is being made regarding whether orientees should be able to review their own evaluations, that decision would not be based on the orientees' right to know or the instructors' right to confidentiality but rather on whether allowing orientees to see their evaluations creates the greatest good for all involved (that is, orientees, staff members, staff development educators, administrators, and patients).

Two major philosophical problems are present with the utilitarian approach to ethical decision making. The first problem is that if only outcomes to determine the rightness of a given act are used, morally reprehensible actions could be supported because their outcomes created the greater good. Thus the end justifies the mean. If behavior is permissible as long as the outcome is acceptable, trust and cooperative action would become limited.

The second problem created is that the outcome of any given action is not predictable. The situations in which staff development educators function are complex and contain multiple variables that can influence the results of an action in unforeseen ways. Thus the use of a predicted outcome as rationale for present behavior is risky. For example, one orientee who reads an evaluation describing serious deficiencies may be motivated to study and improve; another may become discouraged and quit trying. Although doing the greatest good seems to be a desirable and moral aim, several problems arise in applying this broad, optimistic goal as a guide for choosing and justifying behavior. Staff development educators have responsibilities to many groups—learners, patients, patients' families, employers, and other educators. These responsibilities may conflict with one another.[38]

Determining the greatest good is often difficult if not impossible. Good can be interpreted in different ways. An outcome that may be good for one group may not be good for another. For example, staff development educators may be tempted to teach their favorite topics or trendy new issues instead of those classes most required for high-quality care. Although teaching these favored or trendy topics may fulfill the needs of the staff development educator, a disservice may be done to nursing staff and patients if only the educator's needs are met.

Educators should ask themselves the following questions:

- Who becomes the recipient of the greatest good?
- How is the correct portion of good allocated among recipients?
- Does majority rule?
- Is it better to effect a great good for a few people or a moderate good for many?

These are not easy questions to answer and should not be left to each educator to decide unilaterally. Clinical and administrative nursing representatives should participate in discussing and deciding important issues. A committee of educators and administrators should jointly reflect on their philosophies, values, and goals and then clearly articulate them to help guide educational practice.[7]

Deontological/Principled. Deontological or principled ethical theories emphasize the action as the locus for establishing morality. The deed, not the outcome, determines whether a course of action is ethical. The deontological approach to ethics provides the language commonly associated with morality—principles, rights, and duties. Kant's theory of the categorical imperative is the foundation for deontological ethics.[35]

Kant[20] believed acts should be universally valid and followed by people of good will. Moral decisions should be rule bound and rational based on what Kant believed to be objective truths. Each act should appeal to a general rule and remain true regardless of circumstances or possible outcomes. The uniqueness of each situation has less bearing on the ethical decision making in this framework.

Ethical principles require people to act in specific ways. These principles create duties. Perfect duties may never be ignored; imperfect duties allow for flexibility in decision making.[26] At times this distinction between perfect and imperfect duties can lead to unusual circumstances. For example, keeping a promise is a perfect duty for Kant. However, if a group of learners were told they could observe in a specialty unit, but when the scheduled time arrives, the unit has a particularly difficult patient census and several absent staff, should the promise be kept or the opportunity rescheduled? This situation may become more complicated if learners promised an opportunity to observe are unable to participate at the new time. The lack of situational and outcome sensitivity with the categorical imperative and perfect duties is a drawback to using them in practice.

One fundamental concept from Kant's work with strong implications for contemporary health care ethics is the philosophy that each person is an end. This means that ethical people cannot use another person simply as a means to achieve their own goals but that each person must be granted autonomy and treated with dignity and respect.[23]

Guiding Principles of Ethics

Most deontological approaches to ethical theory have multiple principles. The four basic principles in historical order are as follows[23]:
1. Nonmaleficence (avoiding harm)
2. Beneficence (doing good)
3. Autonomy (self-determination)
4. Justice (treating others fairly)

Nonmaleficence. Nonmaleficence can be traced to the Hippocratic oath of ancient Greece. Florence Nightingale also made nonmaleficence a cornerstone of nursing care. Nonmaleficence includes avoiding deliberate harm, risk of harm, and harm that may occur during the act of doing good. The vulnerability of many patients, the relative power of the health care establishment, and the potential for devastating iatrogenic illness and injury make this principle extremely important. The code of ethics of most health care professions are grounded on the principle of doing no harm to patients.[1,3,5]

Avoiding deliberate harm may be a straightforward idea, but avoiding harm or risk of harm that occurs while doing good is not as easy. Harm can encompass emotional, psychological, spiritual, and moral parameters, in addition to physical injury. The increasing invasiveness of health technologies and the diversity of caregivers magnify the potential risk of harm to patients. The expanding complexity of patient care requires interdependent interactions among nursing staff and between nursing staff and other health care providers. Some caregivers may believe they can provide care without receiving help from others, that is, the idea that to ask for help would be a sign of professional weakness and inhibit professional autonomy. During orientation classes, all learners must be impressed with the necessity of asking for consultation or assistance if a patient's care is beyond their knowledge and skills. This should not be presented as a sign of ignorance or deficiency but as professional strength in meeting ethical and legal responsibilities to avoid doing harm.

All patients have a right to high-quality nursing care. Ethical duties for staff development involve the acceptance of responsibility and accountability for the evaluation of learners' performances. Staff development educators must screen newly employed nurses so that deficits in knowledge, skill, and affect are identified during orientation and skill training. If educators have screened new nurses well, patients are more likely to receive high-quality nursing care. This benefits patients and learners.

The primary responsibility of staff development educators is to ascertain whether the instruction provided is correct and provides learners with skills for safe patient care within the organization. An educator is ethically obliged to take action if that educator has reason to believe another educator is incompetent or teaching incorrect or obsolete information.[34] The form of action taken depends on the cause. For instance, incompetence caused by chemical dependency requires different action than incompetence caused by lack of knowledge.

The follow-up of incompetent, unethical, or illegal activity within the staff development department requires the situation to be reported to higher authorities if the situation is not corrected within the department. This "whistle blowing" may have negative individual and departmental consequences, but whistle blowing is required if ethical standards are to be maintained. Also, educators should remember that the consequences of whistle blowing are ultimately less severe than allowing the incompetence to remain unreported until a patient is injured by the actions of a learner who was taught incorrectly or improperly supervised.[3,21,24]

The duty to prevent harm also extends to learners who should be protected from injuring themselves as they attempt to learn new skills or work with new

equipment.[34] Exposure to chemical, microbial, radiological, and other environmental health hazards should be avoided by adequate preparation. The staff
development educator must ascertain that learners have adequate preparation
for the clinical tasks undertaken. Equipment in learning laboratories and on
units must be monitored to ensure safety in its use. Protective garments and other
safety devices must be in use whenever appropriate, and instruction and supervision in the proper use of these garments and safety devices is mandatory.

Beneficence. Beneficence corresponds to the purpose of nursing care in that it
enhances the patient's health status. Most nurses enter nursing because they have
a strong desire to do good for others. The principle of beneficence demands more
of nurses than merely avoiding harm; it requires nurses to do good for their
patients. The demands of this principle can become overwhelming because doing
good is a limitless goal. The line between duty and the ideal is the most difficult
area of beneficence. Doing good is duty, but if that duty does not have bound-
aries, it changes from an expected duty to a rarely attainable heroic ideal. The
American Nurses Association's (ANA's) *Code for Nurses with Interpretive
Statements,*[1] *Standards for Clinical Nursing Practice,*[5] and *Standards for Nursing
Professional Development: Continuing Education and Staff Development*[6] are
important for not only clearly stating the expectations for professional practice
but also setting parameters of expectations.[2,5,7] Staff development educators can
help administrators set reasonable staffing patterns, develop job descriptions
based on levels of expertise, and update policies.

Staff development educators should emphasize the critical elements of a skill
or activity to learners. Once they are working on the unit ("the real world")
nurses may be tempted to "cut corners" to save time. If possible, these short cuts
should be anticipated in teaching, and rationales for not following them should
be provided. Periodic review of care, such as infection control or quality
improvement, may highlight areas in which practice techniques are less than
desirable and remedial instruction is needed. Conversely, staff development educators should work with orientees to help them set realistic self-expectations.
New graduates often come to the organization with highly idealistic goals for
themselves that cannot possibly be achieved. Educators may prevent new
employees from burning out by helping learners develop a more reasonable set
of expectations and realistic time frame for achieving their goals, thereby creating beneficence to colleagues.

Staff development educators, as all nurses, have the responsibility to implement and improve competencies essential for the practice of nursing. These competencies include skills, knowledge, humanitarian concern for others, and
accountability for actions. Educators should also possess the desire to improve
nursing practice for the public. Staff development often plays a major role in the
nursing department's quality improvement plans and the education of future
nurses. The nursing department depends on the staff development department to
design educational interventions in response to deficits revealed by quality-
improvement monitors. In this way the staff development department is critical

in implementing and improving standards of nursing practice.[7] Improved standards demonstrate beneficence for patients.

Advances in nursing research lead to ongoing modification in nursing knowledge and skills.[32] A barrage of new medications, equipment, and protocols must constantly be integrated into current practice. The responsibility of incorporating research educational activities presupposes that staff development educators read research.[32] Educators must be capable of critically analyzing findings and applying these findings to their practice. This competence is not easy to acquire and takes many years to master. However, the integration of knowledge and skills to improve patient care shows another example of beneficence.

Peer review activities are as necessary to teaching as they are to clinical practice. Peer review should include periodic monitoring of others' classes, objective review of anonymous evaluations from learners, an annual review of teaching performance, and an annual plan to increase competencies in specific areas of staff development.[7] The staff development department should also be under constant quality-improvement monitoring and should institute changes as suggested by evaluations. An annual total program evaluation focused on cost-benefit principles should determine program revisions.[7] Adherence of staff development to ethical and legal aspects of instruction is an important part of the total annual evaluation. In addition, the evaluation methods themselves must meet ethical and legal standards regarding such issues as confidentiality and nondiscrimination.[3,7]

Autonomy. *Autonomy* refers to respect for individuals by fostering self-determination, that is, allowing people the personal freedom of choice and action. Because autonomy implies choice, autonomous people must be capable of decision making and have choices. In the patient care setting, autonomy is usually only restricted to prevent harm and is supported through informed consent, right to refuse treatment, lack of deception (veracity), respect of privacy, maintenance of confidentiality, and honoring of commitments (fidelity).[9]

Feelings of helplessness and alienation can occur and hinder a patient's ability to act autonomously if that patient is unsure of who provides the various aspects of care. The public is entitled to know the professional and legal status of the people providing nursing care. As a result, staff development educators should set an example and teach others to always wear identification regarding their legal status as an RN and other academic degrees whenever performing patient care activities. Verbal introduction and identification of staff position is helpful for patients who are visually impaired.

Staff development educators are in the unique position to participate in or facilitate the research of others. In many large organizations, research is included in the staff development department's title, and staff development is responsible for all nursing research carried out within the agency. Research is necessary for all professions because the profession's body of knowledge must continually be expanded and incorporated into clinical practice. Each educator has an obligation to participate in research as a principle investigator, participant, or user of research findings.

Staff development educators must determine whether a research project has received approval from the internal review board, especially when human subjects are involved, before human subjects particpate in the research. Acting ethically requires that the autonomous rights of others (for example, informed consent, confidentiality, veracity, and fidelity) be safeguarded. Subjects must be informed of the risks and benefits of the research and understand that they can withdraw from the study at any time without penalty. If nurses are research subjects, they must also have these rights protected and be provided with the same information.[34]

Respect for each individual and the principle of autonomy also guide the interactions of staff development educators and learners. All people should be treated with respect so that each is seen as a unique individual regardless of differences. Staff development managers should adhere to policies of nondiscrimination in the selection and assignment of learners and instructors.[4,34] Whenever possible, learners should be included in planning and evaluating their learning experiences.

It is an ethical duty to instill in learners an attitude of lifelong self-responsibility for remaining competent in practice.[19] Learners must be taught ways to avail themselves of self-study opportunities to increase their proficiency. Educators occasionally jump on the bandwagons of self-directed learning or competency-based learning without adequately considering the ability of nursing service personnel to be self-directed learners. Establishing a learning center, purchasing audiovisual materials, and constructing pretests and posttests do not fulfill the staff development educators' responsibility for education. Learners must be coached, assisted, and helped until they begin to find satisfaction in moving at their own learning pace.[12]

In staff development, restrictions may be placed on the autonomous decisions of nurses. For example, newly hired nurses may choose the unit or specialty area in which they wish to practice, but they cannot be permitted the autonomy to refuse orientation or fail competence requirements for the unit.

Confidentiality is the respect of privileged information and supports the principle of autonomy. In addition to teaching staff members to safeguard patients' charts, prevent the invasion of patients' privacy, and not divulge patients' diagnoses, educators are responsibile for respecting confidential information about learners. Ethical conduct requires staff development personnel to keep all records pertaining to learners confidential.[34] Such knowledge is disclosed to the appropriate people *only* for evaluation purposes. These reports can direct a continuum of learning experiences so that learners may continue to master skills and become competent. Because staff development educators are often viewed as helpful mentors or preceptors, learners often confide in them. Some of these confidences could be potentially damaging to the individual (for example, past chemical dependency or psychiatric hospitalization). Talking indiscriminately about learners is as reprehensible as talking indiscriminately about patients.

Veracity pertains to truth telling. Truth provides the foundation for relationships with others by forming the basis of trust. If one person lies to another, the deceit is a type of manipulation that demonstrates a lack of respect. Except in extremely rare cases in which telling a patient the truth would cause serious harm, patients have the right to expect that their caregivers are honest in their communications.

If the staff development educators participate in research, they should be certain that scientific misconduct and fraud does not take place. Fry[16] indicates that activities such as fabricating data, manipulating subjects, forcing findings to support a preconceived outcome, plagiarizing in literature reviews, and misinterpreting results must not be condoned. Research that is openly reviewed by trusted colleagues has a better chance of being not only worthwhile but also free from ethical and legal problems.

Veracity is a basic component of an educator's position. Learners must be able to trust their educator's judgment regarding whether they are ready to fulfill the responsibilities of an assigned shift. If learners are deficient in some area, they must be told about their deficiency and, whenever possible, be provided with methods and resources for correcting the problem. Although informing people that their clinical performance is unacceptable in certain areas may be an uncomfortable task, it would be worse for learners to think they have successfully mastered a skill that they may in fact be unable to perform safely. Not only would this be a lie to the learner, but future patients could be placed in jeopardy.

Staff development educators should only use dignified and truthful ways of disseminating information about their services. They should also teach others acceptable means of advertising. Sometimes this involves teaching others the ways to write a resume or assemble a curriculum vitae, interview a prospective employee, or be interviewed for a new position.

When new nurses are hired by an organization, the staff development educators should make certain orientees receive honest information about the job requirements and expectations. Promises made about work hours and conditions should be factual and kept except on rare occasions.

Justice. In health care, justice focuses on a person's efforts to treat others fairly and ensure that the cost and benefits of health care are distributed equitably among individuals and groups.[23] This principle is concerned with the allocation of health resources and general health care delivery policies.

Effectiveness of program planning necessitates that staff development educators reflect the cultural diversity of the organization's patients, families, community, and personnel. Staff development managers have an ethical responsibility to hire staff educators of diverse backgrounds. This diversity should influence the design of classes so that efficient and effective learning occurs for patients and staff members.[7]

Educators play important roles in maintaining employment conditions conducive to high-quality patient care. These educators can impart the principles of problem solving, creativity, assertiveness, self-responsiblity, and accountability, and a powerful image of nursing while teaching employees in clinical and classroom settings.[34] Their attitude of respect for each new employee as an individual and the contribution that each employee can make to high-quality nursing care can be empowering. In this way many problems on the nursing unit can be solved before they become crises.

Staff development educators, through their example and teaching, should stress the responsibility of nurses for the community's health and the need to be active in community efforts to obtain high-quality health care at a reasonable cost. Political awareness and involvement can be fostered during contact with learners in class and clinical areas by discussing community-based health issues and local responses.[8,25]

Adversarial relationships with other disciplines do not contribute to optimal health care delivery, which can be attained only by interdisciplinary planning and cooperation. Because high-quality health care is the goal of nursing, educators must set an example of interdisciplinary collaboration with those in allied health occupations and physicians. Discussion regarding ways to make referrals should be included in orientation so that nursing staff begin with a mindset of collaboration. Communicating patient care information between disciplines through progress notes, reports, referrals, and patient care rounds can be effective.

In this age of entrepreneurs, many staff development educators may have interests in products, services, or activities unrelated to their responsibilities and positions within the organization. Ethically, such entrepreneurs should avoid conflicts of interest by not advocating their products or services while performing their responsibilities as educators. These educators should not take advantage of their responsibility for writing patient education monographs by including their products or services to the exclusion of similar products or services.

Educators should use and teach others to use generic names for referring to medications and products while teaching patients and their families. Families must be aware of all products or medications of similar quality so that the health teaching does not appear biased toward certain manufacturers. Thus patients and their families can maintain their autonomy in making decisions about products to purchase. Similarly, staff development educators should inform staff members about updates on medications and products so that patients receive the latest information. In all instances, nurses should refrain from discussing medications or products in a way that implies endorsement by the nursing profession rather than the opinion of one nurse.

The staff development department's budget should be cost effective but still permit educational activities to improve the clinical practice of nurses. Some staff development departments, in an effort to produce income, can become involved in presenting continuing education programs to nurses who are employed in other facilities. Such practice could lead to the educational neglect of nursing service personnel within the facility because the department's scarce resources are devoted to continuing education programs for learners outside the organization.[7]

Ethical considerations dictate that even in attempts to be cost effective and efficient, educators should make an honest effort to provide high-quality learning experiences. This precludes unethical practices such as entertaining rather than teaching, using general "boiler-plate" lesson plans rather than tailoring lesson plans to meet learners' needs, teaching general principles rather than specific nursing care based on general principles, and dazzling learners with credentials and multisyllabic words so that learners feel embarrassed to ask questions.[7]

Summary of Ethical Theory

The difficulty with ethical theories lies in the resolution of dilemmas occurring if two or more basic principles conflict. If two fundamental principles support mutually exclusive courses of action, determining which takes precedence is difficult. In many instances, patient safety (nonmaleficence) always takes priority.[15] If conflict between deontological principles occurs, a consequentialist viewpoint in the discussion is helpful to consider. The principle of utility brings concerns about outcomes. Although the utilitarian and principled perspectives differ in some respects, in practice, most people use a combination of the two in determining and justifying a course of action. The limitations of each theoretical realm are thus mitigated and the advantages of both are incorporated.[29] Staff development educators could play important roles by becoming members of the organization's ethics committee. Not only can staff development educators provide valuable insights to the ethics committee, but the committee can provide ideas about integrating ethical concerns in classes.

LEGAL ISSUES

Although ethics and law judge behavior and each influences the standards of the other, ethics and law perform different functions. Ethics focuses on the choice of action based on social values that affect human welfare. Law represents the authority and power that people have given their government to control human action. The codified legal standards of behavior are enforceable through a system of established regulations and punishments. Because of this threat of punishment, people are often more concerned with the legality than the ethics of a given action.

The legal system has several limitations as a manner of evaluating and controlling behavior. Many areas of human endeavor are beyond the scope of the law. Although ethically educators should treat their students with respect and dignity, legislation that could direct that to happen would be extremely difficult to draft. In addition, the law usually prevents the occurrence of specific behaviors by the threat of prosecution. People do not act in certain ways to avoid legal penalties; however, sometimes the fear of being caught is not enough to prevent undesirable behaviors because the chance of legal prosecution is slim. For example, if educators break confidentiality and tell their friends detailed information about the performance of orientees, the legal system is not likely to become involved. If society depended solely on the threat of legal action to regulate behavior, there would be chaos without the internalized standards of morality.

The sources of law are twofold—legislative/statutory and judicial/case. The statutory laws are enacted by governing bodies such as Congress. These laws

Table 16-2 Comparison of criminal and civil law

Criminal Law	Civil Law
State prosecutes	Plaintiff must sue
Guilt beyond a shadow of doubt	Preponderance of evidence
Incarceration and fines	Monetary awards to plaintiff
(for example, rape, theft, assault, murder)	(for example, malpractice, negligence, harassment, copyright, libel)

quickly effect change in broad groups of people. For example, in 1990 the federal Patient Self-Determination Act was passed, requiring all states to provide some mechanism for advanced directives such as a living will or health care proxy. When this law went into effect in 1991, every state had to have some form of advanced directive in operation. The legislature, which enacts the statutory laws, governs only specific geographical areas. That is, the laws for one state are only binding in that state. For example, each state has its own mental health code that defines the forms and requirements of commitment. There is a hierarchy to statutory law so that state laws supersede local laws and federal laws supersede state laws.[13]

The judiciary system is also restricted geographically and hierarchically. Local court rulings are only binding within that locality and state. Federal appeals courts can reverse lower court decisions. Judicial law is specific to each case but serves as a precedent to guide people in similar circumstances; therefore judicial law can have far-reaching results.[13]

There are two types of law—criminal and civil. Criminal law deals with acts found by the state to be such a threat to society that the state prosecutes the transgressors. Those people who are found guilty could be required to pay fines or be incarcerated. The evidence to find someone guilty must be proved beyond "a shadow of doubt."

Civil law, also called *tort law*, involves the infringement of legal rights or violation of public or private duties that cause damage to individuals. Unlike criminal acts, which are seen as threats to the public welfare, civil complaints are considered a matter between the defendant and plaintiff. In civil law the state does not bring the case forward, but rather one party sues the other for the legal case to occur. The amount of evidence for rendering a decision does not have to be as definitive as in criminal law. A preponderance of evidence is expected. In civil law the guilty party pays restitution for the harm done to the plaintiff. Civil law carries no threat of incarceration (Table 16-2).[13]

Criminal Law

Criminal offenses include murder, rape, assault and battery, and theft (from individuals and organizations). Although these acts seem far removed from nursing practice, these acts are committed by employees, patients, and visitors in special settings in which patients are vulnerable. For example, some employees view taking home hospital supplies, such as diapers and stock medications, as a "perk" of the job. Organizational mechanisms for prevention, detection, and reporting of crimes must be in place, and staff members must be aware of the way to use these mechanisms. This is especially true of crimes against patients.

Violation in the use of controlled substances is also a criminal offense. Because new graduate nurses may have had limited experience working with controlled substances, they should be instructed regarding the proper way to "waste" narcotics and monitor controlled substances on the units. A review of ways to identify chemically impaired people could also contribute to the management of controlled substances.

Often staff development educators are the first to suspect that an employee has a chemical-dependency problem. Ethical conduct requires judicious validation of suspicions and the involvement of the impaired employee in a rehabilitation program. It is unethical to find another reason to terminate the person's employment because the behavior will continue in another facility's nursing department and place other patients at risk. Also, if impaired employees are not openly and nonjudgmentally confronted about their illness, their denial of their disease will continue. If the organization does not have a program for chemically impaired employees, staff development educators can be the stimulus for establishing such a program. Educators can also provide information about other groups that offer professional peer support for nurses.

Fraud is a criminal offense that could relate to educators who provide programs for a fee but fail to meet advertised expectations. Truth is not only a just and ethical expectation for advertised programs but also a legal one. Sometimes, in their enthusiasm to have learners attend continuing education programs, educators make false claims about the program's benefits. Occasionally, seminars about motivation, assertiveness, case management, or nursing diagnosis are made to sound like cure-alls for the problems in nursing practice. Misrepresentation of faculty, falsely advertised Continuing Education Units (CEU) or approval information, promises of a benefit not provided and promised content not being provided are all unethical and can lead to fraud charges.[31]

Civil Law

Legal Rights. Civil law that focuses on legal rights includes issues of false imprisonment, lack of consent, invasion of privacy, defamation of character, discrimination, harassment, and copyright infringement. If educators instruct learners about informed consent, use of restraints, and involuntary commitment, the educators should include legal information about patients' rights. This is a critical element in the provision and documentation of care. Confidentiality of patient information with health care providers and visitors is especially important for educators to emphasize.

Educators must be certain that only the information needed for job performance is shared with learners and appropriate personnel. Personal facts about learners that are unrelated to job performance should remain confidential. If information is indiscriminately given out, a learner could bring charges against the educator for invasion of privacy, defamation of character, or slander.[34] Educators must be aware of and make others aware of copyright restrictions on materials they use. The Library of Congress has simple monographs available to provide basic information regarding copyright laws. These monographs are Circular 1: *Copyright Basics,* Circular 15: *Duration of Copyright,* Circular R 15: *Extension of Copyright Terms,* and Circular 22: *How to Investigate the Copyright Status of a Work.* These monographs can be obtained free by calling the Copyright Office Hotline at any time ([202]707-9100). As these circulars are updated, the Library of Congress sends the appropriate replacement for the circular requested.

These circulars discuss the "fair use" principle of copyrighted materials and the way to copyright personal materials. In general, fair use of copyrighted material depends on "the purpose of the use, the nature of the copyrighted work, the amount and substantiality of the material used in relation to the copyrighted work as a whole, and the effect of the use on the copyright owner's potential market for his work."[28] Since the copyright laws were revised in 1976, most educational institutions have adopted stringent regulations related to fair use of copyrighted material.[14]

Although reproduction of printed materials or copying films and computer software ordered for preview may seem cost effective during times of budgetary constraints, this practice is unethical and could violate copyright law. Copyright restrictions should be reviewed and followed after computer-assisted instructional software is purchased. Many software programs prohibit copying even for onsite use only. Instruction materials from a variety of media (print, audio, video) should be used in compliance with copyright laws.

At times, educators could be tempted to take materials from courses that they have attended, remove the original name, and use the materials for in-house classes. This is unethical in that it does not truly state the material's source and could violate copyright law. Staff development educators should request permission from the author or only use the material as a resource by combining its ideas with content tailored to the organization. In these cases, ethical practice includes adding a reference list that gives credit to the sources of ideas.

Although the overall design and content of the educational offering may include the work of one or several educators, the materials belong to the organization and not to individuals who wrote the lesson plans. This is called *work for hire.* Such work may not be used by individual instructors if they are hired by others outside the organization to present similar classes. For this latter use, instructors need permission from the original organization. Instructors also may not take these courses with them if they are hired by another organization.[30] The organization for which the educator worked when the courses were developed holds the copyright to the material.[28] Thus the unauthorized use of materials can be unethical *and* illegal.

Title VII of the Civil Rights Act of 1964 makes it illegal to discriminate against an individual with respect to terms and conditions of employment because of that person's race, color, gender, religion, or national origin. Prohibition of sexual harassment is part of the Title VII law. Staff development educators should be sure their teaching, including media being used, does not stereotype individuals or groups. Each educational program should be designed to develop an understanding of bias and harassment and their negative impact on the work environment. Organizational policies regarding discrimination and harassment, in addition to methods of remediation, should be available for all learners.[18]

Careful records documenting a learner's performance in classes and clinical settings are important to maintain. Documentation should be specific, objective, and observable. Evaluation criteria should be applied uniformly to all learners in the same situation and should reflect critical elements in the performance.[34] Learners should be aware of the standards of performance and methods of evaluation. Employment decisions based on capricious or discriminatory evaluations can lead to Title VII action.

Negligence/Malpractice. The second major area of civil law is malpractice law. This part of tort law deals with professional acts of negligence and malpractice. These terms are often used interchangeably but differ in certain aspects. Negligence is the failure to do something that a reasonable person in a similar situation would do (for example, raise the siderails after sedating a patient) or doing something that a reasonable person would not do (for example, giving an infant to the wrong mother). Negligent acts are breaches in duty that require less professional judgment to be carried out properly than acts of malpractice. Malpractice refers to professional misconduct, unreasonable lack of skill, or lack of fidelity in professional duties. Examples of malpractice include the failure to properly assess and intervene in a timely way or perform procedures incorrectly.

The four components of a negligence/malpractice suit are duty, breach of duty, harm, and proximate cause. All four should be present to make a strong case. *Duty* means that a professional relationship must have been established between the nurse and patient. Dereliction or breach of duty implies that the care provided fell below the accepted standards of practice. The patient must show that some harm or damage occurred. (This damage could be emotional or physical.) Finally, the breach in duty must be shown to directly cause or contribute to the patient's harm.[13]

Written documentation is critical in the decision-making process in malpractice cases. A malpractice case may not be filed until years after the care was given. Reconstruction of the events without a solid, written history is extremely difficult. Staff development educators need to be sure that new nurses know the organization's proper charting and reporting policies. The purpose and process of incident reporting should be explained to new nurses. In addition to the legal implications of incidence reporting, the use of these reports to discover patterns of problems should be stressed, thereby decreasing or preventing future occurrences.

If malpractice litigation involves nurses, litigation ordinarily concerns clinical nursing practice and not education provided by staff development. However, malpractice in a clinical situation may be defended by citing that inappropriate instruction in the classroom or supervision on the unit caused the breech in duty. This is especially possible if the nurse's performance involves highly technical skills and judgments.

In determining malpractice, courts ordinarily assume nurses should have performed duties in a manner and with the degree of skill that a reasonable, prudent nurse with similar training and experience would have used under the same or similar circumstances. The circumstances usually considered are "the nature and complexity of the nursing function; and the urgency of the overall situation."[17] The staff development educators may become involved because they are usually the ones who assess each nurse's professional qualifications to function in the assigned unit. Some states allow damages to be apportioned among multiple defendants, and the portion is determined by the extent of each defendant's involvement.

The following guidelines should be followed by educators to avoid liability[17]:
1. Practice within the scope of the nursing practice criteria.
2. Observe the hospital and nursing department's policy and procedure manuals.
3. Practice according to established standards for nursing practice and staff development.
4. Always put the patient's rights and welfare first.
5. Develop and maintain a good interpersonal relationship with all patients and their families.

Staff development educators can be legally held responsible for the actions of those they supervise. Under the doctrine of respondeat superior, an employer is held responsible for the negligent acts of employees. As a supervisor of nurses while they are learners, staff development educators are not automatically held liable for the negligent acts of learners. However, educators could be held liable if they were negligent in supervising the learners or requesting learners to perform tasks outside their scope of nursing practice.[17]

Nurse and medical practice acts are written in broad language. Many actions are not specified as nursing or medical actions; therefore some actions once performed only by physicians are now performed by nurses. Likewise some actions once performed only by RNs are now delegated to LPNs or nursing assistants. Each state or organization has regulations or guidelines governing activities that can be performed by nurses and activities that assistants can provide. Malpractice insurance companies may also have a set of guidelines regarding the scope of nursing practice. There should be joint policy statements from nursing and medicine delineating activities that comprise the "gray areas" not specifically permitted or forbidden in the nurse and medical practice acts. Staff development educators must remain up-to-date on the changes in practice acts, joint policy statements, and guidelines for practice. Educators should be aware if additional instruction is needed for nurses to practice within these gray areas and develop programs to assist the staff in acquiring necessary credentials.[33]

This part of the regulation of nursing practice by nurses is accorded to the profession by the public. Beyond basic licensure, professionals are expected to be individually responsible for their own practice and for the practice of their peers. If nurses assume functions such as the monitoring of high-risk newborns, the interpretation of cardiac dysrhythmias, or peritoneal dialysis, staff development educators assume the responsibility of designing educational programs that upgrade and update the skills of practicing nurses and of ascertaining that nurses who are new to the organization are competent in these skills.

Thus if staff development educators have been careless in assessing the ability of learners to care for certain patients or have made an assignment that exceeds the normal scope of nursing practice, they could be held liable for malpractice under the doctrine of respondeat superior. Similarly, educators must stress the responsibility of nurses in delegating activities to others. There is an ethical and legal obligation to correctly assess the competencies of others before delegating patient care. All nursing staff should receive instruction regarding the delegation of activities also governed by joint policy statements and guidelines of the organization.[17]

Staff development educators should carry their own malpractice insurance. Although some people believe that if staff development educators do not have insurance, they will be less likely to be sued, lawsuits are usually brought against as many people as possible in the current litigious society. The employing organization carries malpractice insurance for all its nursing staff, but individual nurses still find it important to have a lawyer who considers only that nurse's concerns.

SUMMARY

Staff development educators have a responsibility to their learners, their employing organization, and the patients served by the organization to remain current with the legal requirements of nursing practice and incorporate these requirements into learning experiences. Legal concerns are often enmeshed with ethical concerns. As staff development educators plan course content, they have an opportunity to include legal and ethical concerns.

REFERENCES

1. American Nurses Association: *Code for nurses with interpretive statements*, Kansas City, Mo, 1985, The Association.
2. American Nurses Association: *Continuing education in nursing guidelines for staff development*, Kansas City, Mo, 1978, The Association.
3. American Nurses Association: *Guidelines on reporting incompetent, unethical or illegal practices*, Washington, DC, 1994, The Association.
4. American Nurses Association: *Multicultural issues in the nursing workforce and workplace*, Proceedings of invitational meeting, Washington, DC, 1994, The Association.
5. American Nurses Association: *Standards for clinical nursing practice*, Washington, DC, 1991, The Association.
6. American Nurses Association: *Standards for nursing professional development: continuing education and staff development*, Washington, DC, 1994, The Association.
7. American Nurses Association: *Standards for nursing staff development*, Kansas City, Mo, 1990, The Association.

8. Aroska MA: Ethical foundations in nursing for broad health care access, *Sch Inq Nurs Pract* 6(3):201, 1992.

9. Bandman EL, Bandman B: *Nursing ethics through the lifespan*, ed 2, Norwalk, Conn, 1990, Appleton & Lange.

10. Bentham J: *An introduction to the principles of morals and legislation*, New York, 1948, Hafne.

11. Brock D: The nurse-patient relation: some rights and duties. In Spicker SF, Gadow S, editors: *Nursing: images and ideals*, New York, 1980, Springer.

12. Brocket R, editor: *Ethical issues in adult education*, New York, 1988, Teachers College.

13. Cowdrey ML: *Basic law for the allied health professions*, Boston, 1990, Jones & Bartlett.

14. Dorr RC, Munch CH: *Protecting trade secrets, patents, copyrights, and trademarks*, Somerset, NJ, 1990, John Wiley & Sons.

15. Fowler MDM: Ethical decision making in clinical practice, *Nurs Clin North Am* 24(4):955, 1989.

16. Fry ST: Ethical issues in research: scientific misconduct and fraud, *Nurs Outlook* 38(6):296, 1990

17. Goldstein, AR, Perdew S, Pruitt S: *The nurse's legal advisor: your guide to legally safe practice*, Philadelphia, 1989, JB Lippincott.

18. Goodner ED, Kolenich DB: Sexual harassment: perspectives from past, present practice, policy, and prevention, *J Contin Educ Nurs* 24(2):57, 1993.

19. Jameton A: *Nursing practice: the ethical issues*, Englewood Cliff, NJ, 1984, Prentice-Hall.

20. Kant I: *Fundamental principles of the metaphysics of morals*, New York, 1949, Macmillan (Translated by TK Abbott).

21. Kiely MA, Kiely DC: Whistleblowing: disclosure and its consequences for professional nurse and management. In Pence T, Cantral J, editors: *Ethics in nursing: an anthology*, New York, 1990, National League for Nursing.

22. Mill JS: *On liberty*, New York, 1926, Macmillan.

23. Munson R: *Intervention and reflection: basic issues in medical ethics*, ed 4, Belmont, Calif, 1992, Wadsworth.

24. Muyskens JL: The nurse as a member of a profession. In Pence T, Cantral J, editors: *Ethics in nursing: an anthology*, New York, 1990, National League for Nursing.

25. Northrop CE, Kelly ME: *Legal issues in nursing*, St Louis, 1987, Mosby.

26. Nunner-Winkler G: Two moralities? A critical discussion of an ethic of care and responsibility versus an ethic of rights and justice. In Kurtine W, Gerwitz J, editors: *Morality, moral behavior, and moral development*, New York, 1980, John Wiley & Sons.

27. Nursing Ethics Commitee, Department of Nursing, The Mount Sinai Medical Center, New York City: The ethics survey: an important step in promoting nursing ethics, *J NYSNA*, 20(4):4, 1989.

28. Party WF: *The fair use privilege in copyright law*, Washington, DC, 1985, The Bureau of National Affairs.

29. Payton RJ: Pluralistic ethical decison making. In Thompson JO, Thompson HO, editors: *Professional ethics in nursing*, Malabar, Fla, 1990, Robert E Krieger.

30. Pearson GA: Business ethics: implications for continuing education/staff development practice, *J Contin Educ Nurs* 18(1):20, 1987

31. Pearson GA, Kennedy MS: Business ethics: implications for providers and faculty of continuing education programs, *J Contin Educ Nurs* 16(1):4, 1985.

32. Pettengill MM, Gillies DA, Clark CC: Factors encouraging and discouraging the use of nursing research findings, *Image: J Nurs Sch*, 26(2):143, 1994.

33. Quinn CA, Smith MD: *The professional commitment: issues and ethics in nursing*, Philadelphia, 1987, WB Saunders.

34. Rosenkotter MM: A code of ethics for nurse educators, *Nurs Outlook* 31(5):288, 1983.
35. Thompson JE, Thompson HO: *Bioethical decision making for nurses*, Norwalk, Conn, 1985, Appleton-Century-Crofts.
36. Turner SL, Rufo MK: An overview of nursing ethics for nurse educators, *J Contin Educ Nurs* 23(6):272, 1992.
37. White JE: *Contemporary moral problems*, St Paul, 1991, West.
38. Winslow GR: From loyalty to advocacy: a new metaphor for nursing, *Hastings Center Report*, 14(3):32, 1984.

JACQUELINE M. KATZ

Managing the Dual Dimensions of Quality

17

New values and economic necessity are two crucial elements responsible for social change.[20] High quality is a prevalent value of this new era in health care; cost containment is an economic necessity. Managing these elements successfully depends on a dual role of current staff development educators in implementing the new quality initiatives embraced by many health care organizations.

Value, which is the relationship between quality and cost, has become the new objective of health care. In a resource-driven environment the challenge is to keep quality up and costs low. Organizations that achieve cost-effective quality have the competitive edge.

Achieving that competitive edge is intimately linked to the quality of the practitioners providing health care. According to the Joint Commission on Accreditation of Healthcare Organizations (JCAHO),[13] "the ability of a health care professional or other staff to perform or support a patient care activity (i.e., without fault or error) and to perform or support the correct patient care activity (i.e., conforms with or adheres to preestablished guidelines) often has direct bearing on the quality of patient care. These abilities are related to the health care professional or other staff's training, experience and other attributes."[11] Educational services play a critical role in supporting the quality efforts of organizations. The internal quality of educational services must be sound to contribute to any organization's overall quality initiative.

This chapter focuses on the two dimensions of quality involved in the role of staff development educators. These dimensions are the organization's quality, especially in the nursing service department, and the quality the staff development department. Specific characteristics of quality and the responsibility of the staff development department for improving that quality within the organization and staff development department are discussed in relation to the characteristics of high quality and a framework for achieving high quality.

WORKFORCE AND WORKPLACE FACTORS AFFECTING QUALITY

Anything that affects the competence of the health care worker directly affects the quality and cost of service an organization can provide. Staff development educators must confront and overcome many workforce and workplace issues to fulfill their accountability for maintaining the staff's competence. Although not every organization is affected by all these factors, each organization is affected by at least one.

The first factor, illiteracy, is often a hidden saboteur in many current nursing service departments. Approximately 27 million Americans are functionally illiterate; another 45 million are only marginally literate.[1] This problem may lead to an inability to compute medication dosages, write clear patient notes, or comprehend written instructions or procedures. The problem is compounded by the success of many of these individuals at camouflaging their problem. In addition, the employment of foreign-born nurses has added the problems of knowing English as a primarily second language to the literacy issue.

The second factor affecting competence is the "skills gap," that is, the deficit between the skills needed to function as a beginning clinician and those possessed by the new graduate. With dynamic work environments, hospitals are at great risk if a skills gap exists. Patient care suffers if a proportion of the staff members cannot fulfill the responsibilities of their jobs. Preceptor programs require a large investment from the organization to bridge the existing gaps in skills and knowledge.

The third factor is the rapid pace of technologic change. These rapid changes place a strain on the competence of all clinicians, even the experienced. Whether the advances are in the form of new clinical procedures and equipment, such as lithotripsy or streptokinase injection, or systems technology, such as computers and fax machines, the performance pressure increases.

The fourth factor, demographic changes in the workforce, has resulted in increased cultural diversity within the nursing staff. The Bureau of Labor Statistics projects that African-Americans, Hispanics, and other nonwhite groups will account for approximately 53% of the growth in the labor force between 1988 and the turn of the century.[23] Many of these individuals will occupy entry-level positions in health care and require special types of orientation and ongoing enculturation.

The fifth factor involves changes in the operating systems of health care. Shared governance, managed care, continuous quality improvement, and the emphasis on cost containment have profoundly influenced the skills required of clinicians and managers within the nursing service department. The new JCAHO standards for nursing care and the *Agenda for Change* are creating a trend toward a results-oriented, rather than process-oriented, approach to the delivery of nursing services.

All these factors combine to increase the accountability of the staff development department for maintaining and monitoring the competence of nursing service staff. Staff development educators are responsible for ensuring that the nursing service staff are capable of performing consistently and uniformly. The changing workforce and workplace variables challenge the ingenuity and resilience of educators to prepare nursing staff members who are capable of delivering high-quality care in the most efficient and effective way possible.

THE FUTURE OF QUALITY IN HEALTH CARE

Quality management, a discipline concerned with doing the right things correctly, is the economic imperative of the future in health care. High quality gives an organization a competitive edge in the current health care environment; quality management is the means to achieving high quality. Quality management is a systematic method of ensuring that everything happens according to plan. It is the process of working smarter, not harder.

Quality management builds on the premise of continual improvement, a concept akin to the Japanese process called *Kaizen*, which sets progressively higher objectives in the pursuit of incremental improvement.[19] According to Dennis O'Leary, president of JCAHO, quality can never be ensured; at best, quality can only be improved.[21] Attention must be focused on improving norms for performance rather than solely on reacting to performance problems as they arise.

Quality management means that services are planned, implemented, and evaluated to ensure high-quality services for consumers. "The service is defined, standards are set and both accounting and utilization monitoring processes are developed. Building quality into the service is based on the standards for quality service."[4]

Three interrelated components make up quality management—quality awareness, quality appraisal, and quality improvement. Quality awareness is the development of a value system. The organization's written standards explicitly detail the value system of that organization. This value system is composed of commitment to quality, standards development, and staff education. Quality awareness provides the foundation for quality appraisal.

Quality appraisal consists of monitoring and evaluating activities. These activities include quality assurance, performance review, customer satisfaction analyses, and research. Quality appraisal confirms the achievement of results, staff compliance with standards, and the satisfaction of internal and external customers. Quality appraisal provides the data necessary for quality improvement.

Quality improvement is the response system. Crosby[6] emphasizes that the elements found in quality appraisal are not as important as the resulting action. "All the planning, inspection, testing, measuring, and other activities...are a waste of time if they don't lead to preventing a recurrence of a problem." Quality improvement comprises research and action planning, implementation, and follow-up. "Quality improvement means all employees in the institution are trying every day to do their jobs better, not merely trying to attain a minimum level of competence to satisfy QA standards."[8] Quality improvement reinforces the need for ongoing quality awareness.

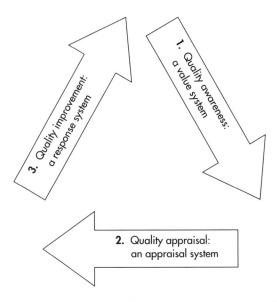

Fig. 17-1   Components of quality management model. (Courtesy Katz JM, Green E, Baltimore, 1991.)

Figure 17-1 illustrates the relationship of these three components. Quality awareness is the value system, quality appraisal is the appraisal system, and quality improvement is the response system.

LINKING NURSING SERVICE QUALITY EFFORTS AND EDUCATION

The staff development department cannot work in isolation nor can it measure success by classroom evaluations. A staff nurse who meets learner objectives used to indicate that educators had done a good job. Currently, staff educators must look beyond their classroom doors to the clinical units to judge whether they have done their jobs well.

Staff development educators have struggled for years to identify their contribution to improved patient outcomes. Evaluating the impact of education on patient care is difficult because many variables other than education affect patient care. If educational activities are linked to nursing service practice, educators can evaluate their activities in terms of improved patient care.

Evidence of the link between educational activities and improved patient care is a necessity. Accrediting bodies demand documentation of educational activities as a means of solving quality problems. Site visitors review the percentage of educational activities devoted to quality improvement. The JCAHO standards for quality assessment and improvement[15] suggest that "the leaders assure that organization staff are trained in assessing and improving the processes that contribute to improved patient outcomes." The administration expects staff development education to support its priorities for high-quality patient care. Ulschak says[25]:

The key for education today is to be doing the work of the organization; the education department's every objective needs to be directly tied to the organization's objectives. All the work of the education department should be on target with the needs of the organization.

Economic survival of the staff development department is contingent on the department's ability to distinguish itself in all three phases of the nursing service department's overall quality management program (that is, quality awareness, quality appraisal, and quality improvement).

Staff Development as a Quality-Awareness Resource

Two major mechanisms are necessary for the staff development department to fully realize its potential role in quality awareness. The first is the role department members play in strategic planning and decision-making; the second is the department's role in providing staff education that focuses on quality.

Of the support-service roles played by the staff development department, no role is more important than the department's involvement in strategic planning. The staff development department should not be notified *after* a new program is initiated or a major change has occurred. The staff development department should not be left out of major decisions because this department is the major facilitator of change within an organization. In the current environment, input from the staff development department members is critical for any new program or major change. This necessitates that the director of the staff development department have a voting position on the nursing executive committee, thereby assuring that the education department is informed of and has input into the nursing service priorities for change.

According to Hefferin,[12] if the educational component is included during the design phase of any major change, traditional problems of educators' lack of authority over line managers may be overcome. If quality is to be built into the design phase of change, educational implications of that change must be considered.

Nowhere is the need for this input more obvious than in the change to a quality-improvement initiative. The most carefully designed and marketed program for monitoring and improving the quality of patient care will be ineffective if staff members are not educationally prepared for the new process. Educating staff regarding the "whys", "how tos", and "whats" of quality improvement is another aspect of using the staff development department as a quality-awareness resource. Quality educational programming should permeate the three major areas of staff development activity—orientation, in-service education, and continuing education.

Bennett and Tibbitts[3] believe that high quality begins with orientation. Instilling quality as the focus of all their patient care activities is the major function of orientation for new staff. This is the first step in the ongoing enculturation of staff regarding their responsibilities and accountability for the quality of patient outcomes. The focus of in-service education should not only be on the specific task or new product, but also on the ways in which this task or new product facilitates the pursuit of high-quality patient care and improves patient outcomes.

Educational programming must not only focus on the technical aspects of monitoring quality, but also on the individual's role in quality analysis and improvement. Bliersbach[5] suggests that classes should deal with attitudes related to quality such as overcoming resistance to change, individual accountability for outcomes, and creating incentives for improving quality.

Staff Development as a Quality-Appraisal Resource

Stanley Randall is credited with saying that the closest to perfection a person ever comes is filling out a job application. Ideal candidates are hired, but something happens to them between the time they are hired and the time they begin work. Those ideal people suddenly become human with all of humanities inherent frailties and flaws.

Generally, whenever nursing staff members display their frailties and make mistakes, someone suggests they need to take a class. These nurses are then sent to an in-service class to correct the problem. If the problem crops up again, some educators will reeducate them again and again. Not only is this process frustrating for the learners and educators, it is a colossal waste of resources. Contrary to popular belief, education is not the golden ticket to eradicating quality problems.

Many administrators are victims of this educational "revolving-door" syndrome because they possess a limited vision of performance. If performance is solely based on competence, education becomes the catchall solution. Performance is actually composed of competence and productivity. A person must possess the knowledge, skills, and attitudes to perform a specified activity and then apply that knowledge appropriately to get the job done. A person's possession of correct knowledge, skills, and attitudes is competence. Application of the knowledge, skills, and attitudes at the right time to effect the right results is productivity. Competence without productivity is useless and recalls the philosophical question, "If a bomb goes off in the desert but there is no one to hear it, did it make a sound?" Likewise, if a person passes all the tests and return demonstrations but does not apply the skills appropriately, is that person productive?

Performance-based quality problems usually result from either individual or organizational factors. The individual factors are either a lack of competence or productivity. The organizational factors are usually either a lack of resources or participation (Fig. 17-2).

Sovie[24] suggests that educators "investigate before you educate" and lists the following four criteria that can be applied while determining whether a problem requires an educational solution.

1. Is there documented evidence of staff skill or knowledge in this area?

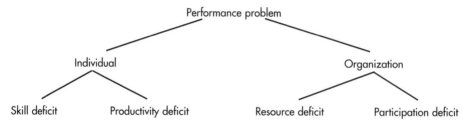

Fig. 17-2   Performance problem tree. (Courtesy Katz JM, Green E, Baltimore, 1991.)

2. Are other departments performing to expected or established standards?
3. Are the organization's policies and procedures written clearly, and do they adequately suit the situation?
4. Does the problem disappear if a policy or procedure is changed or the task is carried out appropriately by a responsible staff member?

If the answer to the first question is yes, there is no need for an educational solution to the problem. One way for educators to ensure that there is documented evidence of competence is to focus on the critical competencies essential for the delivery of high-quality services. Focusing competency checks on the major aspects of clinical practice for specific units and eliminates long lists of competencies required for all nurses. The staff development department focuses on competencies for those aspects of practice of a high priority and requiring most of the nurses' time. Guaranteeing skills and knowledge in the high-priority practice areas directly affects the goals of monitoring and evaluation activities. "The emphasis of monitoring and evaluation activities should progressively shift from individual 'outlier' identification to on-going assessment of the composite performance of key functions."[22] Similarly, the shift in emphasis in staff development must be from validating all competencies to assessing performance of critical competencies necessary to perform those key functions. Only then can education document its link with quality-improvement efforts. Educators can ensure that the answer to Sovie's first question is a resounding "yes" by defining the critical competencies in writing, developing programs to ensure competence in these areas, and documenting competence.

Staff Development as a Quality-Improvement Resource

The challenge for any quality-improvement program is to work smarter not harder. A crucial need to find quicker, smarter, less-expensive methods of achieving high-quality outcomes exists in these times of economic instability and downsizing.

Staff development educators play a critical role in helping the nursing service department offer service quicker, smarter, cheaper, and better. Current and accurate educational programming based on the latest nursing research provides the information that staff members need to change a practice method.

If educators want to play a vital role in the quality-improvement process, they must be able to show ways that education affects the bottom-line. Educators must be able to document the staff development department's contribution to issues of quality and cost. Although education is not the only determining factor in an organization's positive return on investment, educators must increase their visibility and credibility regarding their contributions to high-quality outcomes. The members of the staff development department must look internally and design mechanisms for continuous quality improvement to accomplish increased visibility and credibility.

NEW EMPHASIS ON INTERNAL QUALITY MANAGEMENT

Standard NC.2 of the JCAHO nursing standards states that "all members of the nursing staff are competent to fulfill their assigned responsibilities."[11] Nursing staff positions include RNs, LPNs, LVNs, nursing assistants, and other nursing personnel. Those individuals who provide care must be competent to provide high-quality patient care. Requirements for competence assessment are outlined in standard NC.2 (box).

Specific internal mechanisms must be in place to meet the requirements of this standard. Although the organization may choose the way its competence assessment system is constructed, certain basic elements must be present. The elements necessary for compliance with JCAHO requirements are as follows[14]:

1. Nursing staff members have their competence assessed as part of the initial employment and orientation process.
2. The competence of nursing staff members is maintained through a combination of ongoing competence assessment and educational activities.
3. An objective, measurable performance evaluation system is used to evaluate current competence.

REQUIRED CHARACTERISTICS OF JCAHO STANDARD NC.2

NC.2: All nursing staff members* are competent to fulfill their assigned responsiblities

NC.2.1: Each nursing staff member is assigned clinical and/or managerial responsibilities based on educational preparation, applicable licensing laws and regulations, and an assessment of current competence.

NC.2.1.1: An evaluation of each nursing staff member's competence is conducted at defined intervals throughout the individual's association with the hospital.

NC.2.1.1.1: The evaluation includes an objective assessment of the individual's performance in delivering patient care services in accordance with patient needs.

NC.2.1.1.2: The process for evaluating competence is defined in policy and procedure.

---

*Nursing staff members include RNs, LPNs, LVNs, nursing assistants, and other nursing personnel.

From Joint Commission on Accreditation of Healthcare Organizations, Chicago, 1994.

4. A report about the levels of competence and competence maintenance functions is given at least annually to the governing body.

The competence assessment system must be explained in writing and include objective measurement tools. Examples of objective measurement tools include management-by-objectives techniques, clinical ladders, performance standards, and peer review.

In addition, section four of the latest accreditation manual focuses on the orientation, training, and education of staff members. This content will ultimately be integrated into the human resources segment of the section about organizational functions. Standards in section four include statements such as the following:

1. The organization provides a sufficient orientation for employees related to their individual responsibilities and ways to fulfill these responsibilities. Orientation is necessary for every newly hired person or whenever an individual transfers to a different department or service.
2. The organization provides education and training for all personnel to improve their knowledge and skills. This education is based on a needs assessment that considers the patient population served; the type and nature of the care provided; each staff member's needs; results of performance reviews; peer review data; and findings from plant, technology, safety management, and infection control programs. The education must include learning objectives and effective instructional strategies.
3. The effectiveness of orientation and continuing education efforts are monitored by quality assessment and improvement activities.
4. Staff members are competent as appropriate to their individual responsibilities regarding the knowledge and skills required to carry out those responsibilities, the safe and effective use of equipment required in the pursuit of those responsibilities, infection control, and cardiopulmonary resuscitation (CPR).

ACHIEVING HIGH QUALITY

Evaluation of program effectiveness has been a concern of staff development educators for a long time. Many evaluation models have been developed to assist educators with evaluation. However, now that the current focus is on bottom-line accountability, the need to use an outcome-focused evaluation is more important than ever.

The traditional focus of evaluation efforts has been on whether educational programs meets the identified needs of learners. The current focus must shift to be on whether and how those identified needs of learners significantly contribute to the continuous quality improvement program. The former view of program evaluation must give way to an expanded view of evaluation as part of quality management within the staff development department.

Hefferin's review of the literature[11] about the evaluation of in-service effectiveness indicates little evidence of this type of broad-based evaluation of in-service activities and a total absence of guidelines for conducting such a broad-based evaluation. Her review indicates that the current focus of evaluation is still on learner achievement of behavioral objectives.

As a support service within the department of nursing, staff development is similar to a service subsidiary. Staff development does not exist to fulfill the primary mission of the nursing department but rather to *assist* in the fulfillment of the primary mission. In any service three critical components exist—customer, employee, and system. The customer receives the service, the employee provides the service, and the system is the mechanism by which the service is delivered. Each component is critical to the existence of any business; eliminate one, and no business can exist.[15] In staff development the business is education. The customer is each member of the nursing service department. The employees are the staff development educators hired by the department and educator extenders such as preceptors and clinical specialists who have educational responsibilities as part of their clinical roles. The system is composed of the operating mechanisms used to help the department fulfill its mission. The quality of any service depends on the interplay of these components.

DEFINING QUALITY

Harry S Truman once said, "If you can't convince them, confuse them." This might be the operant slogan for the current state of the quality health care movement. Much lip service has been given to the concept of quality, whereas the word itself has become an enigma. Many definitions for quality in health care exist, although each one is more complex than the other. This lack of consensus regarding the definition of quality has inhibited the pursuit of increased quality by mystifying it. Basically three arenas exist in which to define quality—user-, service-, and system-based quality.

User-Based Quality

Although health care professionals find quality difficult to define, consumers (or users) can easily distinguish the lack of quality. Some definitions of quality refer to it purely as meeting customers' expectations. This user-based definition assumes that quality is in the eye of the beholder.[7] This may work well in the general market in which consumers have become savvy about the workings of a computer or an automobile; however, most patients have not yet achieved the acumen to determine diagnostic effectiveness.

In staff development, consumers (or users) are the learners. Learners are quick to define a high-quality educational offering. A learner-based definition of quality is highly subjective and may vary widely from one learner to the next. Participant evaluations of a learning experience may reveal that for some learners the level of presentation was too advanced, for others it was too basic, and for the remainder the level was just right. This "three bears" response pattern makes the user-based approach to defining the quality of education unreliable. Although the user's perception of quality is important in determining the degree of quality, it is not and cannot be the *only* defining variable.

Service-Based Quality

Much of the focus on quality in health care has been centered on the clinician. In this approach the focus of quality is as a service-based phenomenon. The concentration is on the process of providing health care services. Quality deals with the supply side of the equation and is usually defined as conformance to requirements.[6]

In staff development, service-based quality has also been the focus. The process of applying for program accreditation has focused on questions such as "Were the behavioral objectives clearly stated?" and "Does the content to be presented match the course objectives?" Defining quality by using only service-based quality questions is also too narrow a view. Experienced educators all have stories about beautifully planned and executed programs that were totally ineffective. One reason for this outcome might be that planners of the program failed to consider individual learners differences, for example, differences in learning styles.

System-Based Quality

The third arena of quality is system based. Quality is defined in terms of some ingredient or attribute possessed by the system. In health care the latest technologic advances and the newest equipment might be examples of ingredients or products that contribute to the improved quality of health care. The product of staff development is the curriculum. Having the newest innovation in educational hardware or software does not in and of itself ensure quality. A computer laboratory, interactive videodisks, and a preceptor program do not necessarily make a high-quality educational service. Thus the system-based definition of quality is also too narrow in scope in that it fails to take individual preferences and service applications into account.

User-based, service-based, and system-based quality can conflict with each other. It is possible for individuals within the same department to adopt differing approaches to quality. The results can be less than optimal. Individually, each way of defining quality has limitations. In reality, quality is an amalgam of all three. Trying to devise a succinct statement that incorporates the essence of all three has eluded the best quality experts.

Key Dimensions of Quality

Garvin[7] suggests in his book *Managing Quality* that defining quality by its characteristics is much easier and more precise. He defined the following eight key dimensions or characteristics of quality:
1. Performance
2. Features
3. Reliability
4. Conformance
5. Durability
6. Serviceability

7. Aesthetics
8. Perceived quality

Performance. Performance is the primary operating characteristic of a service and is the primary functioning of the department. It is composed of the functions and responsibilities that make up the essence of the department. Performance influences the outcomes of the service and is composed of the service's capabilities and productivity. It is possible to determine the quality of performance by asking, "Is the service able to achieve quality results and does the service apply the abilities it has to achieve the desired results?" In the airline industry this would include the volume of lost luggage or the on-time flight arrival record. In health care the question might involve the amount of time patients wait between requesting pain medication and receiving it. In education a performance variable might be the response time between identification of a competency deficit and its correction. High-quality performance requires careful attention to design and educators capable of preparing strong designs for educational programs. In education, quality is built into the program development phase.

Features. Features are the secondary characteristics that supplement the service's basic functioning. These are the "bells and whistles" components. Although not essential to the service, features provide extra value by enhancing the efficiency, comfort, or timeliness of the service. For example, double-coupon savings are a feature at supermarkets. In health care, complimentary wine with dinner, 24-hour room service, or color-coordinated sheets may make a patient's hospital stay more pleasant, but these features are not essential to the safe and effective delivery of patient care. Similarly, in education, a continental breakfast and comfortable seats are not essential to effective learning, but they certainly add to the educational experience.

Reliability. Reliability is the accuracy of the service over time, among providers, and across consumers. If a service is reliable, consistent results are obtained regardless of the time that the service is provided, the person providing the service, or the person receiving the service.[16] An example of service reliability is the American Automobile Association (AAA), providing travelers with information and assistance regardless of time, location, or person. In health care, reliability means patients receive the same type and level of care regardless of the unit, nurse, shift, or patient. In education, reliability depends on the ability of learning experiences to achieve consistent results regardless of the instructor, learners, time, or location.

Conformance. Conformance is the degree to which a service meets preestablished industry standards. In a service business, conformance measures are typically related to accuracy and timelessness. For instance, in an accounting firm, conformance might relate to the accuracy with which tax returns are prepared. In health care, compliance occurs if standards set by agencies, such as JCAHO, are put into practice. In education, industry standards are also set by professional organizations and accrediting bodies. The ANA's Council for Professional Development: Continuing Education and Staff Development has developed standards for staff development.[2] The American Nurses Credentialing Center (ANCC) and state nurses' associations have accreditation standards for the awarding of continuing education contact hours. Internal standards are developed within the staff development department that define expectations of the department, its staff members, and the learners.

Durability. Durability is the amount of use consumers receive from a product before that product physically deteriorates. In a service business, durability refers to the length of time a product lasts. In staff development, durability relates to the amount of time a class is effective and the life cycle of a program; that is, the length of time a particular type of program is viable or can be taught before a major revision in design is required.

Serviceability. Serviceability involves speed, courtesy, competence, and the response to problems. Serviceability involves responsiveness because problems arise even with the best of service. Serviceability deals with the manner in which service problems are handled and is closely associated with customer satisfaction. Serviceability in the hotel industry might involve speed with which a broken air conditioner is repaired or a misplaced reservation is found. In the health care industry, cold meals and impersonal service reflect on the organization's serviceability. In staff development, malfunctioning audiovisual equipment, lost attendance records, or speakers who arrive late affect the serviceability. These serviceability problems can contribute to customer dissatisfaction with an educational event.

Aesthetics. Aesthetics include the way a service looks, feels, and sounds. Aesthetics also deal with tastefulness and propriety. This subjective element is clearly a matter of personal preference. In business, aesthetics may involve the cleanliness of the dining room and the coordination of the furnishings. In the health care industry, aesthetics relate to whether the rooms and furniture are well proportioned. In staff development, aesthetics involve the creature comforts of a teaching session (for example, room temperature, food, seating, breaks, acoustics). In reviewing participant evaluations a percentage of learners will inevitably rate the room as too hot, while an equal percentage will indicate that the room was comfortable. Aesthetics also relates to the presentation style and content of the instruction. Occasional profanity used for emphasis may not bother some participants but may insult others. The appearance of promotional materials and the conduct of an educational marketing campaign also rely on aesthetics.

Perceived Quality. Perceived quality is the customer's idea of quality. Reputation is a critical determinant of perceived quality. A staff development program that has ANCC approval is generally considered of high quality because of the ANCC's strong reputation.

These eight dimensions of quality include aspects from the consumer-based, service-based, and system-based arenas. Serviceability, aesthetics, and perceived quality are aspects of the consumer-based approach to quality. Conformance and reliability are part of the service-based approach to quality. Performance, features, and durability involve the system-based approach to quality.

Garvin[7] suggests that businesses compete on the eight dimensions of quality. Distinguishing the staff development department in a few dimensions while maintaining a high level of quality in the other departments is the key to acquiring a quality niche.

As discussed earlier, the major areas of activity in staff development include continuing education, in-service education, and orientation. In these areas of activity the identification of those dimensions of quality critical for program success provides direction for the development of written standards and foundation for a targeted, quality program. The desired result of the orientation program is a safe, competent, functional clinician. Orientation programs must be consistent, effective, and accurate to achieve this result; thus the dimensions of conformance, performance, and reliability are the critical quality dimensions on which educators should concentrate when designing the orientation program.

The combination of the three arenas of quality with the eight characteristics or dimensions of quality should help the staff development department strive for improved quality. If educators incorporate these aspects with the three phases of quality management, high-quality educational services will develop. The focus on quality influences the planning, implementation, monitoring, and improvement of educational programs that become outcome focused and resource driven.

QUALITY AWARENESS
Commitment to Quality

Commitment to quality is the first step in quality awareness. Commitment must come from the highest-ranking staff members and permeate the department. Quality commitment begins with the department's mission. The mission of the staff development department must be clearly defined. "Without a clear sense of mission, the education department will drift from crisis to crisis, often torn between client groups and multitudes of programs."[25] This is to support the achievement of high-quality patient outcomes through cost-effective maintenance of staff competencies. The mission provides the basis for all quality efforts within the staff development department, focuses the department's efforts on outcomes, and addresses the cost and quality imperative. In addition, the mission statement should define those dimensions of quality in which the department wishes to excel. The staff development department, similar to clinical units, must be able to maintain a high quality of services while controlling the costs of providing those services. This creates the department's competitive edge.

Standard Development

Standard development is the second step in quality awareness. The mission of the staff development department sets the direction for all written standards within the organization. Standards make quality a daily goal. Similar standards address the same three arenas as quality (that is, user-, service-, and system-based). As described earlier, these are the critical components of any service business. In the clinical arena, the consumer is the patient, and standards of care are written regarding the services that the patient receives. Standards of practice are written to define the expectations of caregivers; standards of governance are written the way care delivery is organized and managed. The customer of the staff development department is each nursing service staff member. The standards of education outline the services that are or will be provided to each nursing service staff member. Standards of practice define the expected behaviors of the educators and those assisting the educators in the teaching and learning process. Standards of governance define the organization and management of the staff development department.

The written standards must also include structure, process, and outcomes to be comprehensive. Structure standards provide the framework for the service. These structure standards consist of the mission, philosophy, goals, and policies of the department. Process standards focus on the "how tos;" they are the vehicles defining the way in which service will be provided. Process standards consist of procedures, practice guidelines, plans, and documentation. Outcome standards define the results to be achieved by implementing the service; they are the desired results of the process. In an outcome-driven service these desired results are determined first. Only then are the process standards designed to achieve those results.

In the staff development department, mission, philosophy, goals, and policies must define the rules related to learners, educators, and educational management. That is, these standards are user-, service-, and system-based standards. Process standards define the way that the teaching and learning process and management of educational services are carried out. Outcome standards define the learning, teaching, and management results that should follow if educators adhere to the process standards. Table 17-1 describes the relationship between the service arenas (consumer, employee, and system), domains of practice (educational, professional, and administrative), and types of standards (structure, process, and outcomes).

Staff Education

Staff education is the third step in quality awareness. Staff education requires orientation and continuing education of the educators regarding the commitment to quality and value of written standards. This step also involves education regarding the other two phases of quality management (that is, quality appraisal, quality improvement).

Table 17-1   Relationship of service arenas, domains of practice, and types of standards

	Service arena		
	Consumer (learner)	Employee (educator)	System (staff development department)
Domain of practice	Educational domain	Professional domain	Administrative domain
Structure standards	Philosophy of learning Goals Policies	Philosophy of teaching Goals Policies	Philosophy of management Goals Policies
Outcome standards	Learner objectives	Teacher objectives	Departmental objectives

Process standards	Procedures
	Practice guidelines
	Staff development
	  plan
	Lesson plan
	Documentation
		Procedures
		Practice guidelines
		Educator development
		  plan
		Documentation
			Procedures
			Practice guidelines
			Administrative action plan
			Documentation

Courtesy Katz JM, Green E, Baltimore, 1991.

QUALITY APPRAISAL

Quality appraisal in staff development refers to mechanisms for ongoing evaluation of educational services. The appraisal component consists of performance measurement and technology measurement.

Comprehensive quality-assessment activities must not only focus on learners, but also on educators and the system. Experience shows that quality problems may not always fall within the realm of poorly planned educational activities. A well-designed program will flounder if the presenter is inept; the best presenter with great content will not be effective if learner attendance is limited by poor staffing on the units or poor marketing of the program. High-quality educational services will result if the problems are analyzed by considering the presenter's performance and other impeding factors to high quality within the system.

Quality assessment activities are aimed at the service- and system-based dimensions of quality (performance, conformance, features, reliability, durability). Performance and technology measurements focus on these dimensions.

Performance Measurement

Performance is composed of competence and productivity. The department's ability to achieve its desired outcomes determines its competence. The use of its resources to produce those results is the department's productivity.

Performance measurement in staff development includes mechanisms to appraise learner, staff, and administrative performance. The mechanisms include direct measures such as quality monitoring studies, competency assessments, attendance reports, test results, cost analysis, and satisfaction analysis. These direct measures monitor learner, staff, and system outcomes.[9]

Educator and Learner Functioning. Individual performance reviews include learner accomplishments and faculty performances. Examples of standard methods for evaluating the accomplishment of learner objectives are plentiful in the literature. The performance appraisal of staff development educators is usually determined by the personnel appraisal system used by the organization.

Systems. Systems to measure productivity are the tools used to monitor the ways in which resources are used and make decisions about resource allocations. In the current health care environment, productivity systems are an economic necessity. Various productivity systems specific to staff development are currently being developed.[10,18,26]

Another critical tool for reviewing system performance is the cost-benefit analysis. In the current cost-contained environment the economics of education as a support service is paramount. Worth or value is measured by the bottom line. Results must be worth the investment. Just as clinical units must evaluate their cost-benefit, so must the staff development department. Cost-benefit analysis is an essential decision-making tool of staff development educators for deciding whether to develop new programs or improve existing programs. This is a valuable aid for determining resource distribution because it focuses on the outcomes of the educational services.

Customer Satisfaction Analysis

Satisfaction analysis, the third step in quality appraisal, evaluates the user-based dimensions of quality (that is, serviceability, aesthetics, perceived quality). Satisfaction analysis should include learner, educator, and administrative satisfaction indicators. Staff development personnel have a long history of soliciting feedback from learners regarding learners' perceptions of their learning experience and the usefulness of this learning experience in daily practice. Staff development educators and all faculty are also asked to evaluate teaching and learning experiences from their perspective. Administrative staff satisfaction analysis is important because they are the internal customers and their perception of quality in staff development activities is a high priority. The staff development department must not only *have* high productivity, but must be *perceived* by administration to have high productivity.

Technology Measurement

Technology measurement includes research and product evaluation.[9]

Research

Research is an evaluative activity occurring in each of the service domains. In its broadest sense, research is a problem-solving activity involving data collection and analysis. Conducting research within each service domain can provide valuable information about the learning, teaching, and management processes. Examples of learner-centered research include review of the effects of medication-administration testing, courses about the incidence of medication errors, and use of competency-based assessment as a learner evaluation tool. Examples of educator-based studies include the ways in which cognitive styles of preceptors and preceptees affect the success of a preceptor program and the way the staff's perception of the clinical competence of educators affects credibility of these educators. System studies include the investigation of the impact of self-directed learning packages for specific mandatory topics regarding educator productivity and the effect of computerization on record-keeping accuracy. Research provides the groundwork for change.

Product evaluation is a critical component of technology measurement. Many a great presentation has been ruined by faulty equipment, poor photocopying, or an inadequate physical facility. Product evaluation in staff development ensures that the learners, educators, and department have the best resources available to achieve their desired outcomes. Product evaluation consists of evaluating and documenting the effectiveness of equipment, support materials, and physical facilities used in the educational process. This analysis includes a performance component, cost component, and satisfaction analysis. The results of this analysis are used to make future planning and purchasing decisions.

QUALITY IMPROVEMENT

Within the staff development department, quality-improvement activities are also aimed at the three service domains. The steps involved in quality improvement are research utilization, action planning, implementation, and follow-up.

Research Utilization

Research utilization is the first step in quality improvement within the staff development department. Use of research about the processes and management of staff development education is the basis for quality-improvement strategies. Research utilization provides a scientific basis for decision making and ensures a solid foundation for change.

Action Planning

Action planning is the second step in quality improvement. The most effective tools available for problem resolution and service improvement are action planning and an organizational structure that encourages participation in the planning and implementation of change. Action planning uses the same concepts of lesson planning to design a framework for change within the department. No major change should occur without a written action plan. This step serves as documentation of departmental progress.

Implementation

The third step in quality improvement is implementation. Participation of staff development educators and nursing service staff in the decisions, planning, and implementation of educational program changes can be accomplished through shared governance system of the organization and the use of task forces to work on specific program designs or revisions.

Follow-up

Follow-up is the final step of quality improvement. Staff development educators need to spend as much time examining the results of educational programming on learners and patients as they do in the preparation and presentation of their programs.

A QUALITY MANAGEMENT MODEL

An organizing framework helps ensure that quality continues to improve rather than diminish and that the full scope of educational services is of a high quality. A sound quality-management model integrates the three domains of service and the three phases of quality management. Just as a builder uses a blueprint to direct the completion of a skyscraper or a conductor uses a score to direct the symphony, THE BLUEPRINT for quality management in staff development, adapted from Katz and Green's *THE BLUEPRINT for Quality Management*, directs the development of a high-quality staff development program. As shown in Figure 17-3, THE BLUEPRINT is a service-oriented, outcome-focused, and resource-driven model.

Service Domains of Practice

The three service domains are represented vertically in the model. The consumer (or learner) is represented by the first track. This includes those educational standards, appraisals, and improvement systems that focus on learning outcomes. The employees (or educators) are represented by the middle track. This track includes those teaching standards, appraisals, and improvement systems necessary for maintaining teaching excellence. The system is represented by the third track, which includes those administrative standards, appraisals, and improvement systems necessary to ensure the achievement of high-quality operational outcomes. The phases of quality management are integrated into the model horizontally.

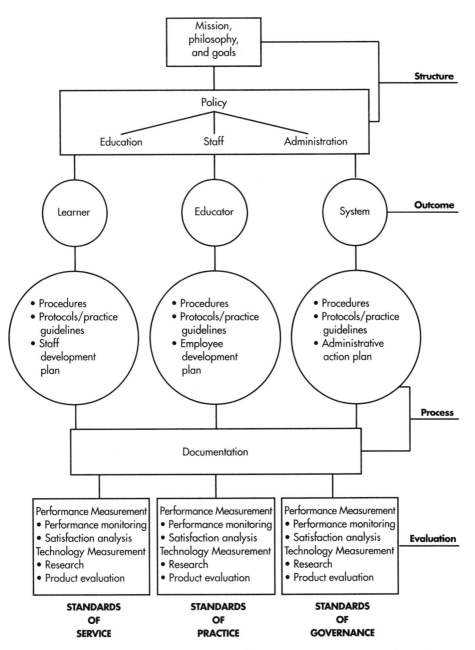

Fig. 17-3   THE BLUEPRINT in staff development. (Courtesy Katz JM, Green E, Baltimore, 1995.)

Quality Awareness

In the model, quality awareness is represented by the structure, process, and outcome standards in each service domain. Standards of education direct the way in which educational activities are organized and carried out, and they define the desired results of the learning process. Standards of professional practice direct the ways that teaching activities are organized and carried out, and they define the desired outcomes of the teaching process. Standards of governance direct the ways in which operations are organized and carried out, and they define the desired results of the administrative system. The standards are divided into structure, process, and outcome standards in each of the service domains.

Structure Standards. Structure standards are the written value statements defining the circumstances under which a service is delivered. These structure standards include the mission, philosophy, goals, and policies of the department. Structure standards are the nonnegotiable standards. These standards must be carried out as written; no room for situational modification exists. Examples include a policy on license validation, meeting the JCAHO's standard for CPR certification, and the record keeping requirements.

Process Standards. Process standards are written value statements that determine the manner in which a service is delivered. These include the procedures, practice guidelines, action plans, and documentation systems of the staff development department. Examples include the procedures for cleaning CPR mannequins, the practice guideline for in-house credentialing, specific lesson plans for teaching CPR, or the process of storing and retrieving records.

Outcome Standards. Outcome standards are the written value statements regarding the results of the staff development department's service delivery. These include learner, staff, and annual department objectives. These outcomes may include the expected impact of staff education on specific clinical outcomes within a future-oriented system.

Quality Appraisal

Quality appraisal is represented by the evaluation component. Each service domain has an evaluation component. Learner evaluation includes activities that monitor compliance with the written standards of education, participant satisfaction analysis, learner performance review, equipment evaluation, and research regarding learning. The educator evaluation includes activities that monitor compliance with the written standards of professional practice, educator satisfaction analysis, educator performance review, equipment evaluation, and research related to teaching. System evaluation includes activities monitoring compliance to the written standards of governance, administrative satisfaction analysis, system performance review, equipment evaluation, and research related to educational administration.

Quality Improvement

Quality improvement is integrated throughout the model through the use of evaluation data to redesign the written standards. Quality improvement uses research to guide the planning and implementation of corrective action. Follow-up activities evaluate the plan's success and identifies needs for modification of the interventions or outcomes outlined within the plan.

THE BLUEPRINT

The following five underlying principles permeate THE BLUEPRINT:
1. Education must be outcome focused. Crosby[6] believes, everything that happens in a quality system must be a result, not a reaction. Staff education must define itself by the results produced, not simply by the teaching and learning process.
2. Individual accountability for continued competence is essential. Individuals must play active roles in maintaining competence within their specific area, whether in clinical practice, education, or management.
3. Controlled decentralization must occur. Mechanisms to ensure the coordination of unit-based education events must exist. Similarly, a master plan must direct the coordination of educational efforts and organizational priorities. Accountability for that coordination should be centralized in the staff development department.
4. A proactive approach to education is crucial. Planning eliminates management by crisis and enables the staff development department to focus on internal mandatory requirements and organizational priorities.
5. Education must be resource driven because economic survival requires this. Resource-driven educational decisions ensure that priority programs not only survive, but also thrive in the face of budget constraints. In a resource-driven educational system, need alone is not the primary issue; rather the need for an educational event is analyzed relative to nursing service priorities. Decisions are based on resource availability, and resources are allocated according to priority rankings.

The following lists six advantages to using THE BLUEPRINT[17]:
1. It organizes system values by organizing the staff development department into three service domains.
2. It facilitates the appraisal of all variables affecting the service rather than focusing only on the learner.
3. It promotes continual improvement by enabling the department to pinpoint the source(s) of a particular problem, whether the source(s) is(are) the learner, educator, system, or some combination of all three.
4. It controls the service through a proactive approach to problem prevention through standards development.
5. It controls costs by reducing duplication of effort and facilitating performance improvement.
6. Accreditation requirements are fulfilled as efforts are synchronized with the latest requirement of the professional and national accrediting bodies.

The major advantage of this framework is its versatility. This organizational framework enables individual staff development departments to integrate their specific values, conceptual frameworks, assessment and appraisal tools, planning devices, and products into a coordinated system to manage the quality of education.

SUMMARY

Quality represents a dual-edged sword for staff development departments on a number of fronts. Quality provides an opportunity to solidify the importance of education in "the big picture" and increase the visibility and credibility of educational services; however, it also increases the responsibility and accountability of education's contribution to patient results. The external role of staff development as a quality resource must be defined. Internal mechanisms to manage quality must be implemented. Staff development educators must become more business-like in their approach to education. The quality of the staff development department's services must remain high and the costs of these services are kept low.

A total quality-management framework is the key to controlling these quality responsibilities. Quality management involves three phases—quality awareness, quality appraisal, and quality improvement. These phases of quality management must be applied to the full scope of educational services (that is, the learner, educator, and system). THE BLUEPRINT for quality management in staff development provides an organizing framework for integrating the phases of quality management and service domains into a coordinated approach to controlling the quality of educational services.

REFERENCES

1. American Hospital Association Division of Public Relations: *Literacy in the workplace: you can't afford not to care*, Chicago, 1990, The Association.
2. American Nurses Association: *Standards for nursing professional development: continuing education and staff development*, Washington, DC, 1994, The Association.
3. Bennett A, Tibbits S: *Maximizing quality performance in health care facilities*, Rockville, Md, 1989, Aspen.
4. Beyers M: Quality: the banner of the 1980s, *Nurs Clin North Am* 23(3):617, 1988.
5. Bliersbach C: Quality assurance in health care: current challenge and future directions, *QRB* 14:315, 1988.
6. Crosby PB: *Quality is free*, New York, 1979, New American Library.
7. Garvin D: *Managing quality*, New York, 1988, The Free Press.
8. Gillem TR: Deming's 14 points and hospital quality: responding to the consumer's demand for the best value health care, *J Nurs Quality Assur* 2(3):70, 1988.
9 Green E, Katz J: *Clinical practice guidelines for the adult patient*, St Louis, 1995, Mosby.
10. Haynes P: The evaluation of a model to measure productivity: implications for the hospital education department. In Martin ED, editor: *Innovation and excellence in health care education*, Chicago, 1984, American Hospital Association.
11. Hefferin EA: Evaluation of in-service effectiveness. In Henry B, editor: *Dimensions of nursing administration*, Boston, 1989, Blackwell Scientific Publications.
12. Hefferin EA: Trends in the evaluation of nursing inservice education programs, *J Nurs Staff Dev* 3(1):28, 1987.

13. Joint Commission on Accreditation of Healthcare Organization: *1994 Accreditation manual for hospitals*, Chicago, 1994, The Joint Commision.
14. Joint Commission on Accreditation of Healthcare Organizations: *An introduction to joint commission on nursing care standards*, Chicago, 1991, The Joint Commission.
15. Joint Commission on Accreditation of Healthcare Organizations: *Quality assessment and improvement proposed revised standards*, Chicago, 1990, The Joint Commission.
16. Katz J, Green E: The blueprint for quality management. In Schroeder P: *Encyclopedia of nursing quality*, vol 2, Gaithersburg, MD, 1991, Aspen.
17. Katz J, Green E: *Managing quality: a guide to monitoring and evaluating nursing services*, St Louis, 1991, Mosby.
18. Kelly K: A productivity measure for nursing staff development, *J Nurs Staff Dev* 6(2):65, 1990.
19. Kerfoot K, Rohe D: Kaizen: innovations for nurse managers to improve productivity, *Nurs Econ* 7(4):228, 1989.
20. Naisbitt J, Aburdene P: *Reinventing the corporation*, New York, 1985, Warner Books.
21. O'Leary D: Characteristics of clinical indicators, *QRB* 15(11):330, 1989.
22. O'Leary D: *Outlook 2000*, BLS bulletin No 2352, Washington, DC, 1990, The Bureau of Labor Statistics.
23. O'Leary D: CQI: a step beyond QA, *QRB* 17(1):4, 1991.
24. Sovie M: Investigate before you educate, *J Nurs Adm* 11(14):15, 1981.
25. Ulschak FL: *Creating the future of health care education*, Chicago, 1988, American Hospital Publishing.
26. Waterstradt C: A productivity system for a hospital education department, *J Nurs Staff Dev* 6(3):139, 1990.

Research in Nursing Staff Development

18

Nursing research is as vital to the practice of nursing as the provision of patient care. Research enhances professional nursing practice by defining the scope of practice, extending the scientific knowledge base of clinicians, and identifying the unique difference nursing makes in the health status of individuals.

Staff development educators play a unique role in nursing research within the hospital environment. Not only may educators be called on to communicate research findings, they may also be asked to conduct research and prepare staff members to participate in the research process. This chapter provides guidelines and suggestions designed to assist educators as they identify research topics and incorporate that research with daily practice in staff development.

IDENTIFYING RESEARCH TOPICS

The Commission on Nursing Research of the American Nurses Association (ANA) identified priorities for nursing research in the 1980s. These priorities included studies generating knowledge related to promoting health and well-being, preventing health problems, and designing and developing cost-effective health care systems. These same topics seem appropriate for the 1990s, although priorities specific for research in staff development need to be designated.

Crucial Areas for Research

Abruzzese identified four crucial areas of research for staff development educators.[1] These include the transfer of learning to practice, clinical teaching methodologies, an increased rate and retention of learning, and effectiveness of teaching strategies.

326

Transfer of Learning to Practice. Patient care coordinators often complain to the staff development educator that members of the nursing staff are unable to perform certain functions. The staff development educator knows, however, that the particular function in question has been taught during orientation or another class. Sometimes nurses do not implement new learning because they do not see the practical value of information that has been learned, or they fear criticism from other staff members who may do things differently. Some research questions that might appropriately be explored in this area include "Did learning actually occur?" and "Is there a knowledge deficit or a performance deficit?" If learning did occur, educators must determine the factors impeding the transfer of that knowledge.

Changes in organizational structure resulting in shared governance and increased professional accountability require educators to create continued opportunities for professional growth and performance improvement.[13] While nurses have always cared about the quality of health care,[20] past efforts of quality improvement programs predominately focused on auditing charts and drafting reports.[21] Research directed toward enhancing continued performance improvement may focus on identifying specific strategies that enhance the transfer of learning from the classroom to the bedside, including strategies to empower first-line managers to reinforce the application of new knowledge.

Clinical Teaching Methodologies. Research can be conducted regarding clinical teaching methodologies. Such research topics include the following:
- Do new graduates who have just completed 2 to 4 years of education, consisting predominately of classroom lecture, benefit from 2 or more weeks of classroom orientation in the hospital?
- Is one-to-one clinical teaching better and more cost-effective than group learning experiences?
- Should new graduates be paired with experienced preceptors or mentors, or do new graduates learn best from each other?
- Would orientees (and their patients) benefit from a 3- to 6-month experience working in a clinical unit staffed only by new graduates?
- What is the best approach to teaching new clinical skills to experienced nurses?

Each of these questions could form the basis of a research study important to staff development.

Increasing Rate and Retention of Learning. Current hospital climates require educators to accomplish more in less time and with less money. Alternate teaching strategies may provide creative, cost-effective solutions. Educators should ask the following questions:
- Does the use of games and simulations enhance learning and retention?
- What type of individual learns best from programmed instruction?
- Do nontraditional teaching strategies facilitate learning for adult learners?

- Can skills be learned more quickly through the use of computer-assisted instruction or interactive video?
- Do leaderless group discussions facilitate retention?
- What impact do environment and social climate have on learning?

Perhaps reading these questions will provoke new, potentially researchable questions. All of these questions, however, reinforce the need to evaluate the effectiveness of teaching strategies.

Evaluating the Effectiveness of Teaching Strategies. Emphasis on evaluation has grown from an increased need for fiscal accountability and from a response to public demands for information about the ways their needs are being met. The ANA defined evaluation as "a systematic process by which a judgment is made about consequences, results, effects, or merit of a continuing education provider unit or continuing education program in order to make subsequent decisions."[4]

Staff development educators can combine evaluation with research through a strategy called *evaluation research*. Evaluation research is an approach to "judge and to improve the planning, monitoring, effectiveness, and efficiency of health, education, welfare, and other human service programs."[19] Evaluation research can assist with decision making, program development, assessment of program use and effectiveness, and determining cost effectiveness.

Rossi and Freeman[19] suggested that the following questions could be answered by the evaluation research approach:

- What is the extent of an identified problem?
- Will the program design enhance attainment of program goals?
- Has the program been implemented as planned?
- Does the program make efficient use of resources?
- Did the program reach the appropriate target group?
- Were the goals obtained as a result of the program or through some other means?
- Was the program cost effective?

Additionally, research can help evaluate the extent to which programs have changed, the knowledge and attitudes of the participants, and the affect programs have had on patient outcomes. Research can be an important tool to assist educators whenever that research is incorporated into daily activities.

INCORPORATING RESEARCH INTO STAFF DEVELOPMENT RESPONSIBILITIES

Nurses in clinical practice are increasingly expected to participate in the research process. Similar to many other nursing activities, research is a skill to be learned and facilitated by staff development educators. Because no agreed on minimum level of educational preparation is required for planning and conducting research,[25] it is helpful for educators to be familiar with guidelines established by the ANA.

Educational Preparation and the Research Process

According to Woods and Catanzaro,[31] "Every nurse, regardless of educational preparation, can be involved in and benefit from nursing research." The ANA recommended that the extent of participation in research should be guided by the educational preparation of the clinician.[3,5] Graduates with associate degrees can understand and appreciate the value of research and assist with identification of researchable problems and collection of data. Nurses with baccalaureate degrees should also be able to read, interpret, and evaluate research findings for their applicability to nursing practice. Clinicians with master's degrees can conduct studies and facilitate research by collaborating with other investigators and providing consultation in their area of expertise. The doctorally prepared nurse provides a leadership role by conducting investigations, developing methodologies, and integrating scientific knowledge to advance the practice of nursing.

Conducting and teaching research can be a challenging task for staff development educators. The challenge need not be overwhelming and can be made more manageable by the identification of available resources.

Resources to Assist with Knowledge Building in Research Design and Statistical Analysis

Although enrollment in formal educational programs in research and statistics is an excellent approach to preparing educators as participants in and facilitators of nursing research, it is only one of many resources available to individuals seeking to develop or enhance their research skills. Colleges and local chapters of Sigma Theta Tau International (the international honor society of nursing) frequently conduct research colloquia and symposia to present research findings, discuss advances in methodology, and explore ethical considerations. Numerous journals, including *Nursing Research, Research in Nursing and Health*, and *Advances in Nursing Science*, are readily available at libraries or by subscription. Advertisements for books related to research can be found in many popular nursing journals; publishers of these texts are often willing to send copies on approval. The departmental budget should include a provision to cover the cost of attendance at conferences and purchase of research journals and texts.

Individuals who can help staff development educators expand their knowledge include nursing colleagues, affiliated faculty, the infection control officer, and other health professionals engaged in research. Staff development educators should seek out nursing staff members who are currently enrolled in collegiate programs in nursing, because most programs include courses in research and statistics. These individuals are usually willing to share course outlines, texts, and bibliographies and are often eager to talk about their own research activities.

Affiliated faculty members are also potential sources of information about research and statistical analysis. Faculty members are usually master's or doctorally prepared and are often involved in research projects. Faculty members frequently look for individuals to assist with literature reviews or data collection. In addition, faculty members who serve as thesis and dissertation advisors might be willing to critique or collaborate with a research proposal designed by the staff development department.

The infection control officer often has expertise in the efficient collection, management, and reduction of data. Reviewing data collected by the infection control officer may also point out problems within the organization that need to be researched. Additionally, reviewing incident reports and consulting with the environmental safety department may lead to opportunities to participate in organizational research.

It might be mutually advantageous to form an informal group with individuals interested in discussing research because this may lead to the design and conduct of a research study. Educators can also gain invaluable experience with research by collaborating with experienced researchers and serving as members of the Institutional Review Board (IRB).

SERVING ON THE ORGANIZATION'S REVIEW BOARD FOR RESEARCH

The IRB is a committee of nurses, physicians, pharmacists, social workers, lawyers, clergy, and consumers charged with the responsibility of reviewing, approving, and monitoring all research within the organization that involves human subjects. The functions of the IRB are directed by federal policies and guidelines established by such agencies as the United States Public Health Service (USPHS), the National Commission for the Protection of Human Subjects of Biomedical and Behavioral Research (NCPHSBBR), and the Department of Health and Human Services (DHHS).[10] Rules and regulations of the DHHS regarding the protection of human research subjects were published in the *Federal Register* of January 26, 1981. The *Federal Register* is available in most hospital libraries. In preparation for becoming an effective member of the IRB, staff development educators should familiarize themselves with the ANA publication entitled *Human Rights Guidelines for Nurses in Clinical and Other Research*.[2]

The nurse's role as a member of the IRB includes reviewing research proposals to determine that subject participation will be voluntary, provisions have been made to obtain an informed consent from subjects, the benefits of participation outweigh the risks, the subject will be free to withdraw from the study without retribution, and the investigator is qualified to conduct the research. The nurse member of the IRB should also ascertain the impact of the investigation on nursing personnel and the delivery of patient care. Because staff development educators understand the functioning of the nursing department, they can suggest changes in research methodology to facilitate the investigation with minimal disruption of patient care.

Many nursing departments have established independent nursing research committees to approve and monitor research activities that affect the nursing department. Staff development educators may assist in the development of this committee or in writing policies and procedures and may serve as committee members.

Participation in the IRB and departmental research committee offers educators the opportunity to learn about types of research, research methodology, and regulations governing the conduct of research.[23] Membership also allows educators to network with others interested in research, identify potential resources and contacts, and distinguish research from problem-solving activities.

DISTINGUISHING RESEARCH FROM PROBLEM-SOLVING ACTIVITIES

Research is similar to the problem-solving process in some respects but has some important differences. The goal of the problem-solving process is to find practical solutions to immediate problems.[7] Although the research process can also be used to solve problems, the goal of nursing research to advance knowledge and theory to enhance patient care.[24]

The problem-solving process includes identifying a problem, determining a goal, listing alternative solutions, selecting the most appropriate alternative, implementing the selected alternative, and evaluating the effectiveness of the action. For example, a staff development educator faced with a slide projector that mysteriously malfunctions during a presentation, uses the problem-solving process to resolve the problem. This staff development educator must decide whether it would be more prudent to find a replacement for the projector, repair the machine, or continue the presentation without audiovisuals. A decision is made by reviewing the options. Later, the impact of that decision is considered while evaluating the effectiveness of the presentation.

Continuous quality improvement (CQI) and evaluation are other problem-solving activities that may be undertaken by the staff development department. The primary focus of quality-improvement activities is "the continuous and practical solution of day-to-day problems in patient care service and administration"[24] through gathering and interpreting objective data. Evaluation, on the other hand, is designed to measure the worth or effectiveness of something or someone by the application of an external test.[6]

The aim of problem solving is to answer a question or resolve an issue.[6] Although similarities exist between the problem-solving and the research processes, "research is more rigorous and broader in scope than problem solving."[27]

The Research Process

Kerlinger defined research as the "systematic, controlled, empirical, and critical investigation of hypothetical propositions about the presumed relations among natural phenomena."[14] The purpose of research is to generate or define new knowledge.[6,22]

The research process, an elaboration of the scientific method, is an orderly method of obtaining and a system of arranging knowledge. The process consists

---

KEY COMPONENTS OF THE RESEARCH PROCESS

Formulate the problem
Review the literature
Identify variables and
   hypotheses
Develop and test
   methodology

Gather and analyze
   data
State conclusions
Communicate findings

---

of a number of interrelated steps that provide an organizing framework to guide the investigator. Although different authors may identify a different number of steps, the key steps of the research process are identified in the box.

Primary distinctions between the problem-solving and research processes include scope, purpose, and time frame. Problem solving seeks to find immediate solutions to well-defined, single-situation problems. Research, on the other hand, is time consuming, broader in scope, more varied in approach, and seeks to generate new knowledge.

APPROACHES TO RESEARCH

Numerous ways exist to pursue knowledge, and the purpose of research is to develop new knowledge, therefore numerous ways to conduct research exist. Stetler[24] identified four strategies appropriate to nursing—original research, replication research, application projects, and special projects. Original research is an investigation undertaken to discover new knowledge that does not substantially duplicate the design or methodology of another study. Replication research is based on previous research by exact duplication or slight modification. Application projects systematically examine the applicability of research findings to nursing practice, management, or education. Special projects involve an assessment or evaluation of current practices or needs. Stetler acknowledged that special and application projects are not true research because these projects are less rigorous than original or replication research. These projects, however, may "provide the basis for development of future research proposals."[24]

Classically, research has been broadly categorized as quantitative or qualitative. Quantitative research is known for its precision, narrow focus, rigid controls, objectivity, and use of numbers in data analysis. A recent study by Good,[11] entitled *A Comparison of the Effects of Jaw Relaxation and Music on Postoperative Pain,* is an example of a quantitative study.

Qualitative research uses a more subjective and holistic approach than quantitative designs. The qualitative approach is broader in scope and usually seeks to develop theory. *The Paradox of Comfort* by Morse, Bottorff, and Hutchinson[15] is an example of a qualitative approach to research. Table 18-1 lists some of the more common research approaches.

Table 18-1   Quantitative and qualitative research approaches

Quantitative approaches	Qualitative approaches
Descriptive	Ethnographic
Correlational	Grounded theory
Experimental	Historical
Methodologic	Phenomenologic

Recently, investigators began to combine elements of qualitative and quantitative research in an approach called *blended research*. Regardless of the research approach taken, some universal elements of the research process exist.

DEMYSTIFYING THE ELEMENTS OF THE RESEARCH PROCESS

The steps of the research process should not be interpreted as intimidating obstacles to be completed consecutively. A process is continuous; therefore the steps can be modified slightly to meet the needs of the specific project. The steps of the research process can be used as a guide to enhance progress with a few helpful pointers discussed in the following sections.

Sources for Formulating Problems to Study

The problem identifies the topic to be investigated. Research topics often stem from ideas an individual wants to know more about or an individual's desire to find improved ways of doing something. Identifying the problem is often an arduous task for educators desiring to begin research but ideas for research topics emanate from a variety of sources.

It is usually best for individuals to investigate problems with which they are familiar. Accordingly, research topics might arise from the practice setting. Nurses are confronted daily with problems requiring solutions or questions needing answers. Solutions or answers might involve the role of educators or learners, management of nursing departments, or provision of patient care. Important research questions educators might ask while planning programs include the following:

- Do the learning needs of nurses with associate degrees differ from those of nurses holding baccalaureate degrees?
- Does the teaching method influence the learner's transfer of knowledge to clinical practice?
- Does the nurse's level of education influence the length of orientation?

While reviewing texts and journals in search of solutions to questions identified in the practice setting, other research problems may also become apparent. Curious readers may also ask about ways recommendations or solutions proposed by the literature may be applied to their own practice. Questions about what would happen if the suggestions were followed or modified to fit individual situations could arise. Also, if recommendations from several authors were combined, would results be similar or new problems arise.

Another excellent source of ideas for research topics comes from research reported by others. A good research study often generates more questions than solutions. Authors usually translate these questions into recommendations for further research, which can generally be found in the last section of a thesis, dissertation, or research article. For example, in the last paragraph of a research study related to substance abuse among RNs, the authors suggest that "future studies should focus on the identification of nurse subgroups that may be at increased risk for substance abuse."[28]

Replication of existing studies, through exact repetition or slight modification, is also an expedient approach to identifying a research problem. Repeating previous studies helps confirm the findings of that study and tests the generalizability of findings to other samples and situations. For example, in a recent project undertaken by Healey and Hoffman,[12] a self-instructional poster was used to instruct nursing staff regarding the care of postoperative vascular patients. Evaluating the project, the authors found that the nursing staff responded favorably to the teaching format and attained scores of 80% or better on the posttest. Replicating this study would allow educators to assess the efficacy of this nontraditional teaching strategy within their own organization.

Potential researchable problems constantly surround all aspects of nursing. Staff development educators wishing to identify a researchable problem can find such problems by reading the existing literature, reviewing research reports, and examining their own professional practice and working environment.

Time-Saving Ways to Review the Literature

The review of literature involves identifying, locating, reading, and summarizing materials related to the research problem.[18] Conducting a literature review can be interesting and exciting; it can also be boring and laborious. It is helpful to develop a plan.

First, a list of key words, synonyms, or concepts related to the topic under investigation should be identified. For example, the staff development educator focusing on rehabilitation nursing may be interested in researching the concept of body image. Utz et al[29] identified key words, including self-concept, self-image, body structure, self-perception, and self-attitudes in their study of body image. These key words will lead to appropriate books and articles in the library and will save time and money.

Second, researchers should identify a system of collecting and recording information, such as using large index cards, which are more suitable for note taking than scraps of paper or notebook pages. The staff development educator should also take time to become familiar with the library by locating reference books and periodicals, in addition to the reference librarian who can arrange for interlibrary loans.

Identifying Resources. Identifying potential sources of information is the first step in reviewing the literature. Potential sources can be obtained by using the list of previously compiled key words to review indexes and abstracts or to conduct a computer search. The box provides a partial listing of some of these resources. Additionally, reviewing the bibliography listed at the end of books and articles can also help identify sources that may have been overlooked.

Each potential source should be cited on its own index card. The full citation should be written on the front of the card as it will appear in the final bibliography. The source of the citation should also be noted, in addition to aids for locating the material in the library. Completed cards should be sorted into separate, alphabetized groups (for example, books, pamphlets, and journals). It might be helpful to cluster articles from the same journal together in individual piles according to year.

Locating Sources. Potential sources can be systematically located and obtained from the library stacks by using the sorted index cards. Arrangements through the librarian for interlibrary loan of materials unobtainable at local libraries can be made at little or no cost.

Reading Obtained Materials. In general, it is best to read materials as they are obtained. This screens out irrelevant materials and helps avoid formation of

---

EXAMPLES OF SOURCES FOR IDENTIFYING LITERATURE PERTINENT TO THE RESEARCH PROBLEM

Abstracts
Abstracts of Hospital Management Studies
Dissertation Abstracts
ERIC (Education Reasearch and Information Center)
Nursing Abstracts
Online Journal of Knowledge Synthesis for Nursing
Psychological Abstracts

Computer Searches
BIOSIS PREVIEWS
DataBase of Nursing Knowledge
ENVIROLINE
HISTLINE
MEDLINE
SCISEARCH

Indexes
Books in Print
Card catalog of the library
Cumulative Index to Nursing and Allied Health Literature
Index of Hospital Literature
Index Medicus
International Nursing Index
Nursing Studies Index

intimidating piles of articles that tend to be moved, unread, from table to chair to floor. Skimming large books and articles helps researchers decide whether the books or articles contribute to the study. It is tempting to photocopy every article, however, only those materials that appear to be key references or may be quoted extensively should be copied.

Summarizing Obtained Materials. As each article is read, the content should be summarized and pertinent quotes recorded with their page number on the back of the index card. If research articles are being summarized, the problem statement, conceptual framework, hypotheses, methodology, instrumentation, sample characteristics, data analysis techniques, and findings should be included on the card.[7]

Guidelines to Identify Variables and Hypotheses

A main focus of research is to investigate the relationship between two or more variables. "A variable is anything that can change or anything that is liable to vary."[27] Thus age, gender, pain, anxiety level, and job satisfaction are all variables. A change in the variable and factors influencing that change are of interest to the investigator. For example, if a researcher is trying to determine whether job satisfaction changes with the age of an employee, variables must be clearly identified and defined before relationships can be tested.

Before testing relationships between variables, the independent and dependent variables must be identified. The independent variable is the factor controlled or manipulated by the investigator. The independent variable, sometimes referred to as the *antecedent* variable, can be thought of as the cause or stimulus for change in the dependent variable. The dependent variable is the presumed effect or response that results from a variation in the independent variable.[14] For example, in Deiriggi's study,[9] entitled "Effects of Waterbed Flotation on Indicators of Energy Expenditure in Preterm Infants," waterbed flotation is the independent variable presumed to influence changes in energy expenditure, which is the dependent variable.

After the variables have been identified, the problem statement can be written. The problem statement describes the topic to be researched and population of interest. The format of the problem statement can be a declarative or an interrogative sentence. The problem statement in Deiriggi's study might have been to investigate the effects of waterbed flotation on energy expenditure among preterm infants or to determine the relationship between waterbed flotation and energy expenditure among preterm infants. Note that in each statement the independent variable precedes the dependent variable and the population of interest has been specified.

The review of the literature leads to the formation of the study hypothesis. A hypothesis is a statement of the purported relationship between the independent and dependent variables. A good hypothesis will be logical, testable, and based on fact or theory and will state the nature or direction of the relationship between the variables. Traditionally, the independent variable appears in the hypothesis before the dependent variable. For example, Deiriggi might form the hypothesis that "preterm infants on waterbed flotation (*the independent variable*) will sleep (*measure of the dependent variable*) for longer periods of time than will infants on standard incubator mattresses (*nature of the relationship*)." After formulating the problem, reviewing the literature, identifying the variables, and stating the hypothesis, the next step is to decide setting and the way in which the study will be conducted.

Developing and Testing Methodology

Methodology involves a determination of how, when, and where the study will be conducted and the way that the data will be measured, collected, and analyzed. Many research texts provide a thorough discussion of research design and methodology.[14,16,18,22,26] Staff development educators should keep three things in mind—feasibility, simplicity, and pilot studies.

Consideration must be given to the feasibility of the study. This involves an assessment of available resources, in addition to other factors such as the following:

- Can permission to carry out the study be obtained?
- Is there enough time to conduct the study?
- Is the study free from actual or potential harm to subjects and their environment?
- Are subjects obtainable?
- Are there tools or instruments available to measure the variables under consideration?
- Can the hypothesis be tested?
- Is there adequate financial support?
- Is there access to libraries, mentors or consultants, and computers for data analysis?
- Does the nature of the study fall within the scope of the investigator's capabilities and area of expertise?

If the project is feasible, another concept, called *KISMIF* (keep it simple, make it fun) should be kept in mind. If the focus of the research problem is too global, hypothesis testing becomes an impossible task. For example, a staff development educator may be interested in studying the effects of teaching strategies on the transfer of knowledge to the clinical setting. Because there are innumerable teaching strategies, this study could take years to complete. Instead, the educator might narrow the study by investigating the effects of programmed instruction or the group-process approach.

Narrowing the scope of the problem facilitates completion of the project. Initially the study may best be limited to one independent and one dependent variable. A series of small studies is more productive than a global study that remains unfinished. Because completing a research study requires the expenditure of a great deal of physical and emotional energy, the topic should be of vital interest to the educator. Whenever boredom occurs, the project is usually abandoned.

The importance of a pilot study cannot be overemphasized. A pilot study's purpose is to detect problems and verify feasibility before large amounts of time, money, and effort are expended. For example, a staff development educator might plan to investigate the attainment of nursing skills by videotaping performance. A pilot study could help identify optimal placement of the video equipment to allow full view of the nurse without restricting the nurse's ability to move.

Efficient Ways to Collect and Analyze Data

Step-by-step procedures for data collection must be planned and tested before the actual data collection. It is wise to establish positive communication patterns and working relationships with staff members who may be affected by the study to avoid resistance to data collection within the organization. Researchers must be flexible and maintain a sense of humor. Whenever subjects or the educator are not tired or rushed, researchers should plan to recruit subjects and collect data. Orientees should be approached at the beginning of class rather than at the end; patients are best approached between visiting hours rather than immediately before or after visiting hours.

The researcher should ascertain that adequate materials are available and equipment is functioning before approaching potential subjects. Instructions to subjects must be specific, complete, and comprehensible. Consistency in the data collection pattern at each data collection event is essential to maintain. Privacy should be provided for subjects, and the reasearcher should verify that all data have been obtained before the subject leaves. All data collection sheets should be kept intact for each subject to aid in identification during the data analysis phase.

If others are going to assist with data collection, training, practice sessions, and follow-up are essential. Assistants should know the way to collect data, the way to obtain answers if a question arises, and the place to return collected data.

The amount of raw data collected may seem overwhelming. Preparing data for analysis as data are collected, rather than after it has all been collected, will facilitate record keeping. Data analysis can be expedited through use of prepackaged computer programs. A computer programmer can assist with selecting and writing appropriate programs. It may be worthwhile to consult a statistician who will suggest appropriate statistical approaches, conduct the analysis and interpretation of the data, or confirm that analyses have been appropriately employed.

Techniques for Writing a Scholarly Report

Scientific communication differs from creative writing in style and format. Wordiness, ambiguity, clichés, and jargon must be avoided. Words should be used with precision, especially words with statistical implications. The casual use of terms such as *significant*, *valid*, or *correlate* should be avoided unless statistical analyses have been conducted that support their use. Also, hypotheses are never proved or disproved; rather, significant differences are found, relationships are demonstrated, the hypothesis is supported, or the findings failed to reject the null hypothesis.

The format of the written report should carry the reader logically through the steps of the research process. Research reports are generally divided into sections, which include the introduction, methodology, results, and discussion. Although the sections are interrelated, the report will have greater clarity if results are not integrated with the method or discussion is not integrated with the results. Authors can replicate the format of published journal articles or consult a resource such as the *Publication Manual of the American Psychological Association* for guidelines and a suggested outline.

Results must be presented clearly, concisely, completely, and accurately. The results section typically begins with a description of the demographic characteristics of the sample including the number, gender, and age of the subjects. Other demographics pertinent to the research topic, such as educational preparation, ethnic background, or birth weight, might also be described. The mean and standard deviation of all quantitative variables are reported; the median, mode, and range are also included if they enhance understanding. Tables can summarize and simplify the presentation of large amounts of information, but tables should supplement, not duplicate, the text. Table 18-2 provides a sample of a table that might appear in the research report.

Data analysis techniques and statistical findings are efficiently reported by first restating the hypothesis and then describing the analyses and results. It is not sufficient to state that the findings were significant at a given probability level; the test symbol, degrees of freedom, and test statistic (obtained value) must be reported, in addition to the probability level. For example, the author might write the following:

It was hypothesized that orientees who worked with preceptors would have higher levels of job satisfaction than orientees without preceptors. Orientees working with preceptors reported a mean job satisfaction score of 23.6 ($SD = 1.25$), whereas orientees without preceptors had a mean job satisfaction score of 18.2 ($SD = 2.89$). Analysis of variance

Table 18-2   Distribution of subjects by age and personality type

Personality type	*n*	Mean	Median	Mode	*SD*
Extrovert	42	28.3	28.5	31	3.6
Introvert	41	31.3	31	31	4.2
Ambivert	34	32.1	32	32	3.9
TOTAL:	117	30.5	30	31	3.9

revealed that orientees working with preceptors had significantly higher levels of job satisfaction than orientees without preceptors (F [1, 42] = 4.37, p = .003).

Avenues to Communicate Findings

The final step in the research process is the communication of findings. Avenues to communicate findings are not limited to written reports published in books or journals, but include verbal and visual presentations.

Verbal Presentations. Research findings can be presented at informal gatherings of colleagues or at more formal meetings or professional conferences. Sponsors of conferences seek conference presenters through a call for abstracts. These calls may appear in research journals and organization newsletters and in letters directed to colleges and universities. A written abstract of 200 to 500 words is submitted for approval. An abstract summarizes the research and includes the problem, purpose, hypothesis, sample, procedures, results, conclusions, and implications for nursing and further research. Customarily, abstracts are single-spaced and limited to one page.

If the abstract is accepted, the researcher agrees to prepare and deliver the research report. Usually, 15 to 30 minutes is allotted for the presentation of the study with an additional 5 to 15 minutes available for questions. As with staff development programs, the presentation will be enhanced by clear organization, attention to effective communication skills, and liberal use of slides or transparencies. It might be helpful for the researcher to attend several conferences to observe and evaluate presentation styles before attempting to be a presenter.

Visual Presentations. The poster session is a visual display of research findings or research in progress. Typically, the session is held in a large room or hall. Presenters are assigned a table or wall space; attendees are free to walk among the displays and stop to read the posters or chat with investigators. The staff development educator might wish to consult with a media specialist for assistance with the layout of the poster and choice of materials. The poster might include a combination of text, graphs, photographs, and tables. The display must be portable, and the observer should be able to review the presentation in 3 to 5 minutes. The educator should be available for discussion and have an ample supply of printed abstracts available for distribution. The name and address of the educator should be included on the abstract.

SOURCES OF FUNDING AND SUPPORT FOR RESEARCH

Successful completion of a research project requires human, material, and financial resources. The staff development educator conducting an investigation must think about the cost of purchasing instruments, clinical supplies, paper, index cards, file folders, and laboratory tests. Additionally, there may be expenses for research assistants, computer time, or a statistician. While some human and material resources may be supplied by the employing organization, financial resources are usually not. Therefore the educator must seek external sources of funds or grants. Grants are issued by family and corporate foundations, voluntary organizations, and private or federal agencies.

Grantsmanship, the skill of writing a good research proposal coupled with the knowledge of the way in which funding is provided and from whom that funding is available, is a skill that can be developed. Continuing education courses in grant writing are offered by many colleges. Serving on research committees, joining research organizations, and collaboration with faculty or physicians conducting funded research are excellent sources of obtaining funding information.

Identifying Funding Sources

Although funds available for research grants have decreased in recent years and competition for these funds has increased, grants are available to staff development educators with knowledge of funding agencies. The computerized information system, *Sponsored Program Information Network (SPIN)*, which can be accessed by most universities, provides information about federal, private, and corporate foundations. *The Foundation Directory*, available at local libraries, provides information about private and corporate funding foundations and their specific research interests and requirements. Additionally, *The Catalog of Federal Domestic Assistance*, available from the US Government Printing Office, identifies federal funding agencies.

Private Funding Agencies. Private agencies that fund nursing research include such organizations as the American Nurses Foundation of the ANA, Sigma Theta Tau International, the Kellogg Foundation, the Robert Wood Johnson Foundation, the American Cancer Society, and the American Heart Association. The American Nurses Foundation offers grants of up to $2500 to beginning nurse researchers investigating problems in clinical nursing or nursing administration. The Robert Wood Johnson Foundation seeks to fund research related to improving access to health care for undeserved populations. The Kellogg Foundation is particularly interested in application of knowledge and gives priority to research for improving human well-being through continuing education.

Staff development educators might also obtain funding from pharmaceutical companies and manufacturers of medical supplies. For example, an enterprising group of nurses investigating pain relief in patients who have undergone open heart surgery was able to secure a grant of $300 from a local chapter of Mended Hearts. Experienced investigators with greater financial requirements may wish to apply for federal grant monies.

Federal Funding Agencies. The federal government is the largest supplier of grant monies. The National Institutes of Health (NIH), which is part of the Public Health Service (PHS) of the DHHS, established the National Center for Nursing Research (NCNR) in 1986. The NCNR was created to support nursing research and research training in the areas of health promotion, prevention of disease, patient care, and mitigation of the effects of chronic illnesses. In 1993 NCNR became a National Institute for Nursing Research.

Funding may be requested to purchase supplies and equipment, hire consultants, pay for travel expenses, and cover part or all of the investigator's salary. Proposals for the same study may be submitted to and receive funding from more than one agency.

Staff development educators can use one of two approaches to seek funds from federal agencies. They can develop a study of interest and seek out the appropriate federal agency, or an agency will identify a problem requiring investigation and send out a request for proposals or a request for applications to which staff development educators may respond. These requests are published in the *Federal Register*.

Applying for Funding

Application for funding is made by submitting a research or grant proposal. The purpose of the proposal is to explain, in detail, all aspects of the proposed investigation. Guidelines and requirements of the proposal can be obtained from the funding agency. These guidelines must be strictly adhered to because proposals can be rejected for failure to comply with typing instructions or submission deadlines.

Generally, the proposal includes the purpose and significance of the study; methodology, including a statement of protection of human rights; data analysis techniques; the staff development educator's educational, professional, and research background; resources available to support the study; and a proposed budget.

The educator should consider the aims and interests of the agency to which the proposal will be submitted. A proposal that is relevant to the program emphases of that foundation is more likely to be approved. Regardless of the source of funding, the educator must be cognizant of ethical factors inherent in the conduct of nursing research.

ETHICS AND RESEARCH

In the research process, nurses have the dual responsibility of supporting the accrual of new knowledge and vigilantly protecting the rights of human subjects.[2] Basic rights of human subjects participating in research include the rights of self-determination; to privacy, anonymity, and confidentiality; fair treatment; and protection from harm or discomfort.

The Right of Self-Determination

As autonomous beings, individuals have the right to freely choose whether they will participate in a research study. Furthermore, subjects have the right to withdraw from participation without fear of reprisal. The researcher must obtain an informed, written consent without resorting to deception or coercion to protect this right. An informed consent includes the purpose of the study; procedures to be followed; a description of the possible benefits or risks of participation; an explanation of the medical treatment to be provided, in the event that injury occurs; provisions to ensure anonymity and confidentiality; the name of the contact person available to answer questions about the study; and the signatures of the subject, researcher, and witness.[7,17]

The Right to Privacy, Anonymity, and Confidentiality

The right to privacy means that private information will not be gathered from subjects without their knowledge or against their will. Invasion of privacy includes the use of hidden cameras or microphones or the observance of subjects through a one-way mirror without their knowledge.[30]

Confidentiality refers to the management of private information so data that have been collected are not divulged to others. Anonymity occurs if the subject cannot be linked to the data and subjects remain nameless in relation to their participation in the study.[7,8] Ways to ensure confidentiality and anonymity include using code numbers, keeping signed consent forms separate from data, and keeping data locked in a secure place.

The Right to Fair Treatment

The selection of subjects for participation in a study must be done in an equitable manner. Investigators should avoid captive audiences (for example, orientees, conference participants, and patients) and individuals in vulnerable or compromised positions (for example, the dying, elderly, and mentally ill) unless their participation is directly relevant to the problem being researched. Random selection of subjects helps eliminate bias in subject selection.

The Right to Protection from Harm or Discomfort

Members of health professions are bound by the principle of nonmaleficence—"above all, do no harm." Accordingly, ethical conduct of nursing research requires the investigator to balance the potential risks of participation against the potential benefits and ensure that the benefits outweigh the risks.[23]

Staff development educators must consider the following ethical dilemmas. Research design often involves the use of a control group, which is the group that does not receive the treatment under investigation. The researcher must evaluate that administration of the treatment will not harm the recipients and that withholding the treatment will not result in physical or emotional harm to members of the control group. Suppose a staff development educator, based on years of education and experience, developed an educational program designed to increase the state board licensing examination passage rate among new graduates. The educator should consider whether this practice would be ethical to provide that program for some graduates and withhold it from others. In another study the educator may need to consider also whether it would be ethical to use a tool to identify a population at risk and then withhold treatment from the "at risk" population to verify the predictive accuracy of that tool. Although no easy answers to these dilemmas exist, staff development educators engaged in research should be guided by the principle of beneficence to protect the human rights of subjects.

SUMMARY

Nursing research fosters professional accountability and autonomy and enhances effective practice through the generation and dissemination of knowledge. This chapter identified resources to assist the staff development educator to gain proficiency with the research process including journals, colloquia, faculty and colleagues, and formal education. Key elements of the research process from formulation of a researchable topic through communication of findings were discussed, and guidelines for efficient completion of each step were outlined. Protection of the rights of human subjects and identification of funding sources were also emphasized.

Nursing research was distinguished from problem-solving activities, and four areas of research crucial to the special focus of staff development were identified. These areas include investigation of transferring learning to practice, studying clinical teaching methodologies, increasing the rate and retention of learning, and evaluating the effectiveness of teaching strategies.

Staff development educators play a unique role in the research process because they may be responsible for conducting research, disseminating research findings, teaching the research process to staff members, and serving as a member of the IRB. This chapter provided a framework for implementing the research functions of the staff development educator.

REFERENCES

1. Abruzzese RS: Personal communication, July 1990.
2. American Nurses Association: *Human rights guidelines for nurses in clinical and other research*, Kansas City, Mo, 1985, The Association.
3. American Nurses Association: *Preparation for nurses for participation in research*, Kansas City, Mo, 1976, The Association.
4. American Nurses Association: *Standards for continuing education in nursing*, Kansas City, Mo, 1984, The Association.
5. American Nurses Association Commission of Nursing Research: *Guidelines for the investigative function of nurses*, Kansas City, Mo, 1981, The Association.
6. Blair C et al: What constitutes nursing research? *J NY State Nurs Assoc* 14(4):42, 1983.
7. Brockopp D, Hastings-Tolsma M: *Fundamentals of nursing research*, Glenview, Ill, 1989, Scott Foresman.
8. Burns N, Grove S: *The practice of nursing research: conduct, critique, and utilization*, ed 2, Philadelphia, 1993, WB Saunders.
9. Deiriggi P: Effects of waterbed flotation on indicators of energy expenditure in preterm infants, *Nurs Res* 39(3):140, 1990.

10. Department of Health and Human Services: Basic HHS policy for the protection of human research subjects, *Federal Register* 46(10):8366, 1981.
11. Good M: A comparison of the effects of jaw relaxation and music on postoperative pain, *Nurs Res* 44(1):52, 1995.
12. Healey K, Hoffman M: Self-instructional posters: one way to save time and money, *J Contin Educ Nurs* 22(3):123, 1991.
13. Houston S, Bevelacqua T: Improving organizational performance: administrative nurse specialist, *JONA* 21(7/8):47, 1991.
14. Kerlinger F: *Foundations of behavioral research*, ed 2, New York, 1973, Holt, Rinehart & Winston.
15. Morse J, Bottorff J, Hutchinson S: The paradox of comfort, *Nurs Res* 44(1):14, 1995.
16. Nieswiadomy RM: *Foundations of nursing research*, ed 2, Norwalk, Conn, 1993, Appleton & Lange.
17. Polit DF, Hungler BP: *Essentials of nursing research*, ed 3, Philadelphia, 1993, JB Lippincott.
18. Polit DF, Hungler BP: *Nursing research: principles and methods*, ed 5, Philadelphia, 1995, JB Lippincott.
19. Rossi P, Freeman H: *Evaluation: a systematic approach*, ed 3, Beverly Hills, Calif, 1985, Sage.
20. Saunders M: Director of quality improvement research, *J Nurs Car Qual* 7(4):39, 1993.
21. Schroder P, Katz J: Educational needs of nursing quality professionals, *J Nurs Car Qual* 7(4):26, 1993.
22. Shelly SI: *Research methods in nursing and health*, Boston, 1984, Little Brown.
23. Silva M: *Ethical guidelines in the conduct, dissemination, and implementation of nursing research*, Washington DC, 1995, American Nurses Publishing.
24. Stetler CB: *Nursing research in a service setting*, Reston, Va, 1984, Reston.
25. Sweeney MA, Olivieri P: *An introduction to nursing research: research, measurement, and computers in nursing*, Philadelphia, 1981, JB Lippincott.
26. Thomas BS: *Nursing research: an experiential approach*, St Louis, 1990, Mosby.
27. Treece EW, Treece JW: *Elements of research in nursing*, ed 4, St Louis, 1986, Mosby.
28. Trinkoff A, Eaton W, Anthony J: The prevalence of substance abuse among registered nurses, *Nurs Res* 40(3):172, 1991.
29. Utz SW et al: Perceptions of body image and health status in persons with mitral valve prolapse, *Image* 22(1):18, 1990.
30. Wilson H: *Introducing research in nursing*, ed 2, Menlo Park, Calif, 1987, Addison-Wesley.
31. Woods NF, Catanzaro M: *Nursing research: theory and practice*, St Louis, 1988, Mosby.

Appendix

Resources for Staff Development Educators

MAGAZINES AND JOURNALS

Adult Learning (formerly *LifeLong Learning*)
American Association for Adult and Continuing Education
1200 19th Street NW, Suite 300
Washington, DC 20036
Published bimonthly. Rate: $27/yr.

American Journal of Nursing
American Journal of Nursing Company
Subscriptions: PO Box 50480
Boulder, CO 80322-0480
Published monthly. Rate: $35/yr.

Journal of Nursing Staff Development
JB Lippincott
12107 Insurance Way, Suite 114
Hagerstown, MD 21740
Published bimonthly. Rate: $54/yr.

Nursing Management
Springhouse Corporation
Circulation Dept 434 W Downer
Aurora, IL 60506
Published monthly. Rate $32/yr.

The Journal of Continuing Education in Nursing
Charles B Slack
6900 Grove Road
Thorofare, NJ 08086
Published bimonthly. Rate: $47/yr.

Training & Development
American Society for Training and Development
1640 King Street, Box 1443
Alexandria, VA 22313-2043
Published monthly. Rate: $85/yr.

Training: The Human Side of Business
Lakewood Publications (A subsidiary of Maclean Hunter)
Lakewood Building
50 S Ninth Street
Minneapolis, MN 55402
Published monthly. Rate: $68/yr.

RESOURCES FOR AUDIOVISUALS AND BOOKS

American Journal of Nursing
Multimedia Catalogue
555 West 57th Street
New York, NY 10019-2961

American Nurses Publishing
Marketing Services
PO Box 2244
Waldorf, MD 20604-2244

Business Games, Training Materials, and Development Tools
Education Research
360 Lexington Avenue
New York, NY 10017

CareerTrack Publications
3085 Center Green Drive
PO Box 18778
Boulder, CO 80308-1778

Crisp Publications
Audios, videos, books, CD-Rom, computer-based
1200 Hamilton Court
Menlo Park, CA 94025-9600

Jossey-Bass Publishers Catalog
350 Sansome Street
San Francisco, CA 94104
Publishes most books about human resources development and continuing education.

Lakewood Publications
50 S Ninth Street
Minneapolis, MN 55402

National Seminars Workshops, Books & Tapes
Rockhurst College Continuing Education Center
6901 W 63rd Street
PO Box 2949
Shawnee Mission, KS 66201-1349

NLN Books & Videos Catalog
National League for Nursing
350 Hudson Street
New York, NY 10014

Nurses Resource Directory
Standards, Monographs, and References
American Nurses Publishing
Distribution Center: PO Box 2244
Waldorf, MD 20604-2244

National Nursing Staff Development Organization (NNSDO)
Publications include: *Quality Indicators for Nursing Staff Development,
Getting Started in Nursing Staff Development, Guidelines for an
Orientation Program for Novice Nursing Professional Development
Educators Blueprint for Competence,* and *Core Curriculum for Nursing
Staff Development*
437 Twin Bay Drive
Pensacola, FL 32534-1350

The HRD Quarterly
Organization Design & Development
2002 Renaissance Boulevard, Suite 100
King of Prussia, PA 19406

The Info-Line Collection
Practical Guidelines for Training and Development Professionals
American Society for Training and Development
1640 King Street, Box 1443
Alexandria, VA 22313-2043

Mosby Great Performance
Motivation, Patient Education, and Posters
11830 Westline Industrial Drive
St. Louis, MO 63146

Training Ideas
Resource Guide and Product Catalog
Talico
2320 S Third Street, Suite 5
Jacksonville Beach, FL 32250

Pfeiffer & Company International Publishers
Contains references for many training and education books including the
Annual *Developing Human Resources*, which contains many valuable cre-
ative learning exercises.
2780 Circleport Drive
Erlanger, KY 41018

Williams & Wilkins
Electronic Media for Healthcare Education
428 East Preston Street
Baltimore, MD 21202

ORGANIZATIONS OF INTEREST

American Nurses Association Council for Professional Nursing Education
and Development
American Nurses Association
600 Maryland Avenue SW
Washington, DC 20024
Phone: (202) 554-4444

American Society for HealthCare Education and Training of the American
Hospital Association
840 N Lake Shore Drive
Chicago, IL 60611
Phone: (312) 280-6000

American Society for Training and Development
1640 Duke Street, Box 1443
Alexandria, VA 22313-2043
Phone: (703) 683-8100

American Association for Adult and Continuing Education
1200 19th Street NW, Suite 300
Washington, DC 20036
Phone: (202) 822-7866

National Nursing Staff Development Organization
437 Twine Bay Drive
Pensacola, FL 32534-1350
Phone: (904) 474-0995

Mosby Division of Continuing Education and Training
11830 Westline Industrial Drive
PO Box 46908
St. Louis, MO 63146-9806
Annual convention for staff development educators (February each year)
Bimonthly News Letter: *Staff Development Insider*

Index